Breast Cancer

Breast Cancer

Edited by

JOHN J. KAVANAGH, MD
Professor of Medicine
Chief, Section of Gynecologic Medical Oncology
The University of Texas–MD Anderson Cancer Center
Houston, Texas

S. EVA SINGLETARY, MD
Professor of Surgery
Chief, Surgical Breast Section
Department of Surgical Oncology
The University of Texas–MD Anderson Cancer Center
Houston, Texas

NINA EINHORN, MD, PHD
Associate Professor of Gynecologic Oncology
Cancer Foreningen
Radiumhemmet
Karolinska Hospital
Stockholm, Sweden

A. DENNY DePETRILLO, MD, FRCS(C)
Professor, Obstetrics/Gynecology and Surgery
Director, Division of Gynecologic Oncology
Department of Obstetrics and Gynecology
University of Toronto
Toronto, Ontario
Canada

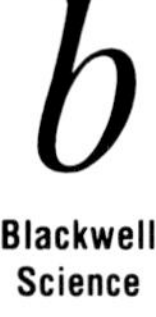

Blackwell
Science

© 1999 by Blackwell Science, Inc.

Editorial Offices:
Commerce Place, 350 Main Street, Malden,
 Massachusetts 02148, USA
Osney Mead, Oxford OX2 0EL, England
25 John Street, London WC1N 2BL, England
23 Ainslie Place, Edinburgh EH3 6AJ, Scotland
54 University Street, Carlton, Victoria 3053, Australia

Other Editorial Offices:
Blackwell Wissenschafts-Verlag GmbH,
 Kurfürstendamm 57, 10707 Berlin, Germany
Blackwell Science KK, MG Kodenmacho Building, 7-
 10 Kodenmacho Nihombashi, Chuo-ku, Tokyo 104,
 Japan

Distributors:

USA
 Blackwell Science, Inc.
 Commerce Place
 350 Main Street
 Malden, Massachusetts 02148
 (Telephone orders: 800-215-1000 or 781-388-8250;
  fax orders: 781-388-8270)

Canada
 Login Brothers Book Company
 324 Saulteaux Crescent
 Winnipeg, Manitoba, R3J 3T2
 (Telephone orders: 204-224-4068)

Australia
 Blackwell Science Pty, Ltd.
 54 University Street
 Carlton, Victoria 3053
 (Telephone orders: 03-9347-0300;
  fax orders: 03-9349-3016)

Outside North America and Australia
 Blackwell Science, Ltd.
 c/o Marston Book Services, Ltd.
 P.O. Box 269
 Abingdon
 Oxon OX14 4YN
 England
 (Telephone orders: 44-01235-465500;
  fax orders: 44-01235-465555)

Originally published in *Cancer in Women* © 1998 by Blackwell Science, Inc.

Acquisitions: Christopher Davis
Production: Irene Herlihy
Manufacturing: Lisa Flanagan
Cover Design: Meral Dabcovich, Visual Perspectives
Typeset by Best-set Typesetter Ltd., Hong Kong
Printed and bound by Braun-Brumfield, Inc.

Printed in the United States of America
99 00 01 02 5 4 3 2 1

The Blackwell Science logo is a trade mark of Blackwell Science Ltd., registered at the United Kingdom Trade Marks Registry

ISBN 0-632-04431-4

Contents

List of Contributors

Sirpa Asko-Seljavaara, MD
Professor and Chief
Department of Plastic Surgery
Helsinki University Central Hospital
Toolo Hospital
Helsinki, Finland

Ahmad Awada, MD
Medical Oncology
Jules Bordet Institute
The University of Brussels
Brussels, Belgium

Aman U. Buzdar, MD
Internist and Professor of Medicine
Deputy Chairman
Department of Breast and Gynecologic
  Medical Oncology
The University of Texas–MD Anderson
  Cancer Center
Houston, Texas

Eleni Diamandidou, MD
Junior Faculty Associate
Department of Medical Breast Oncology
The University of Texas–MD Anderson
  Cancer Center
Houston, Texas

Frankie Ann Holmes, MD
Adjunct Associate Professor of Medicine
Department of Breast Medical Oncology
The University of Texas–MD Anderson
  Cancer Center;
Texas Oncology, P.A.
Houston, Texas

Joseph Kerger, MD
Medical Oncology
Jules Bordet Institute
The University of Brussels
Brussels, Belgium

Stephen S. Kroll, MD
Professor of Plastic Surgery
Department of Plastic Surgery
The University of Texas–MD Anderson
  Cancer Center
Houston, Texas

Lars-Gunnar Larsson, MD
Center of Oncology
University of Umea
Umea, Sweden

Seymour H. Levitt, MD
Professor and Head
Department of Therapeutic Radiology–Radi-
  ation Oncology
University of Minnesota Medical School
Minneapolis, Minnesota

Monica Morrow, MD
Professor of Surgery
Northwestern University Medical School;
Director
Lynn Sage Comprehensive Breast Center
Northwestern Memorial Hospital
Chicago, Illinois

Martine J. Piccart-Gebhart, MD, PhD
Medical Oncology
Head of Chemotherapy Unit
Jules Bordet Institute
The University of Brussels
Brussels, Belgium

Josée-Anne Roy, MD
Medical Oncology
Jules Bordet Institute
The University of Brussels
Brussels, Belgium

S. Eva Singletary, MD
Professor of Surgery
Chief, Surgical Breast Section
Department of Surgical Oncology
The University of Texas–MD Anderson
    Cancer Center
Houston, Texas

Umberto Veronesi, MD
Scientific Director
European Institute of Oncology
Milan, Italy

Victor G. Vogel, MD, MHS, FACP
Professor of Medicine and Epidemiology
Director, Comprehensive Breast Program
The University of Pittsburgh Cancer
    Institute and The Magee-Womens
    Hospital
Pittsburgh, Pennsylvania

Breast Cancer

CHAPTER 1

Breast Cancer Risk Factors and Preventive Approaches to Breast Cancer

VICTOR G. VOGEL

ublic attention and awareness about breast cancer have been heightened by the diagnosis of the disease in prominent political and social figures and by national campaigns that present breast cancer as a public health problem. Programs that promote the benefits of screening mammography also focus attention on breast cancer, as does media coverage of research reports about the genetic basis of the disease. For these and perhaps other reasons, the public is anxious about breast cancer, and many women perceive their risk of dying of breast cancer to be very high in the short term (1). Although for most women the actual risk is significantly lower than the perceived risk, women consult physicians regularly to obtain information to control their risk for breast cancer. Available data suggest that a balanced presentation by health-care professionals about the risk factors for breast cancer and the strategies to lower the risk may reduce anxiety regardless of whether a woman actively adopts measures to reduce her risk.

For clinicians, an understanding of the factors that affect a woman's risk for breast cancer results in better comprehension of the biologic processes that lead to the disease and allows the clinician to give informed, objective responses to patients' questions. This, in turn, reduces patients' anxiety and improves clinical management of the woman at risk. It also facilitates the design and adoption of improved preventive strategies for breast cancer. In this chapter, I review the factors that lead to an increased or decreased risk for breast cancer, examine models that allow clinicians to quantify a woman's risk of developing breast cancer, define techniques for counseling women to decrease their risk, and briefly review clinical methods currently being evaluated for the primary prevention of breast cancer.

Factors That Increase Risk

Clinicians and epidemiologists evaluate risk to identify those women who require special management and to increase understanding of the biologic processes that lead to breast cancer. *Risk* is a relative term derived by comparing the incidence of a disease in a group having a particular risk factor or trait with the incidence of the same disease in a comparison group of individuals who do not carry the risk factor but who are in every other way the same. If risk calculations are derived from retrospective data, risk is expressed as the odds ratio, or the ratio of the odds of having the disease in those with the trait of interest compared with the odds of having the disease in those without the trait. If a trait is evaluated in a prospective study, the risk of disease can be expressed as the ratio of the incidence of the disease in those with the trait divided by the incidence of the disease in those without the trait. This ratio is known as the *relative risk* and can be viewed as the level of increased risk of developing the disease associated with the risk factor. For example, a relative risk (or an odds ratio) of 1.8 means that a person with a given trait or characteristic is 1.8 times more likely to develop the disease than is someone without the trait. A trait associated with a relative risk of this magnitude can also be described as being associated with an 80% increase in risk.

It is important to recognize that the presence of a risk factor does not guarantee the development of a disease just as the absence of a risk factor does not confer absolute protection against the disease. The relationship between a risk factor and the proportion of cases of a disease that it may cause is known as the *attributable risk*. Calculation of attributable risk requires knowledge of the prevalence of a particular risk factor in the population of interest and the relative risk associated with

that risk factor (2). For example, a risk factor that is present in 20% of the population and that has an associated relative risk of 1.5 has an attributable risk of 0.09 or 9%, meaning that the presence of this risk factor explains 9% of the incidence of the disease in the population. Common breast cancer risk factors (3) and their associated relative risks, population prevalence, and attributable risks are shown in Table 1-1.

Few breast cancer risk factors have a population prevalence greater than 10% to 15%, although some are associated with very large relative risks (e.g., mutated genes, cellular atypia), making them important to consider in the clinical management of breast cancer risk (4). Traits associated with large relative risks are rare; common risk factors are associated with relative risks less than 2.0 so that the attributable risk for any particular risk factor is small, as shown in Table 1-1. In addition, because many women possess multiple risk factors for breast cancer and because of the epidemiologic confounding that may occur in evaluating both relative and attributable risks, it may not be pos-

T A B L E   **1-1**

Risk Factors for Breast Cancer, Their Relative Risks, and the Associated Population Attributable Risk

Risk Factor (3)	Comparison Category	Risk Category	Relative Risk	Prevalence (4)	Population Attributable Risk*
Age at menarche	16 yr	Younger than 12 yr	1.3	16%	0.05
Age at menopause	45–54 yr	After 55 yr	1.5	6%	0.03
Age at first live birth	Before 20 yr	Nulliparous or older than 30 yr	1.9	21%	0.16
Benign breast disease	No biopsy or fine-needle aspiration	Any benign disease	1.5	15%	0.07
		Proliferative disease	2.0	4%	0.04
		Atypical hyperplasia	4.0	1%	0.03
Family history of breast cancer	No first-degree relative affected	Mother affected	1.7	8%	0.05
		Two first-degree relatives affected	5.0	4%	0.14
Obesity	10th percentile	90th percentile	1.2	18%	0.03
Alcohol use	Nondrinker	Moderate drinker	1.7	12%	0.08
Estrogen replacement therapy	Never used	Current use ages 50–59 yr	1.5	18%	0.08

*As defined by Lilienfeld and Lilienfeld (2); population attributable risk = (prevalence × relative risk)/[(prevalence × relative risk − 1) + 1].

sible to sum the attributable risks in Table 1-1 to obtain a summary attributable risk. If the risk factors were independent and there were no interactions among them affecting the respective levels of risk associated with them, then the complement of the summary attributable risk (i.e., 1 − attributable risk) would be the product of the complements of the individual attributable risks (5). If this assumption holds, then the summary attributable risk for the risk factors listed in Table 1-1 is 47%. Previously published estimates of the summary population attributable risk for breast cancer range from 21% in premenopausal women to 29% in postmenopausal women (6) to 55% in women in the Breast Cancer Detection and Demonstration Project (BCDDP) (5). Attributable risk does not establish causality, and it is clear that nearly half the attributable risk for breast cancer remains unexplained (7). Nevertheless, it is instructive to examine what is known regarding established risk factors for breast cancer.

Age

All women are at risk for breast cancer, and the most important single risk factor is age. The risk of breast cancer increases throughout a woman's lifetime (4): The annual incidence of breast cancer in U.S. women 80 to 85 years old is 15 times higher than the incidence among women 30 to 35 years old (412 cases/100,000 women/yr at age 80 compared with 27.9 cases/100,000 women/yr at age 30). It is not yet known whether these observed differences are explained by the accumulation of a number of events that occur throughout a woman's lifetime or by a single event that is triggered with greater frequency in older than in younger women.

Race and ethnicity modify the effect of age on the risk of breast cancer. For example, African-American women younger than 50 have a higher age-specific incidence of breast cancer than do their white American counterparts, but older African-Americans have a lower age-specific incidence than do older white Americans (4). There is not yet an adequate explanation for these differences. Furthermore, the breast cancer incidence for Hispanic women living in North America is only 40% to 50% as great as the incidence among non-Hispanic white women. Asian women born in Asia have an extremely low lifetime risk of breast cancer, but their daughters born in North America have the same lifetime risk of breast cancer as do

American white women (8). No explanation, including dietary factors, yet accounts for these observed differences.

Gynecologic Events

The extensive epidemiologic literature about the risk factors for breast cancer is derived from both case-control and cohort studies. Most breast cancer risk factors relate to gynecologic or endocrinologic events in a woman's life (3,9–12). Age at menarche is related to a woman's chance of developing breast cancer: Compared with women who experience menarche at age 16, girls who experience menarche 2 to 5 years earlier have a 10% to 30% greater risk of developing breast cancer later in life. A similar observation has been made for the timing of events at the other end of the reproductive spectrum, the age at menopause. The average age at menopause in the United States is slightly older than 51 years. If women who experience menopause between the ages of 45 and 55 years are used as the referent group, women who experience menopause at age 55 or older have a 50% higher risk of subsequently developing breast cancer, and women who cease menstruating at age 45 or earlier have a 30% lower risk of subsequently developing breast cancer. These data, along with the observations about the age at menarche, indicate that one way of expressing the risk of breast cancer in relation to gynecologic events is simply to count the number of ovulatory menstrual cycles that a woman experiences in her lifetime. Early menarche and late menopause lead to an increased total lifetime number of menstrual cycles and a corresponding 30% to 50% increase in breast cancer risk. Conversely, late menarche and early menopause lead to a reduction in breast cancer risk of similar magnitude. Consistent with this observation is the fact that oophorectomy before the age of menopause (especially before the age of 40) lowers the risk of breast cancer by approximately two thirds (9).

It is tempting to say that the explanation for these observations is the level of circulating estrogen to which a woman is exposed in her lifetime. In an adult woman, the predominant circulating estrogen is estradiol, and most of this is bound to sex hormone–binding globulin (SHBG). A smaller proportion is bound to albumin. Between menarche and menopause, a woman is exposed to higher static levels of circulating estradiol (bound to either SHBG or albumin as well as freely circulating). Cell proliferation is low during the follicular phase of the menstrual cycle and does not increase with the preovulatory peak in estradiol (13). Following ovulation, progesterone stimulates cell proliferation to three times the follicular rates. If fertilization and pregnancy do not occur, progesterone levels fall, breast cell division decreases, and apoptosis follows (14). During pregnancy, circulating levels of both estrogen and progesterone remain elevated. In animal models, progesterone is a potent mitogen to breast cells, possibly making them more susceptible to the effects of breast carcinogens (13). During the second half of pregnancy, however, cell differentiation occurs in the breast, and proliferation decreases.

Pregnancy at a young age, especially before the age of 20, markedly reduces the incidence of subsequent breast cancer (9). Conversely, both nulliparity and age older than 30 at the time of the first live birth are associated with nearly a doubling of the risk of subsequent breast cancer (12). Pregnancies not ending in the birth of a viable fetus do not confer a reduction in the risk of breast cancer (15). For obvious technical, practical, and ethical reasons, there are no data from women that provide a histologic explanation for the protection from breast cancer brought about by early pregnancy.

Benign Breast Disease

Symptomatic changes in the breast are quite common in clinical practice. Various published studies reported that as many as two thirds of women have symptoms and signs variously described as pain, lumps, tenderness, nodularity, or thickening of the breasts (16). Some studies showed a correlation between risk factors for breast cancer and those for benign breast disease (17), while others did not (18). The latter studies raised the possibility that benign breast disease is not a precursor of breast cancer. Few benign lesions show amplification of the HER-2/*neu* oncogene or mutation of the *TP53* tumor suppressor gene (19). The significance of these findings remains to be determined. Although there is some correlation between the presence of nodularity on physical examination and the appearance of the mammogram, benign disease of the breast is not more common in women with other risk factors

for breast cancer such as a family history of the disease. The signs and symptoms of benign breast disease often resolve without treatment and usually do not require breast biopsy for definitive diagnosis; fewer than 20% of women in North America have undergone a biopsy for benign breast disease by age 50 (20). Benign breast disease that results in biopsy does increase the risk of subsequently developing breast cancer (21).

The clinical lexicon is replete with creative, if not accurately descriptive terms for benign breast disease: chronic cystic mastitis, fibroadenoma, fibrocystic disease, and so on. Among women undergoing biopsy for benign breast disease, the risk of subsequent breast cancer is not uniform. The most informative classification schema is based on histopathology: It divides benign disease into proliferative and nonproliferative categories (22). The important subclassifications of proliferative disease are listed in Table 1-2 with their associated relative risks. Proliferative disease accounts for between one fourth and one third of all biopsies for benign disease, and 5% to 10% of the proliferative lesions show cellular atypia, the histologic change associated with the highest risk (22–26). The atypical features are similar to some found in carcinoma in situ. Increasing use of mammographic screening has led to increased identification of women with proliferative lesions of the breast (27).

Cystic disease also increases risk. While early benign disease classification schemes did not include sclerosing adenosis among the lesions that increase risk, recent data indicate that sclerosing adenosis increases the risk of breast cancer by approximately 70%, which justifies its inclusion among proliferative disease without atypia (28). A family history of breast cancer in first-degree relatives has an additive effect on the subsequent risk of breast cancer (22,25,26). While fewer than 5% of women with a biopsy showing no proliferative changes develop breast cancer over the subsequent 25 years, nearly 40% of women with a family history of breast cancer and atypical hyperplasia subsequently develop breast cancer. Biopsy before the age of 50 to 55 years may be associated with a fivefold to sixfold increase in the risk of breast cancer, while biopsy at older ages is associated with only half this risk (21).

Familial breast cancers show an increased prevalence of medullary histology, and it is well established that in younger women invasive

T A B L E **1-2**

Classification of Benign Breast Disease and the Risk for Subsequent
Development of Breast Cancer (22–26)*

		Associated Relative Risk for Breast Cancer	
Benign Lesion	**Description**	**With Family History of Breast Cancer**	**Without Family History of Breast Cancer**
Proliferative disease without atypia	—	2.4–2.7	1.7–1.9
Moderate and florid ductal hyperplasia of the usual type	Most common type of hyperplasia; cells do not have the cytologic appearance of lobular or apocrine-like lesions; florid lesions have a proliferation of cells that fill more than 70% of the involved space	—	—
Additional lesions	Intraductal papilloma, radial scar, sclerosing adenosis, apocrine metaplasia	—	—
Atypical hyperplasia		11.0	4.2–4.3
Atypical ductal hyperplasia	Has features similar to ductal carcinoma in situ but lacks the complete criteria for that diagnosis		
Atypical lobular hyperplasia	Defined by changes that are similar to lobular carcinoma in situ but lack the complete criteria for that diagnosis	—	—
Nonproliferative	Normal glandular histology, cysts, duct ectasia, mild hyperplasia, fibroadenoma	1.2–2.6	0.9–1.0

*Relative risks represent the range of values reported in the published literature.

breast cancer is of higher grade, is more proliferative, has an increased thymidine labeling index and S-phase fraction, and has increased expression of proliferation-associated proteins (29). Early-onset breast cancers also have an excess of invasive ductal carcinoma with a predominant intraductal component, although familial breast cancers do not.

One emerging use of benign breast pathology is in the clinical evaluation of women with a familial predisposition to breast cancer. Among women with normal findings on clinical examination, bilateral fine-needle aspiration of all four breast quadrants yields cytologic evidence of proliferative breast disease in 30% to 40% of patients who have two or more first-degree relatives with breast cancer, compared with only 13% of women without a family history of breast cancer (30,31). The subsequent appearance of breast cancer in some women with these abnormalities suggests that cytohistologic changes may precede the development of breast cancer in women with predisposing risk factors. These changes may also serve as intermediate biologic end points in clinical prevention trials that enroll these women as subjects. Other studies showed an increasing proportion of overexpression of breast cancer–associated biologic markers in fine-needle breast aspirates from women with risk factors for breast cancer (32). More aspirates from women with atypia than from women with proliferative changes only had elevations in epidermal growth factor receptor (EGFR), p53, and aneuploidy. The incorporation of cyto-histologic changes into routine clinical risk assessment awaits the completion of confirmatory studies. Use of these changes in clinical decision making (e.g., the decision to undergo prophylactic mastectomy) has not been evaluated.

It is an extremely interesting observation that estrogen replacement therapy lowers the risk of breast cancer in women with proliferative benign breast disease with or without atypia (33). A history of proliferative benign

T A B L E   **1-3**

Indications for Breast Cancer Risk Counseling

1 More than two first-degree relatives with breast, ovarian, or other cancers
2 Two or more generations affected
3 First-degree relatives with bilateral breast cancer
4 Multiple primary tumors, breast or other
5 Early-onset cancer (younger than 45 years)
6 Sarcomas, adrenocortical carcinomas, or other rare cancers in relatives
7 Ataxia telangiectasia in relatives
8 Premalignant histology on breast biopsy
9 Relative with a known mutation in a susceptibility gene
10 Women considering prophylactic mastectomy or oophorectomy

Source: Reproduced by permission from Peters J. Breast cancer genetics: relevance to oncology practice. *Cancer Control* 1995;2:195–208.

breast disease is not, therefore, a contraindication to estrogen replacement therapy.

Family History of Breast Cancer

Genetic factors contribute to approximately 5% of all breast cancers but to 25% of those diagnosed before age 30 (34). Early-onset breast cancer is that which occurs before age 50, when there is a flattening in the rate of increase in the age-specific incidence rates. A number of factors can indicate a need to explore more fully the history of breast cancer in a family. These factors are listed in Table 1-3 (35). Risk can be quantified rapidly and simply by assessing the number and degree of a woman's relatives affected with breast cancer and their ages at diagnosis. This is illustrated in Table 1-4 (36). Having more relatives diagnosed with breast cancer before the age of 50 increases the cumulative lifetime risk of developing the disease to near 50%, indicating the autosomal dominant behavior of some syndromes of genetically predisposed breast cancer.

Mutation of one gene, *BRCA1*, appears to account for 45% of families with a significantly high incidence of breast cancer and at least 80% of families with an increased incidence of both early-onset breast cancer and ovarian cancer (37,38). *BRCA1* is located on chromosome 17q and appears to encode a tumor suppressor protein that acts as a negative regulator of tumor

Affected Relative	Age of Affected Relative (yr)	Cumulative Breast Cancer Risk by Age 80 (%)
One first degree	<50	13–21
	50	9–11
One second degree	<50	10–14
	50	8–9
Two first degree	Both <50	35–48
	Both ≥50	11–24
Two second degree[b]	Both <50	21–26
	Both ≥50	9–16

[a] Risk estimates are derived by including age extremes from the risk tables calculated by Claus et al (34) as modified by Hoskins et al (36). For example, for affected relatives younger than 50 years, the lower limit is the calculated risk if the affected relative is in the 40- to 49-year age group and the upper limit is the calculated risk for a relative in the 20- to 29-year age group. Thus, these figures represent the range of risk based on age and are not confidence intervals.

[b] Both paternal or both maternal.

Source: Reproduced by permission from Hoskins KF, Stopfer JE, Calzone KA, et al. Assessment and counseling for women with a family history of breast cancer—a guide for clinicians. *JAMA* 1995;273:577–585.

T A B L E   **1-4**

Breast Cancer Risk Estimates for Members of Moderate-Risk Families[a] growth (39,40). It is a large gene containing 5592 nucleotides spread over 100,000 bases of genomic DNA (41). It is composed of 22 coding exons that produce a protein containing 1863 amino acids. At the amino-terminal end of the protein there is a region that is thought to interact with other amino acids or to form protein complexes, suggesting a role for *BRCA1* in regulating DNA transcription. Mutations in *BRCA1* may also play a role in the progression of sporadic breast cancer (40,42). Family studies showed that predisposition to cancer is inherited as a dominant genetic trait, but the associated allele behaves in a recessive way in somatic cells. An inherited copy of the mutant allele causes familial predisposition to cancer, and mutation of the other, paired allele begins the progression toward malignancy.

Reported mutations to the *BRCA1* gene are of several types: frameshift (insertion or deletion of two or more nucleotides resulting in altered translation of the protein), nonsense (nucleotide substitution producing a stop codon and termination of protein translation), missense (change of a single amino acid), and splice-site (which also causes production of an aberrant protein) (41). Mutations result in a truncated protein in 86% of the patients tested to date. All of these mutations appear to be rare in the general population, occurring in somewhere between 1 in 200 and 1 in 500 persons. One particular mutation (185delAG), however, appears to occur in as many as 1% of Ashkenazi-Jewish individuals (43). Confirmatory studies of these preliminary findings are necessary, as are precautions to guard against the unethical or inappropriate use of testing in narrowly targeted populations (44).

The presence of a mutated *BRCA1* gene with a resultant truncated protein has important clinical consequences, as shown in Table 1-5

(45). The relative risk of breast cancer associated with a *BRCA1* mutation is greater than 200 before the age of 40 but drops to 15 in the seventh decade of life (45). The penetrance of the phenotype in carriers of mutated genes is estimated to be 87% for breast cancer and 44% for ovarian cancer by age 70. There is also evidence of allelic heterogeneity, with 29% of *BRCA1* mutations conferring a high risk of ovarian cancer and 71% conferring a moderate risk. If these observations hold true, the average lifetime risk of ovarian cancer in *BRCA1* mutation carriers will be approximately 40%.

Young women with a diagnosis of breast cancer who have multiple affected relatives have a higher likelihood of being mutation carriers. Approximately 45% of families with increased susceptibility to breast cancer carry mutations of *BRCA1* (37). Hoskins et al (36) divided these women into two groups. The first group, those from moderate-risk families, are characterized by a "less striking" family history, an absence of ovarian cancer, and an older average age at diagnosis. High-risk families are generally characterized by the occurrence of breast cancer in at least three close relatives that follows an autosomal dominant pattern. Available data show that 26% of families with three affected members diagnosed before age 60 and 60% of families with four or more members show *BRCA1* mutations (37). The presence of even one case of ovarian cancer in the family makes a *BRCA1* mutation more likely, and a case of male breast cancer makes a *BRCA1* mutation less likely (46). Breast cancer is often diagnosed at an early age (<45 years), and there may be cases of ovarian cancer as well. A description of the evaluation of moderate-risk families is beyond the scope of this chapter; the reader is referred to the appropriate quantitative models (47,48) and review articles (36) for guidance.

T A B L E   **1-5**

Estimated Cumulative Risks of Breast and Ovarian Cancer in *BRCA1* Gene Carriers

| | **Cumulative Risk** | | |
Age (yr)	**Breast Cancer**	**Ovarian Cancer**	**Either Cancer**
30	0.032	0.0017	0.034
40	0.191	0.0061	0.195
50	0.508	0.227	0.619
60	0.542	0.298	0.678
70	0.850	0.633	0.945

Source: Reproduced by permission from Easton DF, Ford BP, Bishop DT, the Breast Cancer Linkage Consortium. Breast and ovarian cancer incidence in BRCA1-mutation carriers. *Am J Hum Genet* 1995;56:265–271.

Current technology permits sequencing of the entire *BRCA1* gene in individuals with an increased likelihood of carrying a mutated gene, particularly in women with breast cancer. Once a woman with a diagnosis of breast cancer is identified by DNA sequencing methodology as having a mutated *BRCA1* allele, additional women at risk in her family may be screened using allele-specific oligonucleotides that efficiently screen for the known mutation (41). Families can also be screened with assays that evaluate the presence of a truncated *BRCA1* protein (49), but these assays are investigational, and precise estimates of test-related sensitivity and specificity are not yet available. Furthermore, the predictive value of a positive test result will depend significantly on the prior probability of carrying a mutation in the individual being tested. A negative test result is only informative in a woman from a family where a known *BRCA1* mutation exists. Her risk of breast cancer would then be equal to that of a woman in the general population. In a family undergoing genetic testing where no *BRCA1* mutation is found, risk should be calculated using quantitative models just referenced and described elsewhere in this chapter.

Because *BRCA1* is an autosomal gene, it can be carried and transmitted by men in the affected families. Although the risk of breast cancer in the male carriers appears to be negligible, there is a threefold risk of prostate cancer and a fourfold risk of colon cancer in male mutation carriers. A second breast cancer gene, *BRCA2*, which localizes to chromosome 13, confers risks for breast and ovarian cancer in women similar to those conferred by *BRCA1* and is associated with an increased risk of breast cancer in male carriers (36,50). Several other genetic syndromes (e.g., the Li-Fraumeni syndrome, caused by mutations in the *TP53* gene) predispose carriers to an increased risk of developing breast cancer, but they are rare and beyond the scope of this chapter. The reader is referred to a comprehensive review of familial cancer risk for details and management recommendations (51).

Women without a diagnosis of breast cancer with increased pretest probabilities of carrying a *BRCA1* mutation can be identified on the basis of the number of their relatives diagnosed with breast cancer and their ages at diagnosis (36,47,48,52). Not all women who are at risk for breast cancer because of a family history of the disease will elect to undergo genetic testing, however. Women who have regular breast examinations by a physician, who believe that mammography effectively detects early breast cancer, and who believe that breast cancer is curable report that they would accept genetic susceptibility testing for breast cancer (53). The proportion of women who actually choose to have testing following counseling is the focus of several ongoing research studies. Guidelines for the responsible use of genetic testing are outlined in Table 1-6 (54–58). All subjects who

T A B L E   **1-6**

Responsible Use of Presymptomatic Genetic Testing for Cancer Susceptibility (54–58)

Cancer susceptibility testing is currently investigational and not routine.
Testing should be voluntary and free from professional and family pressure to participate.
Persons have the right to know the results of their testing.
Persons have the right *not* to know their genetic predispositions.
Participation in genetic testing should be based on understanding and should require fully informed consent.
Testing can have long-lasting and profound psychosocial consequences.
Cancer risk counseling is a prerequisite for testing.
Predisposition testing is most appropriate for diseases that are preventable or treatable.
Results of genetic testing must be private and confidential.
Regulation may be necessary to avoid employment and insurance discrimination.
Vulnerable populations such as minors and incompetent adults need extra protections.
Resources and access to testing should be equitably distributed.
Additional research is needed on specific criteria for test sensitivity, specificity, and effectiveness.
Research into clinical and psychological implications of susceptibility testing is needed.
Ethical consultation and supervision of testing programs are helpful at the current stage of test development.
Quality assurance should include standards for laboratories and professional personnel.

undergo genetic susceptibility testing should undergo counseling. Counseling is necessary to educate the subject about risk, to explain the process and limitations of genetic testing, to assess and manage anxiety and other psychopathology, and to review clinical management options. There are also important legal and ethical complexities that must be considered. The counseling process is complex, and the reader is referred to appropriate reviews (35,36,55,56,59). Patients should be referred to trained and experienced genetics counselors whenever possible.

Management options for women who carry *BRCA1* mutations include mammographic screening, prophylactic mastectomy, and participation in investigational chemoprevention trials, all discussed later in this chapter. The effect of either oral contraceptives or estrogen replacement therapy on the risk of breast cancer in carriers of *BRCA1* mutations is unknown. Ovarian cancer screening with CA-125 antigen and transvaginal ultrasound remains investigational.

Mammographic Parenchymal Pattern

In 1976, Wolfe (60) proposed a classification system for mammograms based solely on the radiographic appearance of the breast parenchyma. Four parenchymal patterns (N1, P1, P2, DY) were associated with a stepwise increase in breast cancer risk. Meta-analysis of multiple published studies revealed a fivefold increase in risk for high-risk parenchymal patterns in prospective cohort studies and a twofold increase in risk in retrospective case-control studies (61). High-risk patterns are more prevalent in countries with an increased incidence of breast cancer than in countries with a lower incidence (62). Women showing the P1 pattern (mostly fat with <25% prominent duct pattern) or the DY pattern (sheet-like areas of increased density) are more likely to have a finding of lobular carcinoma in situ in breast biopsy specimens (63).

Because Wolfe's original classification scheme was somewhat subjective, other investigators sought to assess breast density more quantitatively. Using a compensating polar planimeter, Saftlas et al (64) measured breast densities in mammograms taken prior to a diagnosis of breast cancer. There was a linear increase in the risk of breast cancer with increasing breast density. Using a referent group in whom less than 5% of the mammogram area was dense, they calculated the odds ratio for subsequent development of breast cancer to be 4.3 for women in whom more than 65% of the breast area was dense. In a recent follow-up study of participants in the BCDDP, mammographic densities were evaluated using a computerized planimeter prior to the development of breast cancer in 1880 women who subsequently developed breast cancer (65). High densities with either the P2 (prominent linear and nodular ductal densities that occupy 25%–100% of the breast area) or the DY pattern of Wolfe were associated with odds ratios of 3.2 and 2.9, respectively, of developing breast cancer. Women who had a quantitative breast density of 75% or greater by planimetry had a fivefold increased risk of breast cancer. In the BCDDP, 28% of the incident breast cancer cases were associated with a breast density of 50% or greater. This technique appears to be an independent measure of breast cancer risk although it has not gained wide acceptance in clinical practice.

A mechanistic explanation for the differences in radiographic breast density may lie in plasma lipid levels. In one study, mammographic density was associated with plasma levels of high-density lipoprotein (HDL) cholesterol, low-density lipoprotein (LDL) cholesterol, triglycerides, and apoprotein B, and urinary excretion of the mutagen malondialdehyde (66). The relationship of these observations to breast cancer risk remains to be defined.

Few correlations between mammographic appearance and histopathology have been published. One autopsy study that allowed comparison of breast histopathology with whole breast mammograms of formalin-fixed mastectomy specimens showed that in most women the mammographic parenchymal pattern is confounded by obesity, the normal aging process, and genetic factors (67). Correspondingly, the correlation of the mammographic pattern with the amount of breast parenchyma and the presence of fibrocystic changes was poor. Mammographic lucency was closely associated with age, obesity, and large breast size. These observations suggest that parenchymal pattern may not, in fact, be an independent predictor of the risk of breast cancer.

Risk Factors of Uncertain Significance

Body Size and Obesity

Although body weight and measures of body size are positively associated with the risk of developing breast cancer in postmenopausal women, a negative association between weight and breast cancer risk has been found in premenopausal women (11,68–71). On the other hand, data about height as an independent risk factor are conflicting, and no plausible mechanism has been proposed that would explain the interactive effect of body size and menopausal status on the risk of breast cancer. Some studies reported either that a weight gain in adulthood is associated with increased risk of breast cancer or that the ratio of central to peripheral fat distribution affects risk (68,70). Whether this is related to endogenous estrogen production by adipose tissue remains speculative. The effect of obesity on other risk factors for breast cancer is not well studied, with the exception of the association of obesity or large body size with early age at menarche. It is not clear whether significant weight reduction has a substantial protective effect on breast cancer risk.

Exercise

That physical exercise may be biologically linked to breast cancer risk is plausible because strenuous physical activity is associated with an increase in luteal-phase defects, anovulation, and depressed serum estradiol levels (72). Exercise may also influence the prevalence of obesity, but large body mass has actually been associated with reductions in the risk of premenopausal breast cancer, as noted earlier. Both the timing of weight change in adulthood and body fat distribution may be important determinants of risk, but additional studies are needed to clarify the hormonal consequences of physical activity and obesity.

Studies showing that moderate physical activity can have a protective effect against the development of breast cancer (73) have been difficult to confirm (74,75). Various studies of different designs showed nonsignificant protection afforded by physical activity, or an unexpected increased risk among the most physically active women, either premenopausal (76) or postmenopausal (72). Studies of women with nonsedentary occupations suggested that physical activity at work may lower the risk of dying of breast cancer by approximately 15% (77), but results have been inconsistent (78).

Some of these earlier studies may have been handicapped by an inability to control for other breast cancer risk factors, to accurately measure physical activity, or to account for changes in activity over time. More recent research done with greater methodologic rigor did show that the average number of hours spent in physical exercise activities per week from menarche to early middle age is a significant predictor of reduced breast cancer risk. In one study, women who spent 1 to 3 hours per week in physical activity reduced their risk of breast cancer by 30% relative to inactive women, and those who exercised at least 4 hours per week reduced the risk by 50%. The effect was greatest for women who had at least one child, and the effect was not lost among obese women (79). The interaction of physical activity with other breast cancer risk factors is not yet clear, and more information is required. It is not known, for example, whether physical activity can reduce the risk associated with genetic predisposition or proliferative benign breast disease. Women with these conditions should be counseled that there is uncertainty about the protective effect of physical exercise in the setting of their risk factor profiles.

Diet

Fat consumption in the diet was thought to influence the risk of breast cancer, largely on the basis of the observation that the age-adjusted incidence rates for breast cancer are highest in countries with the highest levels of dietary fat consumption (80). Case-control and prospective cohort studies, however, showed either weak or nonexistent associations between dietary fat and the risk of breast cancer (3). For example, the Nurses' Health Study, a prospective evaluation of more than 90,000 registered nurses in the United States, found equal risks for breast cancer across all levels of dietary fat and fiber consumption for both premenopausal and postmenopausal women (81). The explanation for these apparently conflicting observations may lie in the micronutrient components of the diets consumed rather than in the levels of total fat or calories.

Supporting the view that dietary subcomponents may affect cancer risk more than fat or total calories consumed is the fact that some polyunsaturated fatty acids can serve as substrates for prostaglandin synthesis and are implicated in tumorigenesis (82). Other polyunsaturated fatty acids have a double bond between the third and fourth carbon atoms (so-called omega-3 fatty acids) and are competitive inhibitors of prostaglandin endoperoxidase synthetase. It is possible, therefore, that the omega-3 fatty acids (such as eicosapentaenoic or docosahexaenoic acids) may act as dietary inhibitors of carcinogenesis. This protective effect is suggested by the lower age-standardized breast cancer incidence rates from countries around the world where the consumption of fish oil (a rich source of omega-3 fatty acids) is high (83,84). These data suggest a protective effect from fish oils, but additional studies in women are needed before dietary modification or supplementation can be recommended as a proven breast cancer prevention strategy.

Similar suggestive but unconfirmed data exist for populations with increased dietary consumption of soybeans. Increased soy protein consumption is significantly correlated with a reduction in the risk of breast cancer (85). Asians, for example, eat diets rich in soybean products and have breast cancer death rates one third to one half those of women in the West (86). Foods made from soybeans contain large quantities of isoflavones, which are phytoestrogens with weak estrogen agonist activity and may interfere with the breast cancer–promoting effects of physiologic estrogen (87). These promising compounds merit additional clinical investigations. Until these studies are completed, it is not yet appropriate to suggest to women that they can significantly lower their risk of breast cancer by increasing their consumption of soybean products.

Vitamins

The antioxidant vitamins A, C, and E have potential preventive properties because endogenous production of hydrogen peroxide has been associated with tumor cell proliferation, may confer a growth advantage to tumor cell populations, and may contribute to the malignant phenotype (88). Antioxidant vitamins may reduce the risk of cancer through their functions as free radical scavengers and as blockers

of nitrosation reactions (89). Despite these plausible hypotheses, the epidemiologic evidence demonstrating a significant relationship between either serum levels or dietary intake of vitamins C and E and reduced risk of breast cancer is limited and inconsistent (89,90). The epidemiologic and prospective cohort data for vitamin A intake suggest a modest protective effect against breast cancer among women in is highest intake quartiles (91,92), but it is not yet known whether supplemental vitamin A will reduce the risk of breast cancer for women with average dietary intakes of vitamin A. While clinical studies are in progress to address that question, women should be cautioned not to exceed the recommended daily doses of vitamins—particularly the fat-soluble vitamins A and E—that have known and potentially serious toxicities at higher doses.

Alcohol

There are several mechanisms through which ethanol may increase the risk of breast cancer. It may 1) induce increased levels of circulating estrogen, 2) stimulate hepatic metabolism of carcinogens such as acetaldehyde, 3) facilitate transport of carcinogens into breast tissue, 4) stimulate pituitary production of prolactin, 5) modulate cell membrane integrity with an effect on carcinogenesis, 6) aid production of cytotoxic protein products, 7) impair immune surveillance, 8) interfere with DNA repair, 9) promote production of toxic congeners, 10) increase exposure to toxic oxidants, or 11) reduce intake and bioavailability of protective nutrients (93–95). Few of these mechanisms have been studied, however, either in experimental animals or in humans, with the exception of the effect of alcohol consumption on plasma and urinary hormone concentrations in premenopausal women. When female volunteers aged 21 to 40 years were given a controlled diet that included 30 g of alcohol daily (equivalent to about two drinks) through three menstrual cycles, significant increases were seen in periovulatory plasma levels of dehydroepiandrosterone sulfate, estrone, and estradiol. Luteal-phase increases in levels of urinary estrone, estradiol, and estriol were also recorded (96). Although no changes were found in the percentage of bioavailable estradiol, the increased total estradiol levels in the periovulatory phase suggest elevated absolute amounts of bioavailable estradiol. These results imply that there are major effects of alcohol on both estrogen production and metabolism. It is not clear whether increased levels of bioavailable estradiol increase either the risk of breast cancer or the chance that a breast cancer will contain measurable estrogen receptors, but it is clear that alcohol may play some role.

Individual studies of the effect of alcohol intake on breast cancer risk showed no increase in risk for daily ethanol intakes of less than 6 g, with the risk increasing linearly to an odds ratio of 2.4 for intakes between 33 and 45 g/day (97). Studies also showed little effect on risk from alcohol consumption in early adult life, and a relative risk of approximately 1.2 for consumption of each 13 g/day in later adult life (98).

Meta-analysis of the published literature relating alcohol consumption and breast cancer revealed strong evidence of a dose-response relationship with a very modest slope (99). The relative risks of breast cancer associated with consumption of one, two, or three drinks per day are 1.11, 1.24, and 1.38, respectively. Although nearly all studies in the meta-analysis were adjusted for known breast cancer risk factors and socioeconomic factors, the individual studies remain confounded by a number of biases (95). The data do not support a recommendation that women should abstain from alcohol to reduce their breast cancer risk. Furthermore, the beneficial effects of light to moderate alcohol consumption on overall mortality must be taken into consideration before abstinence can be recommended as a breast cancer control strategy (100,101). Nevertheless, women who are at increased risk for breast cancer and at low risk of heart disease may wish to consider limiting their alcohol consumption.

Oral Contraceptives

The relationship between oral contraceptive use and breast cancer risk has been the subject of numerous epidemiologic investigations over the past several decades (102–107). Earlier studies (102,103) showed little relationship between oral contraceptive use and breast cancer, but recent studies (106) demonstrated an increased risk among certain subsets of users, especially among women diagnosed with breast cancer before age 35 or who have used oral contraceptives for 10 years or longer. Relative risks are as high as threefold for women who began oral contraceptive use before age 18 and continued usage for more than 10 years. Increased risk is also observed for women who used oral contraceptives within 5 years of their cancer diagnosis or who had cancers diagnosed at advanced stages. Oral contraceptive use in the reported case-control studies appears to increase the risk of premenopausal, bilateral breast cancer (108). It is not clear whether the reported increased risk in younger women is due to patterns of use or to specific disease characteristics of the breast cancers such as hormone receptor status or proliferative activity.

With data from eight population-based case-control studies of oral contraceptive use and breast cancer risk among women younger than 45 years, it is possible to estimate that there is a 3.1% increase in breast cancer risk per year of oral contraceptive use (107). This risk increases to 3.8% per year of oral contraceptive use before a first birth. Nevertheless, the absolute risk of breast cancer among younger women in the general population is small, and oral contraceptive use might add one or two additional cases for every 100,000 women in this age group.

Among older women, some studies showed a decreasing risk with either increasing intervals since first or last use of oral contraceptives. This may indicate that oral contraceptives merely advance the presentation of disease rather than acting as a true causal factor (109). Taken together, these studies showed inconsistent patterns of use among those women with excess risk. Because the relative risks in these studies were usually twofold or less, there is the possibility that the positive findings might have been influenced by the selective use of screening among the users with the introduction of both detection and lead-time biases. This possibility is supported by multiple studies showing that oral contraceptive users tend to have tumors that are smaller and less often of late stage than do nonusers (110–112).

In summary, the risk of breast cancer associated with oral contraceptive use is small and is greatest among younger women who use oral contraceptives for prolonged periods of time. There is little evidence to indicate that elimination of oral contraceptive use would have an important effect on breast cancer incidence rates.

Estrogen Replacement Therapy

It is generally accepted that endogenous estrogens play some role in the causation of breast cancer (10,11), but the risk of breast cancer among women using estrogen replacement therapy after menopause is the subject of controversy and conflicting data in the medical literature (113). Although steroid hormones are not known to act as tumor-initiating agents, in postmenopausal women obesity is positively associated both with elevated concentrations of endogenous estrogens (114) and with moderate elevations in the risk of breast cancer. Obesity is characterized by increased peripheral aromatization of precursor androgens to estrogens (115), which is the main source of estrogens in postmenopausal women (116). Intake of replacement hormones in doses adequate for relief of postmenopausal symptoms usually produces serum estradiol levels equivalent to those of the midfollicular phase of the normal menstrual cycle in a premenopausal woman (117) and plasma estradiol levels up to five times higher than those in an untreated postmenopausal woman. Although direct epidemiologic evidence linking endogenous estrogen levels to breast cancer is limited, serum levels of estrogen appear to be related to the risk of developing breast cancer after adjusting for body mass. The odds ratio for the highest quartile of estradiol serum levels is 1.8 when compared with the lowest quartile, and the odds ratios for the highest quartile of estrone are threefold higher (118). Both free estradiol and that bound to albumin appear to increase risk, while estradiol bound to SHBG does not, possibly because it is less biologically active. These observations indicate that factors that either increase the endogenous production of estrogen or reduce the binding of estradiol to SHBG may increase a woman's risk of developing breast cancer.

Our understanding of the effect of progestational agents on the breast is incomplete. Animal studies indicated that the administration of progestagens before a chemical carcinogen inhibits tumor production, while treatment with progestagens after the initiating agent has the opposite effect (119). Human breast epithelial cells proliferate in response to estrogens, and the presence of progesterone further increases cell division (120). Despite these laboratory observations, combined estrogen and progestin hormone replacement therapy in middle-aged women did not increase the risk of breast cancer in some studies (121), but increased it slightly in others (122). The epidemiologic data related to this association are limited, however,

because addition of progestins to hormone replacement regimens is a relatively recent practice and the observation times for women taking progestins are short. It is reassuring that depot medroxyprogesterone acetate, a potent, long-acting injectable progestagen contraceptive, does not increase the risk of breast cancer overall, although the remote possibility exists that it might accelerate the growth of occult cancers (123). More human observational data are required before the effect of combined estrogen and progestin therapy on the breast can be completely understood.

Most studies that evaluated estrogen replacement therapy following menopause and its possible role in the development of breast cancer found no overall increase in risk (33,124–129), though several studies demonstrated a modest overall increase (130,131). Such studies may be confounded, however, by a bias in treatment selection that denies hormone replacement therapy to women with a family history of breast cancer (132). If physicians are less likely to prescribe estrogen for women with a family history of breast cancer, a lack of association or a spurious inverse relationship between estrogen use and breast cancer risk may appear.

Despite methodologic rigor and careful selection of subjects, individual reports about the effect of estrogen replacement therapy on breast cancer risk provide conflicting results. Because individual studies may be subject to serious limitations owing to small numbers of subjects and short observation times, meta-analyses have been done to combine available data and to increase the power of the analyses. Meta-analysis is a systematic and quantitative statistical method of combining data across studies to increase statistical power and to generalize results. Meta-analyses of the effect of estrogen replacement therapy on the risk of breast cancer have yielded mixed results.

At least three meta-analyses to determine the effect of noncontraceptive estrogen replacement therapy on breast cancer risk have been published (133–135). None of the studies found a positive association between estrogen replacement therapy and risk of breast cancer when women who had ever used estrogen were compared with women who had never used it. One study (135) was unable to conclude whether there was an effect of duration of use on the risk of breast cancer, and one study found no effect (134). In a third meta-analysis that used studies published in the English-language literature between 1966 and 1989, Steinberg et al (133) found that the risk of breast cancer did not increase for women who experienced any type of menopause until after at least 5 years of estrogen use. After 15 years of use, the risk of breast cancer increased 30% (relative risk = 1.3), but the increase in risk was largely due to studies that included premenopausal women or women using estradiol with or without progestin, for whom the relative risk was 2.2 after 15 years. Of greatest concern was the finding that the relative risk was 3.4 among women with a family history of breast cancer (at least one first-degree relative) who had used estrogen replacement therapy compared with 1.5 for women with a family history who had not used estrogen replacement therapy. However, the increased risk among women with a family history may be due to the difference in preparations of estrogen used in the United States and Europe.

These results do not provide definitive evidence that hormone replacement therapy with low-dose conjugated estrogens, including therapy in high-risk women, increases the risk of breast cancer. The possibility remains, however, that the risk may be moderately increased with long durations of use (>5 years), with higher doses, and with unconjugated estrogens (e.g., estradiol). Because the data were derived from analyses of retrospectively constructed subsets, the risk of estrogen replacement therapy for women with a family history of breast cancer is unclear.

Unlike the studies of replacement hormones given after menopause, most studies of oral contraceptive use, as noted earlier in this chapter, showed no associated increase in the risk of breast cancer (136–138), and one study suggested a reduced risk in oral contraceptive users (139).

The morbidity and mortality associated with estrogen deficiency in postmenopausal women are substantial. Estrogen deficiency causes hot flashes, mood swings, and genital atrophy with resultant dyspareunia. These symptoms are relieved by estrogen replacement therapy. More importantly, the risk of death from cardiovascular disease increases 18-fold after menopause (140), and elevated levels of total cholesterol and LDL cholesterol have been causally related to an increased risk of coronary vascular disease. Cohort studies indicated reductions in total mortality, coronary heart disease mortality,

and hip fracture incidence among current users of estrogen replacement therapy (141). Increased incidences of breast and endometrial cancers appear to be offset by reduced risks of other neoplasms.

The use of estrogen replacement therapy after menopause has a favorable influence on HDL cholesterol, LDL cholesterol, and total cholesterol levels. Estrogen supplementation reduces the risk for coronary heart disease (142), and estrogen replacement therapy has a vascular protective effect (143). In addition, numerous studies demonstrated that all-cause mortality and mortality from coronary heart disease and cerebrovascular disease are reduced in women who have used estrogen replacement therapy (144). Estrogen supplementation can also reduce or prevent trabecular bone loss and the development of osteoporosis (145,146), another cause of significant postmenopausal morbidity.

Contrary to these arguments for the use of estrogen replacement therapy, there are data showing that breast cancer risk is lower among women who experience menarche at a later age, who have fewer ovulatory menstrual cycles during their lifetime, or who are younger at menopause, whether the menopause is natural or surgically induced (147,148). Despite these observations, the lower risk of breast cancer among women who have lower endogenous estrogen levels does not necessarily imply an increased risk of breast cancer in women who receive estrogen replacement therapy at menopause.

In light of the published benefits of estrogen replacement therapy with regard to quality of life, reduction of cardiovascular morbidity and mortality, and reduction of morbidity and mortality attributable to osteoporosis, estrogen replacement therapy must be considered in postmenopausal women. It is unreasonable to reject such therapy as inappropriate for women at increased risk (149–151). One useful strategy is to assist a woman in weighing the risks and benefits of estrogen replacement therapy in her personal clinical situation. For example, postmenopausal women taking hormone replacement therapy can expect a 35% reduction in the risk of coronary heart disease and a 25% reduction in the lifetime risk of hip fracture (144). The change in life expectancy associated with taking hormone replacement therapy is related to the underlying risks of heart disease, osteoporosis, and breast cancer in each individual and varies from 8 months to more than 2 years. Net benefit may be derived from hormone replacement therapy even if it is associated with a small increase in the risk of breast cancer. Published evaluations of individual risks and benefits are available (144) and should be consulted to assist in clinical decision making. Discussion of the effect of hormone replacement therapy on overall quality of life should be included in the clinical discussion. Estrogen replacement therapy should then be offered to women who accept the potential risks and known benefits (144,152).

Environment (Radiation)

Few environmental exposures have been definitely associated with increased risk of breast cancer, but exposure to ionizing radiation is known to increase the risk. Exposure to atomic bomb irradiation, chest fluoroscopy for tuberculosis, treatment of postpartum mastitis, diagnostic roentgenography for scoliosis, and therapeutic irradiation for breast cancer are all associated with an increased risk of subsequent breast cancer (153). Relative risks vary from 1.2 to 2.4 and are related to both total dose and age at exposure, with younger women being at greater risk than older women (153,154).

Of particular concern are individuals who are heterozygotes for the ataxia telangiectasia (*ATM*) gene, who make up about 1% of the general population. Female AT heterozygotes who are exposed to ionizing radiation have nearly a sixfold increased risk of developing breast cancer compared with nonexposed control subjects (155). This observation raises concerns about the safety of mammographic screening in women who are AT heterozygotes, but there are no current public health recommendations regarding screening of these women. Recent cloning of the gene (156) makes it likely that AT heterozygotes can be identified, but a strategy to systematically identify and counsel these women remains to be defined.

Quantitative Risk Assessment

Women who are at increased risk for breast cancer can be identified using individual risk factors one at a time (see Table 1-1). This approach does not permit combining risk factors, however, nor does it lend itself readily to calculating a woman's lifetime probability of developing breast cancer. Multivariate risk models allow determination of composite relative risk for breast cancer along with a cumulative lifetime risk adjusted both for all risk factors taken together and for competing causes of mortality, expressed as the percentage chance that a woman will ever develop breast cancer. Published data are derived largely from studies of white women, and the generalizability of the data to other racial and ethnic groups is uncertain.

The model developed by Gail et al (21) is a widely used method of quantifying a woman's risk of developing breast cancer. It is being used for risk evaluation in the Breast Cancer Prevention Trial, a clinical study to determine the worth of tamoxifen in preventing breast cancer in women who are at increased risk (157). The model allows estimation of the likelihood that a woman of a given age with certain risk factors will develop breast cancer over a specified interval. The model was derived using 4496 matched pairs of subjects from the BCDDP, a mammography screening project carried out between 1973 and 1980 involving more than 280,000 women. Each pair of subjects included a woman with breast cancer and a matched control subject. Using logistic regression techniques, Gail et al examined a number of possible risk factors for breast cancer including the use of various medications, including hormones; cigarette smoking and alcohol consumption; height; gynecologic history, including a woman's age at menarche and at first childbirth; history of breast biopsy; and family history of breast cancer in first-degree relatives (i.e., mother, sisters, or daughters). The risk factors were adjusted simultaneously for the presence of the other risk factors, and only five factors were shown to be significant predictors of the lifetime risk of breast cancer:

Current age

Age at menarche

Number of breast biopsies

Age at first live birth

Family history of breast cancer in first-degree relatives

Each risk factor is grouped into categories as shown in Table 1-7. The procedure to determine a woman's risk is straightforward. Age at menarche is considered alone, and its associated relative risk is referenced in the table. Next, a woman's age and the number of breast biopsies (incisional, excisional, or fine-needle aspirations but not cyst aspirations) performed for benign breast disease are then considered together, and a second relative risk is derived from Table 1-7. A breast biopsy showing atypical hyperplasia doubles the risk estimate shown in the table. To obtain the final relative risk for the model, a woman's age at the time of first live birth is considered together with the number of first-degree relatives with breast cancer.

Consider, for example, a 45-year-old woman who reports menarche at age 12, one breast biopsy, no children, and a sister with breast cancer. Table 1-7 shows that the relative risk associated with menarche at age 12 is 1.099. For a woman younger than 50 having one biopsy, the associated relative risk is 1.698. Finally, a nulliparous woman with one affected first-degree relative with breast cancer has an asso-

ciated relative risk of 2.756. These three relative risks are then multiplied together to obtain a summary relative risk: $1.099 \times 1.698 \times 2.756 = 5.14$, or 5.0 for practical purposes.

This number, 5.0, represents this woman's lifetime relative risk of developing breast cancer when compared with a woman of the same age without any of the identified risk factors. A relative risk is not very useful, however, for providing information about an individual's risk of breast cancer. Recognizing this, Gail et al calculated lifetime probabilities of developing breast cancer with a given relative risk and adjusting for competing causes of death (a woman cannot develop breast cancer if she first dies of another disease). These data are shown in Table 1-8, which contains estimates of developing breast cancer during 10, 20, or 30 years of follow-up. The table shows an "initial rela-

T A B L E   1-7

Gail's Risk Model and Associated Relative Risks (21)*

Risk Factor (Code No.)		Associated Relative Risk	No. of Cases (n = 2852)	No. of Controls (n = 3146)
Age at menarche (yr)				
≥14 (0)		1.000	790	926
12–13 (1)		1.099	1554	1735
<12 (2)		1.207	508	485
No. of biopsies				
Age <50 yr				
0 (0)		1.000	635	794
1 (1)		1.698	113	93
≥2 (2)		2.882	66	24
Age ≥50 yr				
0 (0)		1.000	1551	1817
1 (1)		1.273	312	300
≥2 (2)		1.620	175	118
Age at first live birth (yr)	No. of relatives			
<20 (0)	0 (0)	1.000	167	285
	1 (1)	2.607	44	40
	2 (2)	6.798	8	0
20–24 (1)	0 (0)	1.244	708	1042
	1 (1)	2.681	208	123
	2 (2)	5.775	25	5
25–29 or nulliparous (2)	0 (0)	1.548	968	1106
	1 (1)	2.756	247	178
	2 (2)	4.907	46	20
≥30 (3)	0 (0)	1.927	307	291
	1 (1)	2.834	87	50
	2 (2)	4.169	19	6

*Relative risk compared with that of an individual of the same age without any risk factors is estimated by locating the person's associated relative risk for age at menarche, number of biopsies, and the combination of age at first live birth and number of relatives and multiplying these three numbers together.

Source: Gail MH, Brinton LA, Byar DP, et al. Projecting individualized probabilities of developing breast cancer for white females who are being examined annually. *J Natl Cancer Inst* 1989;81:1879–1886.

T A B L E **1-8**

Projected Probability (%) of Developing Breast Cancer within 10, 20, or 30 Years of Follow-Up (21)

Initial Age (yr)	Years of Follow-Up	Later Relative Risk[a]	Initial Relative Risk[a,b]					
			1.0	2.0	5.0	10.0	20.0	30.0
20	10	—	0.0	0.1	0.2	0.5	1.0	1.4
	20	—	0.5	1.0	2.5	4.9	9.5	14.0
	30	—	1.7	3.4	8.3	15.9	29.3	40.5
30	10	—	0.5	0.9	2.3	4.4	8.7	12.8
	20	—	1.7	3.3	8.1	15.6	28.8	39.9
	30	1.0	3.2	4.8	9.5	16.9	29.9	40.8
		2.0	4.7	6.3	10.9	18.2	30.9	41.7
		5.0	8.9	10.4	14.9	21.8	34.0	44.3
		10.0	15.6	17.1	21.2	27.6	38.8	48.3
		20.0	27.6	28.8	32.3	37.8	47.4	55.5
		30.0	37.7	38.7	41.8	46.4	54.7	61.7
40	10	—	1.2	2.5	6.1	11.8	22.2	31.3
	20	1.0	2.8	4.0	7.5	13.1	23.4	32.4
		2.0	4.3	5.5	8.9	14.5	24.5	33.4
		5.0	8.6	9.7	13.1	18.3	28.0	36.4
		10.0	15.4	16.4	19.5	24.4	33.3	41.1
		20.0	27.4	28.4	30.9	35.2	42.7	49.5
		30.0	37.7	38.5	40.7	44.3	50.8	56.6
	30	1.0	4.4	5.6	9.1	14.6	24.6	33.5
		2.0	7.4	8.6	11.9	17.3	27.0	35.6
		5.0	15.9	17.0	20.0	24.9	33.7	41.5
		10.0	28.3	29.2	31.8	35.9	43.4	50.0
		20.0	47.5	48.1	50.0	53.1	58.5	63.4
		30.0	61.2	61.6	63.1	65.3	69.3	72.8
50	10	—	1.6	3.1	7.6	14.6	27.1	37.7
	20	—	3.2	6.4	15.1	27.9	47.8	61.9
	30	—	4.4	8.5	19.9	35.5	57.8	71.7
60	10	—	1.8	3.6	8.6	16.5	30.1	41.5
	20	—	3.0	5.9	14.0	25.9	44.6	58.2
70	10	—	1.4	2.7	6.7	12.9	24.1	33.7

[a] The initial relative risk corresponds to the initial age. If the initial age is <50 and if the initial age plus the follow-up specified is >50, then a later relative risk at age 50 should also be specified. If the initial age is ≥50, only the initial relative risk is required. If the initial age is <50 and if the initial age plus the years of follow-up does not exceed 50, then only an initial relative risk is required.

[b] Values in columns are projected probabilities expressed as percentages.

Source: Gail MH, Brinton LA, Byar DP, et al. Projecting individualized probabilities of developing breast cancer for white females who are being examined annually. *J Natl Cancer Inst* 1989;81:1879–1886.

tive risk" and a "later relative risk." As explained in the footnote to Table 1-8, the initial relative risk corresponds to the subject's initial age (i.e., her age at evaluation). If the initial age is less than 50 and the woman will be older than 50 at the end of the specified follow-up period, then a later relative risk should be specified using the age term in Table 1-7. For the woman illustrated above, her initial relative risk is 5.0, but she becomes older than 50 during the first follow-up interval of 10 years, indicating that a later relative risk must be calculated. In Table 1-7, we see that the associated relative risk for a woman older than 50 with one biopsy is 1.273. The later relative risk then becomes: $1.099 \times 1.273 \times 2.756 = 3.85$.

The probabilities in Table 1-8 are approximations, at best. For our 45-year-old patient, we begin in the initial relative risk column labeled 5.0. Looking down the column to the line that corresponds to an initial age of 40 years and 10 years of follow-up, we find a 10-year probability of developing breast cancer of 6.1%. For 20 years of follow-up, we calculated a later relative risk of 3.85, which is between 2.0 and 5.0. The 20-year probability of breast cancer with an initial relative risk of 5.0 and a later relative risk of 2.0 is 8.9%; for an initial relative risk of 5.0 and a later relative risk of 3.8 the 20-year probability is 13.1%. Therefore, this woman's 20-year probability of developing breast cancer is approximately 12%. Finally, her 30-year probability is between 11.9% and 20%, or about 17%.

There are limitations to the use of the Gail model. Investigators who have attempted to validate the model found that it overpredicted absolute breast cancer risk by 33% among women aged 25 to 61 years who did not receive annual screening (158). Most of the overprediction is confined to premenopausal women who do not adhere to guidelines for annual mammographic screening (159) and to women with extensive family histories of breast cancer in whom other risk models may be more appropriate. I consider one of those models later in this chapter. Critics of the Gail model also suggest that there are ethical questions regarding the value of individual breast cancer risk prediction in the absence of safe and effective preventive regimens. Conversely, it may be unethical not to offer counseling to women who overestimate their risk and live with inappropriate anxiety or elect unnecessary procedures such as prophylactic mastectomy.

Alternatives to the Gail model are available. These models offer the advantage of counting the number of first- or second-degree relatives affected with breast cancer and considering their ages at diagnosis (36,48,52). Both of these factors are known to affect the risk of developing breast cancer and are not considered in the Gail model. A practical modification of one of these models is shown in Table 1-4. More complete risk assessment tables are available in the literature (36,48,52), and all permit calculation of a lifetime probability of developing breast cancer.

Any valid estimate of a woman's lifetime probability of developing breast cancer can be used for counseling purposes and for making decisions about clinical management of risk. The clinician should be positive in his or her recommendations and deliver clear messages regarding risk management, emphasizing that risk calculations should be used only to estimate the probability of developing the disease and not the risk of dying of breast cancer (36). Previous research suggests that counseling about risk may have unwanted psychological effects (160), so counseling should include an assessment of risk perception. Women younger than 50 who are at increased risk for breast

cancer tend to overestimate their risk, even as much as 20-fold (1). A substantial proportion of women who have abnormal-appearing mammograms but not cancer report significant impairments in mood and daily functioning (161,162), and more than one fourth of high-risk women may have clinically elevated levels of psychological distress (163). Psychological distress may, in turn, interfere with adherence to recommended breast screening (162–166) or other preventive behaviors. While the preliminary studies showed a greater likelihood of having prior mammograms among women with higher self-perceived risks of breast cancer (167), more research is needed to define at what level risk perception becomes inhibitory rather than motivating. Because of these recognized concerns about psychological issues, it is important to explore a woman's fears about breast cancer, and the clinician should ask each patient if her worries about breast cancer impede her daily functioning. If simple reassurance and encouragement do not relieve anxiety or the patient cannot participate in making clinical decisions because of her anxiety, psychological consultation is warranted.

Management of Women at Increased Risk

Optimal preventive strategies for breast cancer have not yet been identified, although a great deal of research is being conducted in this area. In this section, I highlight current information about mammographic screening prescriptions, prophylactic mastectomy, and primary prevention that will guide clinicians in selecting interventions for women who are at increased risk. Clinicians are referred to several excellent reviews that cover clinical management strategies in greater detail (168–170).

Mammographic Screening Prescriptions

Annual mammographic screening in women 50 years and older reduces mortality by 25% to 30% (171), and there is little debate that screening should be employed in postmenopausal women. There is also growing evidence that screening offers benefit in women between the ages of 40 and 49 years (172), but uncertainty about the magnitude of the benefit remains (173). Only one prospective, randomized comparison of mammographic screening in women younger than 50 years has been published (174), but technical limitations prevent acceptance of the trial's negative findings as definitive (175).

The performance profile of any screening test is related not only to the clinical characteristics of the test (e.g., the sensitivity and specificity of the test), but also to the prevalence of the disease in the population being screened (176). In a population of women younger than 50 years who are at increased risk of breast cancer, the prevalence of the disease is increased, and therefore the performance outcomes of screening mammography should not differ from the outcomes of mammographic screening in older populations who have the same breast cancer prevalence (177). In fact, imaging breast cancers appears to be as efficient in very young women as in older women (178). These observations support annual mammographic screening for women 40 to 49 years old who are at average risk for breast cancer, but the data do not address the question of screening women younger than 40 years who are at increased risk. I review that question next.

Mammographic screening offers several benefits as well as potential risks. The benefits include a demonstrated decrease in mortality for women older than 50 years, the ability to use conservative surgery for smaller, less advanced breast cancers, and the psychological reassurance gained by a woman after negative mammography findings (161). The drawbacks of screening include physical discomfort from compression techniques and the fact that screening increases the likelihood of women having to undergo additional investigations including breast ultrasound, fine-needle aspiration, needle biopsy, or open biopsy. In addition, there is the possibility of overtreating lesions that are actually benign clinically and that would not have come to clinical attention in the absence of screening (179). Unnecessary surgery and radiation therapy may be used to treat these lesions that impose no true threat to health. Screening mammography has inherent limitations in its sensitivity: As many as 15% of negative mammography results may be false negative (180). The false reassurance that follows a negative mammography result may lead to decreased compliance with attendance at future scheduled screenings, and this issue has not been investigated in women who are at increased risk. There is also some psychological morbidity associated with undergoing mammographic screening (161,162).

There are more than 20 million women between the ages of 30 and 39 in the United States, and as many as 20% of these women may be at increased risk for breast cancer (173). Anecdotal reports indicated that mammography visualizes 90% of breast cancers occurring in younger women (178). Although there are no data about the outcome of mammographic screening in women younger than 40, these anxious patients often demand that clinicians do something to help them manage their risk. This is a challenge in the absence of a proven benefit from any specific screening regimen. To do no screening until age 40 in women who are at increased risk may miss an opportunity to prevent mortality from breast cancer, yet it is also possible that screening women before age 40 will incur expense without offering benefit. Clinicians must discuss these uncertainties with patients who request screening before age 40, and they must also inform patients that their health insurance carrier may not cover the cost of their screening mammograms even though mammograms in older women are paid for.

If a clinician decides that screening should begin at age 30, the initial consideration is whether the younger woman is attempting to become pregnant, is pregnant, or is lactating. Although the radiation dose to a fetus from a screening mammogram is minimal, the exposure must be avoided. Equally important, the benign nodular densities that appear in the breasts of lactating and pregnant women generate an increased number of false-positive mammographic readings that must also be avoided. Pregnant and lactating women who are at increased risk of breast cancer must delay initiation of screening mammography until they are no longer attempting to conceive children. Equally important, any symptomatic breast lesion in a pregnant woman must be evaluated aggressively to rule out the possibility of malignancy.

If a woman age 30 or older is not pregnant and there is evidence of genetic predisposition or familial clustering of breast cancer or an increased risk profile for breast cancer, annual mammographic screening may begin. In a woman without a genetic predisposition to breast cancer but who has had a breast biopsy showing either lobular carcinoma in situ or proliferative disease with or without atypia, initiation of annual mammographic screening is warranted after the biopsy that establishes the diagnosis. In women with none of these findings but who have Gail model risk scores of 5 or higher, initiation of annual mammographic screening at age 30 is advised, on the basis of the disease prevalence considerations explained previously. Most of the women with elevated Gail model risk scores will have multiple affected first-degree relatives with breast cancer or a history of breast biopsy or both (21).

Because adequate mammographic visualization can be difficult in young women with dense breasts (178), ultrasonography should accompany screening mammography to distinguish the frequent cystic lesions that occur in these young women from the solid lesions that require biopsy for diagnosis. This strategy will minimize the number of biopsies performed in young women who receive regular screening.

Prophylactic Mastectomy

There are several possible reasons why prophylactic mastectomy might appear to be a desirable clinical strategy for the control of breast cancer. These include elimination of the risk of developing breast cancer, removal of occult carcinomas, and improvement of psychological distress related to unreasonable fears about the risk of developing breast cancer. Indications for prophylactic mastectomy may include genetic risk, proliferative benign breast disease with or without atypia, and lobular carcinoma in situ. A prophylactic mastectomy is an operation that removes the total breast, tail of Spence, lower axillary lymph nodes, areola, and nipple (181,182). It is typically followed by a reconstructive procedure for cosmetic reasons.

Experimental studies of prophylactic mastectomy in rats given chemical carcinogens showed that tumors occur despite total mastectomy (183), and similar observations have been made in mice that develop spontaneous breast malignancies without mammary carcinogens (184). Pathologic examination of the chest wall and axilla in women undergoing mastectomy for breast cancer shows extension of breast tissue well into the axilla and pectoral fascia (185), indicating that total extirpation of the breast requires even more extensive surgery than a total mastectomy. Less extensive subcutaneous mastectomies are known to be followed by invasive carcinomas in up to 1% of patients (186–188). Although as many as 5% of prophylactic mastectomy specimens contain occult carcinomas (187), there are no data comparing the outcomes of patients managed with prophylactic mastectomy with a similar group of women at increased risk who are followed with close surveillance including mammographic screening and timely biopsy when clinically indicated. Nonrandomized, prospective data do show, however, that prophylactic mastectomy does reduce the subsequent incidence of invasive breast cancer to less than 1% of patients (189). Because of these facts, prophylactic mastectomy for women at increased risk of breast cancer must still be recommended with caution.

Available data also indicate that rather than relieving anxiety, prophylactic mastectomy may increase it and cause other adverse psychological consequences. After prophylactic mastectomy and reconstruction, 20% of women believe their breasts are either too small or in the wrong position, 100% lose erogenous sensitivity in the nipple-areola complex, and 60% report markedly negative changes in their sexual lives (190). Based on these observations, it is difficult to argue in favor of prophylactic mastectomy as an effective preventive procedure with satisfactory clinical and psychological outcomes.

Even though the decision to undergo prophylactic mastectomy may have profound physical and psychological implications for the woman at increased risk, it may be appropriate in a small subset of patients. There are published recommended criteria for third-party payer coverage of prophylactic mastectomy. These include lobular or ductal carcinoma in situ; severe dysplasia; personal history of breast cancer or personal history of breast cancer in the opposite breast; one first-degree relative with bilateral, premenopausal breast cancer; desmoid tumor of the breast or giant fibroadenoma; cystosarcoma phyllodes; significant virginal hypertrophy; or postinjection silicone mastopathy (191). These criteria may be overly aggressive, and not all clinicians would recommend prophylactic surgery for these conditions. Slightly more conservative considerations leading to a decision for prophylactic mastectomy are reviewed in Table 1-9. The presence of lobular carcinoma in situ or atypical lobular or ductal hyperplasia in the setting of a history of breast cancer in first-degree relatives increases the risk of breast cancer significantly (21,192). In these patients, the physician may initiate discussion of the possibility of prophylactic mastectomy with the understanding that one half or more of the patients with these predisposing histologic lesions will never develop breast cancer, making the procedure unnecessary for them. There are currently no validated clinical markers available to determine which patients with these predisposing conditions will develop malignancy.

Women who carry genes that increase the risk of breast cancer (e.g., *BRCA1*, *BRCA2*, *TP53*, *ATM*, etc.) have more than a 60% chance of developing breast cancer by age 50 and may want to consider prophylactic mastectomy (38,55). In women whose risk profiles show them to be at increased risk of breast cancer but who have negative results on genetic testing, a history of repeated breast biopsies in the presence of dense breast parenchyma, a history of proliferative benign breast disease on biopsy, or manifestations of extreme anxiety about developing breast cancer should lead the clinician to discuss prophylactic mastectomy with the patient. The physician should never force the decision on the patient and should carefully explore the relative advantages and disadvantages of the procedure, including the lack of certainty that the patient will develop breast cancer and the rare chance that a prophylactic procedure will not prevent breast cancer from occurring (56). For some patients at increased risk, careful consideration of these risks and benefits will lead to a decision to have prophylactic mastectomy and will reduce anxiety.

Primary Prevention

The optimal strategy to control breast cancer is to prevent it from ever occurring, but there are no proven strategies for the primary prevention of breast cancer. Table 1-10 lists the approaches that are currently under investigation for the prevention of breast cancer. Several strategies

T A B L E   **1-9**

Considerations in the Decision for Prophylactic Mastectomy

Carriers of *BRCA1*, *BRCA2*, *p53*, ataxia-telangiectasia, or other predisposing genes

In the absence of genetic testing, a family history that makes a genetic syndrome likely (e.g., bilateral, premenopausal breast cancer in one or more first-degree relatives or multiple affected relatives in several generations)

Women with a multivariate relative risk score >10 or a lifetime probability of breast cancer >20%

Family history of breast cancer in first-degree relative(s) *plus* a breast biopsy showing atypical hyperplasia

Lobular carcinoma in situ *plus* a family history of breast cancer in first-degree relatives

Increased objective risk *plus* repeated breast biopsies with significant scarring resulting in a difficult physical examination and/or multiple nodular densities on the mammogram

Psychological disability due to extreme fear of cancer

T A B L E   **1-10**

Strategies for Detection and Prevention of Breast Cancer

Method	Example	Limitation
Initiation of screening at an early age	Begin annual mammography at age 30	No demonstrated benefit
Prophylactic mastectomy	In a woman with family history, atypical hyperplasia, etc.	Psychological, physical implications; questionable effectiveness
Antiestrogens	Tamoxifen	Investigational; endometrial carcinoma, thrombosis, menopausal symptoms
Retinoids	Fenretinide	Investigational; night blindness, hepatic toxicity
Gonadotropin-releasing hormone agonists	Leuprolide	Investigational; limited human data
Progestogen antagonists	RU 486	Investigational; limited experience with long-term administration
Phytoestrogens	Soy products	Unknown bioavailability; no controlled observations

that may eventually be employed to prevent breast cancer are reviewed later in the chapter. All of these pharmacologic approaches remain investigational, however, and should not be used for the clinical management of women at increased risk of breast cancer until ongoing investigations of the agents are completed.

Tamoxifen

Prevention of Contralateral Breast Cancer Detailed information on the incidence of second primary breast cancers is available from a comprehensive overview of the world's literature on the use of tamoxifen as adjuvant therapy for breast cancer (193). An unexpected observation from these trials was the reduction in the incidence of contralateral breast cancers in patients receiving tamoxifen. The overview presents data from more than 18,000 women enrolled in 42 separate randomized, placebo-controlled trials for whom information is available about second primary breast cancers occurring as long as 10 years after the initial diagnosis. There were 184 women (2.0%) with second primary breast cancers among 9135 women treated with placebo versus 122 with second primary breast cancers (1.3%) among 9128 women who received 10 to 40 mg of tamoxifen for a median of 2 years (193). A dose-response relationship was observed for the duration of tamoxifen therapy: For women who received therapy for less than 2 years, the reduction in the actuarial odds of a second primary breast cancer was only 26%, compared with a 37% reduction for women with therapy for exactly 2 years and a 56% reduction for women who received adjuvant tamoxifen for more than 2 years. Other studies demonstrated that tamoxifen adjuvant therapy for short durations (e.g., 48 weeks) may not be sufficient to provide protection against the development of second primary breast cancers (194).

Tamoxifen is an antiestrogen that binds to the estrogen receptor, resulting in altered RNA transcription, decreased cell proliferation, and partial estrogen agonist activity. Tamoxifen may also cause apoptosis of potentially malignant cells; modulation of production of transforming growth factors; decreases in circulating insulin-like growth factor I; increases in circulating levels of SHBG that may decrease the availability of free estrogen, removing a stimulus for tumor cell growth; and increases in levels of circulating natural killer cells (195).

Cardiovascular Effects In addition to these observed reductions in the odds of developing a second primary breast cancer, the overview data demonstrate a 12% reduction in nonbreast cancer deaths, a 25% reduction in deaths from vascular disease, and a 9% reduction in other causes of death. A major proportion of the reduction in noncancer deaths is due to a reduction in cardiovascular disease mortality (196,197), and these results are due, in part, to decreases in LDL cholesterol observed as early as 2 months after the initiation of tamoxifen therapy. These reductions are followed at 6 months by either no change or an increase in HDL cholesterol, a fall in LDL cholesterol, and an increase in triglyceride levels (198,199). Tamoxifen's estrogenic effect on the liver may lead to increased synthesis of very-low-density-lipoprotein cholesterol and increased triglyceride levels, decreased levels of apolipoprotein B synthesis, and increased levels of apolipoprotein A-I synthesis, with resultant increased levels of HDL cholesterol (200,201). Longitudinal observations of women at risk for heart disease are limited, but available data indicate that a 15% to 20% decrease in LDL cholesterol may result in a 6% to 20% decrease in coronary heart disease (202,203).

The effect of tamoxifen on the development of atherosclerotic cardiovascular disease may also relate to its antithrombotic properties. Postmenopausal women taking tamoxifen show an average drop of only 10% in antithrombin III levels during therapy, while fibrinogen levels decline 16% or more (204). Population studies demonstrated a relationship between fibrinogen levels, myocardial infarction, and stroke, with lower fibrinogen levels associated with lower cardiovascular risk (205,206). Concerns about the durability of these effects arise from studies of former users of tamoxifen that show reversal of the increases in HDL cholesterol at the cessation of tamoxifen therapy (207). A final assessment of the effect of tamoxifen on the risk of morbidity and mortality from cardiovascular disease in healthy women awaits completion of ongoing studies.

Effects on Bone Bone loss in postmenopausal women is caused primarily by loss of estrogen production by the ovaries. Decreased concentrations of circulating estrogen lead to increased bone resorption, decreased bone density, and osteoporosis with fractures, a major cause of morbidity in women older than 55 (208).

Tamoxifen decreases rates of resorption of trabecular bone in experimental animals, with a resultant net preservation of bone density (209–212). In rats that have undergone oophorectomy, tamoxifen also blocks both bone loss (209) and an increase in osteoclast number and activity (211).

Tamoxifen appears to preserve bone mineral density in postmenopausal women (213,214), presumably because of its estrogenic effect on osteoclasts, which slows bone resorption. Experimental data in vitro showing that tamoxifen blocks bone resorption induced by parathyroid hormone, prostaglandin E_2, and 1,25-dihydroxyvitamin D_3 support these clinical observations of benefit (215). Of some concern is the observation that tamoxifen may reduce bone mineral density in premenopausal women by 1.9% annually while increasing bone density in postmenopausal women by 1.8% (216). Prospective, randomized studies of women taking tamoxifen for the primary prevention of breast cancer will clarify this issue.

Toxicity Associated with Tamoxifen Tamoxifen therapy is associated with a variety of symptomatic toxicities including gynecologic symptoms (particularly hot flashes and vaginal discharge in perimenopausal women) (157). Early reports of an increased risk of thrombotic events were not confirmed in subsequent prospective trials with prolonged periods of observation (197), and no hepatic neoplasms have been reported in women taking the usually prescribed 20 mg daily despite preliminary reports of hepatic neoplasms in women taking 40 mg daily (217). Isolated reports of an increased incidence of gastrointestinal neoplasms occurring in women exposed to tamoxifen (218) were not confirmed in the overview analysis that showed a reduction in all second primary malignancies except endometrial cancer among women taking tamoxifen for the adjuvant treatment of breast cancer (193). Similar negative conclusions were also reached when early reports of ocular toxicity associated with tamoxifen were investigated with properly conducted prospective studies.

A well-established consequence of tamoxifen therapy is an increased incidence of endometrial carcinoma. In a randomized trial from Sweden that used 40 mg of tamoxifen daily, the incidence of uterine tumors (both endometrial carcinomas and uterine sarcomas) was 6.5-fold higher in the women who received tamoxifen than in those who received placebo, and the cumulative frequency of uterine tumors was 0.4% in the control group, 0.9% in women who received tamoxifen for 2 years, and 5.5% in women treated with tamoxifen for 5 years (217,219). In another trial using tamoxifen, 30 mg daily for 48 weeks, the incidence ratio for endometrial carcinomas was 1.9, with cumulative incidences after 10 years of 0.3% and 1.0% in the patients receiving placebo and tamoxifen, respectively (194,220).

Additional data are available from the National Surgical Adjuvant Breast and Bowel Project trial B-14 that included 1419 women randomly assigned to receive tamoxifen, 1220 who entered the study after randomization had been performed but who were taking tamoxifen, and 1424 women randomly assigned to receive placebo (control patients). After an average time of study between 5 and 8 years, 2 patients in the placebo group and 24 in the tamoxifen group developed endometrial carcinoma (221). A number of women in both groups had used estrogen replacement therapy for various periods of time, and the relative contribution of the estrogen therapy to the risk of endometrial carcinoma in these women is unknown. The hazard rate in the placebo group was 0.2 per 1000 women compared with 1.6 per 1000 women in the tamoxifen group (relative risk = 7.5). Occurrences of endometrial carcinoma in the placebo group subsequent to the initial publication of the study have lowered the estimated relative risk to approximately 4.0. Endometrial sampling and abdominal or vaginal ultrasound examination of the endometrium before and during tamoxifen therapy are currently being investigated for their ability to detect early malignancy and to lower the chance of dying of endometrial cancer after exposure to tamoxifen.

Breast cancer patients enrolled in clinical trials may be different in many ways from healthy women in the population who might use tamoxifen for the primary prevention of breast cancer. Population-based studies of breast cancer patients who have used tamoxifen for less than 2 years showed a 50% reduction in the risk of contralateral breast cancer and no increase in the risk of either ovarian or endometrial cancer (222). Such studies also showed a twofold risk of endometrial cancer with cumulative tamoxifen doses higher than 15 g (i.e., 2 years of 20 mg daily) (223). The effect of prolonged administration of tamoxifen to healthy women can only be addressed in a clinical trial.

Retinoids

Retinyl acetate and the synthetic retinoid *N*-(4-hydroxyphenyl)-retinamide (4-HPR, fenretinide) are effective inhibitors of chemically induced breast cancer in rats (224). Fenretinide reduces the incidence and time to appearance of these tumors, and doses up to 200 mg daily with a 3-day drug holiday monthly can be administered chronically to humans, without significant toxicity. The effect of fenretinide is enhanced in rats by oophorectomy, but the drug does not affect circulating levels of estradiol, testosterone, dehydroepiandrosterone sulfate, prolactin, luteinizing hormone, follicle-stimulating hormone, or SHBG.

Retinoids induce the synthesis of transforming growth factor-α, a growth factor that negatively modulates cancer growth, and they lower the levels of insulin-like growth factor I, a potent mitogen for transformed breast epithelium, in both breast cancer cell lines and breast cancer patients (225).

Gonadotropin-Releasing Hormone Agonists

Many risk factors for breast cancer (e.g., age at menarche, age at menopause, age at first live birth) are biologic events mediated by estrogen and progesterone. Both hormones induce growth of the breast epithelium, and this sex steroid–driven breast epithelial proliferation may increase the risk of carcinogenesis by accelerating the occurrence of somatic genetic errors (13,226). Although breast cell proliferation increases in early pregnancy, cell proliferation decreases during the second half of pregnancy when cell differentiation occurs (227). This may account for the small protective effect conferred by pregnancy and delivery that occur at an early age. Some investigators hypothesized that any genetic damage acquired by breast cells during the premenopausal period is not lost following menopause and that this is reflected in the rising breast cancer incidence rates that are observed with advancing age (13), but this hypothesis has not been confirmed.

If one accepts this hypothesis, then suppression of ovarian steroidogenesis should have a favorable effect on breast cancer risk. Optimally, this suppression should occur after the first full-term pregnancy and before age 40. The potentially adverse long-term consequences of such suppression are not yet known. If this were to be done for durations as long as 15 years, the theoretical predicted reduction in the lifetime risks of cancer of the breast, ovary, and endometrium are 70%, 45%, and 84%, respectively, based on a published model (228).

Other Agents

Epidemiologic observations show that breast cancer incidence rates are significantly lower in Asia than in the West (229). These differences may be related to high intakes of polyunsaturated fatty acids, β-carotene, or soy protein, or a combination of these. Breast cancer incidence rates are 40% to 50% lower among Asian women with the highest levels of consumption of soy proteins than among Western women (230). This may be related to the presence of naturally occurring phytoestrogens found in soy products. Phytoestrogens may suppress either the production or the activity of endogenous estrogens and may, thereby, function as inhibitors of hormone-dependent carcinogenesis. No controlled investigations for the prevention of breast cancer with these agents are being conducted yet.

Clinical Trials in Chemoprevention of Breast Cancer

Chemoprevention is the use of specific natural or synthetic chemical agents to reverse, suppress, or prevent carcinogenic progression to invasive cancer (231,232). The ability of tamoxifen to prevent breast cancer, lower cardiovascular mortality, and prevent bone fractures is being evaluated in the Breast Cancer Prevention Trial, a randomized, prospective clinical trial comparing tamoxifen with placebo in women at increased risk of breast cancer (157). The trial began in 1992 and will follow 13,000 women during 5 years of drug administration and 2 additional years of observation. The trial is conducted by the National Surgical Adjuvant Breast and Bowel Project with support from the National Cancer Institute and other government agencies. Eligible women include all those age 60 or older and women between the ages of 35 and 59 who are at increased risk of breast cancer as determined by the Gail model. Participants may not take oral contraceptives or replacement hormones during the trial, but non-hormonal medications are permitted for the management of elevated blood lipid levels or prevention of osteoporosis. The study will evaluate the effect of tamoxifen on both lipids and bone mineral density. The utility of endometrial screening is also being investigated. Results from the Breast Cancer Prevention Trial will not be available for several years, and until the studies in progress are completed and demonstrate a definite benefit from the active agent compared with placebo along with an acceptable toxicity profile, it is inappropriate to prescribe tamoxifen or any other agent with potential for the chemoprevention of breast cancer.

Several investigators conducted a pilot trial of ovarian steroid suppression using leuprolide acetate depot as the gonadotropin-releasing hormone agonist along with replacement doses of conjugated estrogen and medroxyprogesterone acetate to eliminate the hypoestrogenic side effects of the gonadotropin-releasing hormone agonist (226). Symptoms with this regimen are tolerable, but loss of bone density in the lumbar region of the spine necessitates addition of an androgen to the regimen. Favorable changes in mammographic density have been reported with this regimen, but it is not known whether this approach will result in the predicted lowering of the risk of breast cancer. It is certainly too early to apply this prevention strategy outside the context of a clinical trial.

A prospective clinical trial is being conducted in Italy to investigate the ability of 4-HPR to reduce the incidence of second primary breast cancers in women with a first breast cancer (233). Eligible women are 35 to 65 years old with T1 or T2 primary breast cancers, axillary lymph nodes negative for cancer, and no evidence of distant disease who did not receive either adjuvant endocrine therapy or chemotherapy. The results of that study will be important for many obvious reasons, as is the observation in rats that tamoxifen and 4-HPR result in enhanced inhibition of mammary carcinogenesis and reduction in tumor-related mortality (234). If both retinoids and tamoxifen are shown individually to prevent breast cancer in women, additional clinical trials of combination therapy will be warranted.

Finally, a very large clinical trial is being conducted in the United States to evaluate the effect of several interventions on chronic diseases in women. The Women's Health Initiative is both a prospective, randomized trial and an observational study that will evaluate the effect of diet on the risks of breast cancer, colon cancer, and cardiovascular disease; the effect of estrogen replacement therapy on the risk of cardiovascular disease, osteoporosis, and breast cancer; and the effect of calcium supplementation and vitamin D on osteoporosis and other risk factors (235). The trial, which began in 1994, will ultimately enroll more than 100,000 participants and will continue as long as 15 years or until significant end points are achieved.

Conclusions

The ultimate goal when studying breast cancer epidemiology is to identify effective strategies for primary prevention. Potentially effective interventions that may significantly reduce the incidence of breast cancer in the near future are being evaluated. Interim management options can be employed until effective primary prevention is available.

REFERENCES

1. Black WC, Nease RF Jr, Tosteson ANA. Perceptions of breast cancer risk and screening effectiveness in women younger than 50 years of age. *J Natl Cancer Inst* 1995;87:720–731.

2. Lilienfeld AM, Lilienfeld DE. *Foundations of epidemiology.* New York: Oxford University Press, 1980:217, 346–347.

3. Harris JR, Lippman ME, Veronesi U, et al. Breast cancer. *N Engl J Med* 1992;327:319–328.

4. Dawson DA, Thompson GB. Breast cancer risk factors and screening: United States, 1987. National Center for Health Statistics. *Vital Health Stat 10* 1989;172:1–60.

5. Bruzzi P, Green SB, Byar DP, et al. Estimating the population attributable risk for multiple risk factors using case-control data. *Am J Epidemiol* 1985;122:904–914.

6. Seidman H, Stellman SD, Mushinski MH. A different perspective on breast cancer risk factors: some implications of the nonattributable risk. *CA Cancer J Clin* 1982;32:301–313.

7. Madigan MP, Ziegler RG, Benichou J, et al. Proportion of breast cancer cases in the United States explained by well-established risk factors. *J Natl Cancer Inst* 1995;87:1681–1685.

8. Buell P. Changing incidence of breast cancer in Japanese-American women. *J Natl Cancer Inst* 1973;51:1479–1483.

9. Kelsey JL. A review of the epidemiology of human breast cancer. *Epidemiol Rev* 1979;1: 74–109.

10. Kelsey JL, Berkowitz GS. Breast cancer epidemiology. *Cancer Res* 1988;48:5615–5623.

11. Kelsey JL, Gammon MD. Epidemiology of breast cancer. *Epidemiol Rev* 1990;12:228–240.

12. Kelsey JL, Gammon MD, John EM. Reproductive factors and breast cancer. *Epidemiol Rev* 1993;15:36–47.

13. Spicer DV, Krecker EA, Pike MC. The endocrine prevention of breast cancer. *Cancer Invest* 1995;13:495–504.

14. Anderson TJ, Ferguson DJP, Raab GM. Cell turnover in the "resting" human breast: influence of parity, contraceptive pill, age, and laterality. *Br J Cancer* 1982;46:376–382.

15. Daling JR, Malone KE, Voigt LF, et al. Risk of breast cancer among young women: relationship to induced abortion. *J Natl Cancer Inst* 1994;86: 1584–1592.

16. Ernster VL. The epidemiology of benign breast disease. *Epidemiol Rev* 1981;3:184–202.

17. Black MM, Modan B, Lubin F, et al. A nationwide study of breast disease. *Cancer* 1988;61: 2547–2551.

18. Yu H, Rohan TE, Howe GR, et al. Risk factors for fibroadenoma: a case-control study in Australia. *Am J Epidemiol* 1992;135:247–258.

19. Millikan R, Hulka B, Thor A, et al. p53 mutations in benign breast tissue. *J Clin Oncol* 1995;13:2293–2300.

20. Vogel VG. High-risk populations as targets for breast cancer prevention trials. *Prevent Med* 1991;20:86–100.

21. Gail MH, Brinton LA, Byar DP, et al. Projecting individualized probabilities of developing breast cancer for white females who are being examined annually. *J Natl Cancer Inst* 1989;81: 1879–1886.

22. Dupont WD, Page DL. Risk factors for breast cancer in women with proliferative breast disease. *N Engl J Med* 1985;312:146–151.

23. Page DL, Dupont WD, Rogers LW, et al. Atypical hyperplastic lesions of the female breast: a long-term follow-up study. *Cancer* 1985;55: 2698–2708.

24. Carter CL, Corle DK, Micozzi MS, et al. A prospective study of the development of breast cancer in 16,692 women with benign breast disease. *Am J Epidemiol* 1988;128:467–477.

25. London SJ, Connolly JL, Schnitt SJ, et al. A prospective study of benign breast disease and the risk of breast cancer. *JAMA* 1992;267: 941–944.

26. Dupont WD, Parl FF, Hartman, WH, et al. Breast cancer risk associated with proliferative disease and atypical hyperplasia. *Cancer* 1993;71: 1258–1265.

27. Rubin E, Visscher DW, Alexander RW, et al. Proliferative disease and atypia in biopsies performed for nonpalpable lesions detected mammographically. *Cancer* 1988;61:2077–2082.

28. Jensen RA, Page DL, Dupont WD, et al. Invasive breast cancer risk in women with sclerosing adenosis. *Cancer* 1989;64:1977–1983.

29. Marcus JN, Watson P, Page DL, et al. Pathology and heredity of breast cancer in younger women. *Monogr Natl Cancer Inst* 1994;16:23–34.

30. Skolnick MH, Cannon-Albright LA, Goldgar DE, et al. Inheritance of proliferative breast disease in breast cancer kindreds. *Science* 1990;250: 1715–1720.

31. Ward JH, Marshall CJ, Schumann GB, et al. Detection of proliferative breast disease by four-quadrant fine-needle aspiration. *J Natl Cancer Inst* 1990;82:964–966.

32. Fabian CJ, Kamel S, Kimler BF, et al. Potential use of biomarkers in breast cancer risk assessment and chemoprevention trials. *Breast J* 1995;1:236–242.

33. Dupont WD, Page DL, Rogers LW, et al. Influence of exogenous estrogens, proliferative breast disease, and other variables on breast cancer risk. *Cancer* 1989;63:948–957.

34. Claus EB, Risch N, Thompson WD. Genetic analysis of breast cancer in the Cancer and Steroid Hormone Study. *Am J Hum Genet* 1991;48:232–242.

35. Peters J. Breast cancer genetics: relevance to oncology practice. *Cancer Control* 1995;2: 195–208.

36. Hoskins KF, Stopfer JE, Calzone KA, et al. Assessment and counseling for women with a family history of breast cancer. A guide for clinicians. *JAMA* 1995;273:577–585.

37. Easton DF, Bishop DT, Ford D, Crockford GP, the Breast Cancer Linkage Consortium. Genetic linkage analysis in familial breast and ovarian

cancer: results for 214 families. *Am J Hum Genet* 1993;52:678–701.

38. Miki Y, Swensen J, Shattuck-Eidens D, et al. A strong candidate for the breast and ovarian cancer susceptibility gene BRCA1. *Science* 1994;266:66–71.

39. Merajver SD, Pham TM, Caduff RF, et al. Somatic mutations in the BRCA1 gene in sporadic ovarian tumors. *Nat Genet* 1995;9:439–443.

40. Thompson ME, Jensen RA, Obermiller PS, et al. Decreased expression of BRCA1 accelerates growth and is often present during sporadic breast cancer progression. *Nat Genet* 1995;9:444–450.

41. Shattuck-Eidens D, Mclure M, Semerd J, et al. A collaborative survey of 80 mutations in the BRCA1 breast and ovarian cancer susceptibility gene. Implications for presymptomatic testing and screening. *JAMA* 1995;273:535–541.

42. Chen Y, Chen C-F, Riley DJ, et al. Aberrant subcellular localization of BRCA1 in breast cancer. *Science* 1995;270:789–791.

43. Struewing JP, Abeliovich D, Peretz T, et al. The carrier frequency of the BRCA1 185delAG mutation is approximately 1 percent in Ashkenazi Jewish individuals. *Nat Genet* 1995;11:190–200.

44. Goldgar DF, Reilly PR. A common BRCA1 mutation in the Ashkenazim. *Nat Genet* 1995;11:113–114.

45. Easton DF, Ford BP, Bishop DT, the Breast Cancer Linkage Consortium. Breast and ovarian cancer incidence in BRCA1-mutation carriers. *Am J Hum Genet* 1995;56:265–271.

46. Stratton M, Ford DF, Bishop DT, et al. Familial male breast cancer is not linked to the BRCA1 locus on chromosome 17q. *Nat Genet* 1994;7:103–107.

47. Slattery ML, Kerber RA. A comprehensive evaluation of family history and breast cancer risk—the Utah population database. *JAMA* 1993;270:1563–1568.

48. Claus EB, Risch N, Thompson WD. Autosomal dominant inheritance of early-onset breast cancer: implications for risk prediction. *Cancer* 1994;73:643–651.

49. Hogervorst FBL, Cornelius RS, Bout M, et al. Rapid detection of BRCA1 mutations by the protein truncation test. *Nat Genet* 1995;10:208–212.

50. Wooster R, Neuhausen SL, Mangion J. Localization of a breast cancer susceptibility gene BRCA2 to chromosome 13q12-13. *Science* 1994;265:2088–2090.

51. Offit K, Brown K. Quantitation of familial cancer risk: a resource for clinical oncologists. *J Clin Oncol* 1994;12:1724–1736.

52. Anderson DE, Badzioch MD. Risk of familial breast cancer. *Cancer* 1985;56:383–387.

53. Chaliki H, Loader S, Levenkron JC, et al. Women's receptivity to testing for a genetic susceptibility to breast cancer. *Am J Public Health* 1995;85:1133–1135.

54. Li FP, Garber JE, Friend SH, et al. Recommendations on predictive testing for germ line p53 mutations among cancer-prone individuals. *J Natl Cancer Inst* 1992;84:1156–1160.

55. Biesecker BB, Boehnke M, Calzone K, et al. Genetic counseling for families with inherited susceptibility to breast and ovarian cancer. *JAMA* 1993;269:1970–1974.

56. King M-C, Rowell S, Love SM. Inherited breast and ovarian cancer: What are the risks? What are the choices? *JAMA* 1993;269:1975–1980.

57. Statement of the American Society of Human Genetics on genetic testing for breast and ovarian cancer predisposition. *Am J Hum Genet* 1994;55:i–iv.

58. National Advisory Council for Human Genome Research. Statement on the use of DNA testing for presymptomatic identification of cancer risk. *JAMA* 1994;271:785.

59. Vogel VG. Counseling the high-risk woman. In: Stoll BA, ed. *Reducing breast cancer risk in women.* Boston: Kluwer Academic, 1995:69–80.

60. Wolfe JN. Risk for breast cancer development determined by mammographic parenchymal pattern. *Cancer* 1976;37:2486–2492.

61. Warner E, Lockwood G, Tritchler D, Boyd NF. The risk of breast cancer associated with mammographic parenchymal patterns: a meta-analysis of the published literature to examine the effect of method of classification. *Cancer Detect Prev* 1992;16:67–72.

62. Gravelle IH, Bulbrook RD, Wang DY, et al. A comparison of mammographic parenchymal patterns in premenopausal Japanese and British women. *Breast Cancer Res Treat* 1991;18(suppl 1):S93–S95.

63. Beute BJ, Kalisker L, Hutter RVP. Lobular carcinoma in situ of the breast: clinical, pathological, and mammographic features. *AJR Am J Roentgenol* 1991;157:257–265.

64. Saftlas AF, Hoover RN, Brinton LA, et al. Mammographic densities and risk of breast cancer. *Cancer* 1991;67:2833–2838.

65. Byrne C, Schairer C, Wolfe J, et al. Mammographic features and breast cancer risk: effects with time, age, and menopause status. *J Natl Cancer Inst* 1995;87:1622–1629.

66. Boyd NF, Connelly P, Byng J, et al. Plasma lipids, lipoproteins, and mammographic densities. *Cancer Epidemiol Biomarkers Prev* 1995;4:727–733.

67. Bartow SA, Pathak DR, Mettler FA, et al. Breast mammographic pattern: a concatenation of confounding and breast cancer risk factors. *Am J Epidemiol* 1995;142:813–819.

68. Tretli S. Height and weight in relation to breast cancer morbidity and mortality: a prospective study of 570,000 women in Norway. *Int J Cancer* 1989;44:23–30.

69. London S, Willett WC. Diet, body size and breast cancer risk. *Rev Endocr Related Cancer* 1988;31:19–25.

70. Willett WC, Browne ML, Bain C, et al. Relative weight and risk of breast cancer among premenopausal women. *Am J Epidemiol* 1985;122:731–740.

71. Brinton LA. Ways that women may possibly reduce their risk of breast cancer. *J Natl Cancer Inst* 1994;86:1371–1372. Editorial.

72. Dorgan JF, Brown C, Barrett M, et al. Physical activity and risk of breast cancer in the Framingham Heart Study. *Am J Epidemiol* 1994;139:662–669.

73. Frisch RE, Wyshak G, Albright NL, et al. Lower prevalence of breast cancer and cancers of the reproductive system among former college athletes compared to non-athletes. *Br J Cancer* 1985;52:885–891.

74. Paffenbarger RS Jr, Hyde RT, Wing AL. Physical activity and incidence of cancer in diverse populations: a preliminary report. *Am J Clin Nutr* 1987;45:312–317.

75. Paffenbarger RS Jr, Lee I-M, Wing AL. The influence of physical activity on the incidence of site-specific cancers in college alumni. *Adv Exp Med Biol* 1992;322:7–15.

76. Albanes D, Blair A, Taylor PR. Physical activity and risk of cancer in the NHANES I population. *Am J Public Health* 1989;79:744–750.

77. Vena JE, Graham S, Zielezny M, et al. Occupational exercise and risk of cancer. *Am J Clin Nutr* 1987;45:318–327.

78. Pukkala E, Poskiparta M, Apter D, Vihko V. Life-long physical activity and cancer among Finnish female teachers. *Eur J Cancer Prev* 1993;2:369–376.

79. Bernstein L, Henderson BE, Hanisch R, et al. Physical exercise and reduced risk of breast cancer in young women. *J Natl Cancer Inst* 1994;86:1403–1408.

80. Prentice RL, Sheppard L. Dietary fat and cancer: consistency of the epidemiologic data, and disease prevention that may follow from a practical reduction in fat consumption. *Cancer Causes Control* 1990;1:81–97.

81. Willett WC, Hunter DJ, Stampfer MJ, et al. Dietary fat and fiber in relation to the risk of breast cancer: an eight-year follow-up. *JAMA* 1992;268:2037–2044.

82. Jurkowski JJ, Cave WT Jr. Dietary effects of menhaden oil on the growth and membrane lipid composition of rat mammary tumors. *J Natl Cancer Inst* 1984;74:1145–1150.

83. Kaizer L, Boyd NF, Kriukov V, et al. Fish consumption and breast cancer risk: an ecological study. *Nutr Cancer* 1989;12:61–68.

84. Hursting SD, Thornquist M, Henderson MM. Types of dietary fat and the incidence of cancer at five sites. *Prev Med* 1990;19:242–253.

85. Lee HP, Gourley L, Duffy SW, et al. Dietary effects on breast cancer risk in Singapore. *Lancet* 1991;337:1197–2000.

86. Shimizu H, Ross RK, Bernstein L, et al. Cancer of the prostate and breast among Japanese and white immigrants in Los Angeles County. *Br J Cancer* 1991;63:963–966.

87. Barnes S, Peterson G, Grubbs C, et al. Potential role of dietary isoflavones in the prevention of cancer. *Adv Exp Med Biol* 1994;354:135–147.

88. Djuric Z, Evertt CK, Luongo DA. Toxicity, single-strand breaks, and 5 hydroxymethyl-2′-deoxyuridine formation in human breast epithelial cells treated with hydrogen peroxide. *Free Radic Biol Med* 1993;14:541–547.

89. Knekt P. Vitamin E and cancer: epidemiology. *Ann NY Acad Sci* 1992;669:269–279.

90. Garland M, Willett WC, Manson JE, et al. Antioxidant micronutrients and breast cancer. *J Am Coll Nutr* 1993;12:400–411.

91. Hunter DJ, Manson JE, Colditz GA, et al. A prospective study of the intake of vitamins C, E, and A and the risk of breast cancer. *N Engl J Med* 1993;329:234–240.

92. Willett WC, Hunter DJ. Vitamin A and cancers of the breast, large bowel, and prostate: epidemiologic evidence. *Nutr Rev* 1994;52:S53–S59.

93. Schatzkin A, Longnecker MP. Alcohol and breast cancer: where are we now and where do we go from here? *Cancer* 1994;74:1101–1110.

94. Blot WJ. Alcohol and cancer. *Cancer Res* 1992;52:2119s–2123s.

95. Rosenberg L, Metzger LS, Palmer JR. Alcohol consumption and risk of breast cancer: a review of the epidemiologic evidence. *Am J Epidemiol* 1993;15:133–144.

96. Reichman ME, Judd JT, Longscope C, et al. Effects of alcohol consumption on plasma and urinary hormone concentrations in premenopausal women. *J Natl Cancer Inst* 1993;85:722–727.

97. Longnecker MP, Paganini-Hill A, Ross RK. Lifetime alcohol consumption and breast cancer risk among postmenopausal women in Los Angeles. *Cancer Epidemiol Biomarkers Prev* 1995;5:721–725.

98. Longnecker MP, Newcombe PA, Mittendorf R, et al. Risk of breast cancer in relation to lifetime alcohol consumption. *J Natl Cancer Inst* 1995;87:923–929.

99. Longnecker MP. Alcoholic beverage consumption in relation to risk of breast cancer: meta-analysis and review. *Cancer Causes Control* 1994;5:73–82.

100. Friedman LA, Kimball AW. Coronary heart disease mortality and alcohol consumption in Framingham. *Am J Epidemiol* 1986;124:481–489.

101. Klatsky AL, Friedman GD, Siegelaub AB. Alcohol and mortality. A ten-year Kaiser-Permanente experience. *Ann Intern Med* 1981;95:139–145.

102. Vessey MP, Doll R, Jones K, et al. An epidemiological study of oral contraceptives and breast cancer. *BMJ* 1979;1:1755–1758.

103. Pike MC, Henderson BE, Krailo MD, et al. Breast cancer in young women and use of oral contraceptives: possible modifying effects of formulation and age at use. *Lancet* 1983;2:926–930.

104. McPherson K, Vessey MP, Neil A, et al. Early oral contraceptive use and premenopausal breast cancer in Sweden and Norway: possible effects of different pattern of use. *Int J Epidemiol* 1989;18:527–532.

105. Kay CR, Hannaford PC. Breast cancer and the pill—a further report from the Royal College of General Practitioners' oral contraception study. *Br J Cancer* 1988;58:675–680.

106. Brinton LA, Daling JR, Liff JM, et al. Oral contraceptives and breast cancer risk among younger women. *J Natl Cancer Inst* 1995;87:827–835.

107. Henderson BE, Bernstein L. Endogenous and exogenous hormonal factors. In: Harris JR, Lippman ME, Morrow M, Hellman S, eds. *Diseases of the Breast.* Philadelphia: Lippincott-Raven, 1996:185–200.

108. Ursin G, Aragaki CC, Paganini-Hill A, et al. Oral contraceptives and premenopausal bilateral breast cancer: a case-control study. *Epidemiology* 1992;3:414–419.

109. Wingo PA, Lee NC, Ory HW, et al. Age-specific differences in the relationship between oral contraceptive use and breast cancer. *Cancer* 1993;71:1506–1517.

110. Rookus MA, van Leeuwen FE. Oral contraceptives and risk of breast cancer in women aged 20–54 years. The Netherlands Oral Contraceptives and Breast Cancer Study Group. *Lancet* 1994;344:844–851.

111. WHO Collaborative Study of Neoplasia and Steroid Contraceptives. Breast cancer and combined oral contraceptives: results from a multinational study. *Br J Cancer* 1990;61:110–119.

112. Schesselman JJ, Stadel BV, Korper M, et al. Breast cancer detection in relation to oral contraception. *J Clin Epidemiol* 1992;45:449–459.

113. Hulka BS. Hormone-replacement therapy and the risk of breast cancer. *CA Cancer J Clin* 1990;40:289–296.

114. Cauley JA, Gutai JP, Kuller LH, et al. The epidemiology of serum sex hormones in postmenopausal women. *Am J Epidemiol* 1989;129:1120–1131.

115. Hershcopf RJ, Bradlow HL. Obesity, diet, endogenous estrogens, and the risk of hormone-sensitive cancer. *Am J Clin Nutr* 1987;45:283–289.

116. Grodin JM, Siiteri PK, MacDonald PC. Source of estrogen production in postmenopausal women. *J Clin Endocrinol Metab* 1973;36:207–214.

117. Adami H-O, Persson I. Hormone replacement and breast cancer a remaining controversy? *JAMA* 1995;274:178–179. Editorial.

118. Toniolo PO, Levitz M, Zeleniuch-Jacquotte A, et al. A prospective study of endogenous estrogens and breast cancer in postmenopausal women. *J Natl Cancer Inst* 1995;87:190–197.

119. Russo J, Tay LK, Russo IH. Differentiation of the mammary gland and susceptibility to carcinogenesis. *Breast Cancer Res Treat* 1982;2:5–73.

120. Key TJ, Pike MC. The role of oestrogens and progestagens in the epidemiology and prevention of breast cancer. *Eur J Cancer Clin Oncol* 1988;24:29–43.

121. Stanford JL, Weiss NS, Voigt LF, et al. Combined estrogen and progestin hormone replacement therapy in relation to risk of breast cancer in middle-aged women. *JAMA* 1995;274:137–142.

122. Colditz GA, Hankison SE, Hunter DJ, et al. The use of estrogens and progestins and the risk of breast cancer in postmenopausal women. *N Engl J Med* 1995;332:1589–1593.

123. Skegg DCG, Noonan EA, Paul C, et al. Depot medroxyprogesterone and breast cancer—a pooled analysis of the World Health Organization and New Zealand Studies. *JAMA* 1995;273:799–804.

124. Gambrell RD Jr, Maier RC, Sanders BI. Decreased incidence of breast cancer in postmenopausal estrogen-progestogen users. *Obstet Gynecol* 1983;62:435–443.

125. Brinton LA, Hoover R, Fraumeni JF Jr. Menopausal estrogens and breast cancer risk: an expanded case-control study. *Br J Cancer* 1986;54:825–832.

126. Lippman ME, Swain SM. Endocrine-responsive cancers of humans. In: Wilson JD, Foster DW, eds. *Williams textbook of endocrinology.* 8th ed. Philadelphia: WB Saunders, 1992:1577–1597.

127. Bergkvist L, Adami H-O, Person I, et al. The risk of breast cancer after estrogen and estrogen-progestin replacement. *N Engl J Med* 1989;321:293–297.

128. Kaufman DW, Palmer JR, de Mouzon J, et al. Estrogen replacement therapy and the risk of breast cancer: results from the case-control surveillance study. *Am J Epidemiol* 1991;134:1375–1385.

129. Newcomb PA, Longnecker MP, Storer BE, et al. Long-term hormone replacement therapy and risk of breast cancer in postmenopausal women. *Am J Epidemiol* 1995;142:788–795.

130. Mills PK, Beeson WL, Phillips RL, Fraser GE. Prospective study of exogenous hormone use and breast cancer in Seventh-Day Adventists. *Cancer* 1987;64:591–597.

131. Hunt K, Vessey M. Long-term effects of postmenopausal hormone therapy. *Br J Hosp Med* 1987;38:450–453, 456–460.

132. Barrett-Connor E. Postmenopausal estrogen replacement and breast cancer. *N Engl J Med* 1989;321:319–320. Editorial.

133. Steinberg KK, Thacker SB, Smith SJ, et al. A meta-analysis of the effect of estrogen replacement therapy on the risk of breast cancer. *JAMA* 1991;265:1985–1990.

134. Armstrong BK. Oestrogen therapy after the menopause—boon or bane? *Med J Aust* 1988;143:213–214.

135. Dupont WD, Page DL. Menopausal estrogen replacement therapy and breast cancer. *Arch Intern Med* 1991;151:67–72.

136. Schlesselman JJ, Stadel BV, Murray P, Lai S. Breast cancer in relation to early use of oral contraceptives—no evidence of a latent effect. *JAMA* 1988;259:1828–1833.

137. Lipnick RJ, Buring JE, Hennekens CH, et al. Oral contraceptives and breast cancer—a prospective cohort study. *JAMA* 1986;255:58–61.

138. Sattin RW, Rubin GL, Wingo PA, et al. Oral-contraceptive use and the risk of breast cancer. *N Engl J Med* 1986;315:405–411.

139. The Centers for Disease and Control Cancer and Steroid Hormone Study: long-term oral contraceptive use and the risk of breast cancer. *JAMA* 1983;249:1591–1595.

140. Carr BR. Disorders of the ovary and female reproductive tract. In: Wilson JD, Foster DW, eds. *Williams textbook of endocrinology.* 8th ed. Philadelphia: WB Saunders, 1992:733–798.

141. Folsom AR, Mink PJ, Sellers TA, et al. Hormonal replacement therapy and morbidity and mortality in a prospective study of postmenopausal women. *Am J Public Health* 1995;85:1128–1132.

142. Barrett-Connor E, Bush TJ. Estrogen and coronary heart disease in women. *JAMA* 1991;265:1861–1867.

143. Paganini-Hill A, Ross RK, Henderson BE. Postmenopausal oestrogen treatment and stroke: a prospective study. *BMJ* 1988;297:519–522.

144. Grady D, Rubin SM, Petitti DB, et al. Hormone therapy to prevent disease and prolong life in postmenopausal women. *Ann Intern Med* 1992;117:1016–1037.

145. Ettinger B, Genant HK, Conn CE. Postmenopausal bone loss is prevented by treatment with low-dose estrogen with calcium. *Ann Intern Med* 1987;106:40–45.

146. Kiel DP, Felson DT, Anderson JJ, et al. Hip fracture and the use of estrogens in postmenopausal women. *N Engl J Med* 1987;317:1169–1174.

147. Henderson BE, Ross R, Bernstein L. Estrogens as a cause of human cancer: the Richard and Hinda Rosenthal Foundation Award Lecture. *Cancer Res* 1988;48:246–253.

148. Bernstein L, Ross RK, Henderson BE. Prospects for the primary prevention of breast cancer. *Am J Epidemiol* 1992;135:142–152.

149. Stoll BA. Hormone replacement therapy in women treated for breast cancer. *Eur J Cancer Clin Oncol* 1989;25:1909–1913.

150. Theriault RL, Sellin RV. A clinical dilemma: estrogen replacement therapy in postmenopausal women with a background of primary breast cancer. *Ann Oncol* 1991;2:709–717.

151. Cobleigh MA, Berris RF, Bush T, et al. Estrogen replacement therapy in breast cancer survivors—a time for change. *JAMA* 1994;272:540–545.

152. American College of Physicians. Guidelines for counseling postmenopausal women about preventive hormone therapy. *Ann Intern Med* 1992;117:1038–1041.

153. Boice JD, Harvey EB, Blettner M, et al. Cancer in the contralateral breast after radiotherapy for breast cancer. *N Engl J Med* 1992;326:781–785.

154. Hoffman DA, Lonstein JE, Norin MM, et al. Breast cancer in women with scoliosis exposed to multiple diagnostic x-rays. *J Natl Cancer Inst* 1989; 81:1307–1312.

155. Swift M, Morrell D, Massey RB, Chase CL. Incidence of cancer in 161 families affected by ataxia telangiectasia. *N Engl J Med* 1991;325:1831–1836.

156. Savitsky K, Bar-Shira A, Gilad S, et al. A single ataxia telangiectasia gene with a product similar to PI-3 kinase. *Science* 1995;268:1749–1753.

157. Nayfield SG, Karp JE, Ford LG, et al. Potential role of tamoxifen in prevention of breast cancer. *J Natl Cancer Inst* 1991;83:1450–1459.

158. Spiegelman D, Colditz GA, Hunter D, Hertzmark E. Validation of the Gail et al model predicting individual breast cancer risk. *J Natl Cancer Inst* 1994;86:600–607.

159. Bondy ML, Spitz MR, Halabi S, et al. Low incidence of familial breast cancer among Hispanic women. *Cancer Causes Control* 1992;3:377–382.

160. Lerman C, Rimer BK, Engstrom PF. Cancer risk notification: psychological and ethical implications. *J Clin Oncol* 1991;9:1275–1282.

161. Lerman C, Rimer B, Trock B, et al. Psychological and behavioral implications of abnormal mammograms. *Ann Intern Med* 1991;114:657–661.

162. Lerman C, Trock B, Rimer B, et al. Psychological side-effects of breast cancer screening. *Health Psychol* 1991;10:259–267.

163. Kash JM, Holland JC, Halper MS, et al. Psychological distress and surveillance behaviors of women with a family history of breast cancer. *J Natl Cancer Inst* 1992;84:24–30.

164. Lerman C, Schwartz M. Adherence and psychological adjustment among women at high risk for breast cancer. *Breast Cancer Res Treat* 1993;28:145–155.

165. Alagna SW, Morokoff PJ, Bevett JM, et al. Performance of breast self-examination by women at high risk for breast cancer. *Women Health* 1987;12:29–46.

166. Lerman C, Rimer B, Trock B, et al. Factors associated with repeat adherence to breast cancer screening. *Prev Med* 1990;19:279–290.

167. Vogel VG, Graves DS, Vernon SW, et al. Mammographic screening of women with increased risk of breast cancer. *Cancer* 1990;66:1613–1620.

168. Vogel VG, Yeomans A, Higginbotham E. Clinical management of women at increased risk for breast cancer. *Breast Cancer Res Treat* 1993;28:195–210.

169. Morrow M. Identification and management of women at increased risk for breast cancer development. *Breast Cancer Res Treat* 1994;31:53–60.

170. Bilimoria M, Morrow M. The woman at increased risk for breast cancer: evaluation and management strategies. *CA Cancer J Clin* 1995;45:263–278.

171. Hurley SF, Kaldor JM. The benefits and risk of mammographic screening for breast cancer. *Epidemiol Rev* 1992;14:101–130.

172. Smart CR, Hendrick RE, Rutledge JH, et al. Benefit of mammography screening in women ages 40 to 49 years—current evidence from randomized controlled trials. *Cancer* 1995;75:1619–1626.

173. Vogel VG. Screening younger women at risk for breast cancer. *Monogr Natl Cancer Inst* 1994;16:55–60.

174. Miller AB, Baines CJ, To T, et al. Canadian National Breast Screening Study. I. Breast cancer and death rates among women aged 40 to 49 years. *Can Med Assoc J* 1992;147:1459–1476.

175. Sickles EA, Kopans DB. Deficiencies in the analysis of breast screening data. *J Natl Cancer Inst* 1993;85:1621–1624.

176. Sackett DL, Haynes RB, Guyatt GH, Tugwell P. *Clinical epidemiology—a basic science for clinical medicine.* Boston: Little, Brown, 1991:69–152.

177. Mettlin C. Breast cancer risk factors—contributions to planning breast cancer control. *Cancer* 1992;69:1904–1910.

178. Meyer JE, Kopans DB, Oot R. Breast cancer visualized by mammography in patients under 35. *Radiology* 1983;147:93–94.

179. Lantz PM, Remington PL, Newcomb PA. Mammography screening and increased incidence of breast cancer in Wisconsin. *J Natl Cancer Inst* 1991;83:1540–1546.

180. Svane G, Potchen EJ, Siena A, Azavedo E. How to interpret a mammogram. In: *Screening mammography—breast cancer diagnosis in asymptomatic women.* St. Louis: CV Mosby, 1993:148.

181. Bland KI, O'Neal B, Weiner LJ, et al. One-stage simple mastectomy with immediate reconstruction for high-risk patients. *Arch Surg* 1986;121:221–225.

182. Rubin LR. Prophylactic mastectomy with immediate reconstruction for the high-risk woman. *Clin Plast Surg* 1984;11:369–381.

183. Wong JH, Jackson CF, Swanson JS, et al. Analysis of the risk reduction of prophylactic partial mastectomy in Sprague-Dawley rats with 7,12-dimethylbenzathracene-induced breast cancer. *Surgery* 1986;99:67–71.

184. Nelson H, Miller SH, Buck D, et al. Effectiveness of prophylactic mastectomy in the prevention of breast tumors in C3H mice. *Plast Reconstr Surg* 1989;83:662–669.

185. Temple WJ, Lindsay RL, Magi E, et al. Technical considerations for prophylactic mastectomy in patients at high risk for breast cancer. *Am J Surg* 1991;161:413–415.

186. Goodnight JE Jr, Quagliana JM, Mortoan DL. Failure of subcutaneous mastectomy to prevent the development of breast cancer. *J Surg Oncol* 1984;26:198–201.

187. Pennisi VR, Capozzi A. Subcutaneous mastectomy data: a final statistical analysis of 1500 patients. *Aesthetic Plast Surg* 1989;13:15–21.

188. Ziegler LD, Kroll SS. Primary breast cancer after prophylactic mastectomy. *Am J Clin Oncol* 1991;14:451–454.

189. Hartmann L, Jenkins R, Schaid D, et al. Prophylactic mastectomy: preliminary retrospective cohort analysis. Proc Am Assoc Cancer Res 1997;38:A168.

190. Wapnir IL, Rabinowitz B, Greco RS. A reappraisal of prophylactic mastectomy. *Surg Gynecol Obstet* 1990;171:171–184.

191. American Society of Plastic and Reconstructive Surgeons. *Position paper on prophylactic mastectomy.* Arlington Heights, IL: American Society of Plastic and Reconstructive Surgeons, 1989.

192. Claus EB, Risch N, Thompson WD, et al. Relationship between breast histopathology and family history of breast cancer. *Cancer* 1993;71:147–153.

193. Early Breast Cancer Trialists' Collaborative Group. Systemic treatment of early breast cancer hormonal, cytotoxic, or immune therapy. *Lancet* 1992;339:1–15.

194. Andersson M, Storm HH, Mouridsen HT. Carcinogenic effects of adjuvant tamoxifen treatment and radiotherapy for early breast cancer. *Acta Oncol* 1992;31:259–263.

195. Vogel VG. Tamoxifen for the prevention of breast cancer. In: De Vita VT Jr, Helman S, Rosenberg SA, eds. *Important advances in oncology—1995.* Philadelphia: JB Lippincott, 1995:187–200.

196. McDonald CC. Fatal myocardial infarction in the Scottish adjuvant tamoxifen trial. *BMJ* 1991;303:435–437.

197. Rutqvist LE, Mattson A. Cardiac and thromboembolic morbidity among postmenopausal women with early-stage breast cancer in a randomized trial of adjuvant tamoxifen. *J Natl Cancer Inst* 1993;85:1398–1406.

198. Bruning PF, Bonfrer JMG, Hart AAM, et al. Tamoxifen, serum lipoproteins and cardiovascular risk. *Br J Cancer* 1988;58:497–499.

199. Love RR, Newcomb PA, Wiebe DA, et al. Effects of tamoxifen therapy on lipid and lipoprotein levels in postmenopausal patients with node-negative breast cancer. *J Natl Cancer Inst* 1990;82:1327–1332.

200. Windler E, Kovanen PT, Chao YS, et al. The estradiol stimulated lipoprotein receptor of rat liver: a binding site that mediates uptake of rat lipoproteins containing apoproteins B and E. *J Biol Chem* 1980;255:10464–10471.

201. Stacls B, Anwer J, Chan L, et al. Influence of development, estrogens, and food intake on apolipoproteins A-I, A-III, and E in RNA in rat liver and intestine. *J Lipid Res* 1989;30:1137–1147.

202. Bush T, Fried LP, Barrett-Connor E. Cholesterol, lipoprotein and coronary heart disease in women. *Clin Chem* 1988;34:60–70.

203. Yusuf SA, Wittes J, Friedman L. Overview of results of randomized clinical trials in heart disease. II: unstable angina, heart failure, primary prevention with aspirin and risk factor modification. *JAMA* 1988;260:2259–2263.

204. Love RR, Wiebe DA, Newcomb PA, et al. Effects of tamoxifen on cardiovascular risk factors in postmenopausal women. *Ann Intern Med* 1991;115:860–864.

205. Kannel WB, Wolf PA, Castelli WP, et al. Fibrinogen and risk of cardiovascular disease. *JAMA* 1987;258:1183–1186.

206. Hoffman CJ, Miller RH, Lawson WE, et al. Elevation of factor VII activity and mass in young adults at risk of ischemic heart disease. *J Am Coll Cardiol* 1989;14:941–946.

207. Cuzick J, Allen D, Baum M, et al. Long-term effects of tamoxifen—Biological Effects of Tamoxifen Working Party. *Eur J Cancer* 1993;29:15–21.

208. Barrett-Connor E. Postmenopausal estrogen, cancer and other considerations. *Women Health* 1986;11:179–195.

209. Jordan VC, Phelps E, Lingren JU. Effect of anti-estrogens on bone in castrated and intact female rats. *Breast Cancer Res Treat* 1987;10:31–35.

210. Turner RT, Wakley GK, Hannon KS, et al. Tamoxifen prevents the skeletal effects of ovarian hormone deficiency in rats. *J Bone Miner Res* 1987;2:449–456.

211. Turner RT, Wakley GK, Hannon KS, et al. Tamoxifen inhibits osteoclast-mediated resorption of trabecular bone in ovarian hormone deficient rats. *Endocrinology* 1988;122:1146–1150.

212. Wakley GK, Hannon KS, Bell NA, et al. The effects of tamoxifen on the osteopenia induced by sciatic neurotomy in the rat: histomorphometric study. *Calcif Tissue Int* 1988;43:383–388.

213. Love RR, Mazess RB, Borden HS, et al. Effects of tamoxifen on bone mineral density in postmenopausal women with breast cancer. *N Engl J Med* 1992;326:852–856.

214. Kristensen B, Ejlertsen B, Dalgaard P, et al. Tamoxifen and bone metabolism in postmenopausal low-risk breast cancer patients: a randomized study. *J Clin Oncol* 1994;12:992–997.

215. Stewart PJ, Stern PH. Effects of the antiestrogens tamoxifen and clomiphene on bone resorption in vitro. *Endocrinology* 1986;118:125–131.

216. Powles TJ, Hickish TF, Kanis JA, Ashley S. Tamoxifen preserves bone mineral density in post-menopausal women but causes loss of bone density in premenopausal women. *Proc Am Soc Clin Oncol* 1995;14:A165.

217. Fornander T, Rutvqvist LE, Cedermark B, et al. Adjuvant tamoxifen in early breast cancer: occurrence of new primary cancers. *Lancet* 1989;1:117–120.

218. Rutqvist LE, Johansson H, Signomklao T, et al. Adjuvant tamoxifen therapy for early stage breast cancer and second primary malignancy. *J Natl Cancer Inst* 1995;87:645–651.

219. Fornander T, Hellstrom A-C, Moberger B. Descriptive clinicopathological study of 17 patients with endometrial cancer during or after adjuvant tamoxifen in early breast cancer. *J Natl Cancer Inst* 1993;85:1850–1855.

220. Andersson M, Storm HH, Mouridsen HT. Incidence of new primary cancers after adjuvant tamoxifen therapy and radiotherapy for early breast cancer. *J Natl Cancer Inst* 1991;83:1013–1017.

221. Fisher B, Costantino JP, Redmond CK, et al. Endometrial cancer in tamoxifen-treated breast cancer patients: findings from the National Surgical Adjuvant Breast and Bowel Project (NSABP) B-14. *J Natl Cancer Inst* 1994;86:527–537.

222. Cook LS, Weiss NS, Schwartz SM, et al. Population-based study of tamoxifen therapy and subsequent ovarian, endometrial, and breast cancers. *J Natl Cancer Inst* 1995;87:1359–1364.

223. van Leeuwen FE, Benraadt J, Coebergh JW, et al. Risk of endometrial cancer after tamoxifen treatment of breast cancer. *Lancet* 1994;343:448–452.

224. Vogel VG, Lippman SM, Boyd N. Is breast cancer preventable? *Can J Oncol* 1991;1:28–37.

225. Torrisi R, Pensa F, Orengo, MA, et al. The synthetic retinoid fenretinide lowers plasma insulin-like growth factor I levels in breast cancer patients. *Cancer Res* 1993;53:4769–4771.

226. Spicer DV, Pike MC. Breast cancer prevention through modulation of endogenous hormones. *Breast Cancer Res Treat* 1993;28:179–193.

227. Battersby A, Anderson TJ. Proliferative and secretory activity in the pregnant and lactating human breast. *Virchows Arch A Pathol Anat Histopathol* 1988;413:189–196.

228. Pike MC. Age-related factors in cancers of the breast, ovary, and endometrium. *J Chronic Dis* 1987;40(suppl):59s–69s.

229. Vogel VG. Early detection, epidemiology, and prevention of breast cancer. *Curr Opin Oncol* 1992;4:1017–1026.

230. Lee HP, Gaurley L, Duffy SW, et al. Dietary effects on breast cancer risks in Singapore. *Lancet* 1991;337:1197–1200.

231. Sporn MB. Carcinogenesis and cancer: different perspectives on the same disease. *Cancer Res* 1991;51:6215–6218.

232. Lippman SM, Benner SE, Hong WK. Cancer chemoprevention. *J Clin Oncol* 1994;12:851–873.

233. Costa A, Formelli F, Chiesa F, et al. Prospects of chemoprevention of human cancers with the synthetic retinoid fenretinide. *Cancer Res* 1994;54:2032s–2037s.

234. Ratco TA, Detrisac CJ, Dinger NM, et al. Chemopreventive efficacy of combined retinoid and tamoxifen treatment following surgical excision of a primary cancer in female rats. *Cancer Res* 1989;49:4472–4476.

235. Rossouw J, Finnegan L, Pottern L, et al. The evolution of the Women's Health Initiative: perspectives from the NIH. *J Am Med Wom Assoc* 1995;150:50–55.

CHAPTER 2

Controversies in Breast Cancer Screening Guidelines

LARS-GUNNAR LARSSON

*I*n parts of the world with a Western lifestyle, such as the United States, Canada, Europe, Australia, and New Zealand, breast cancer is very common and constitutes 20% to 30% of all incident cancers in women. In these regions, breast cancer is usually also the most frequent cause of cancer death among women. In the United States, where lung cancer during recent years has replaced breast cancer as the leading cause of cancer-related death, breast cancer is still—because of its age distribution—the malignancy that causes the most lost woman-years of life. In the regions mentioned above, about 1 woman in 10 will develop breast cancer during her lifetime, and the disease is sufficiently common to be felt as a real threat by most women.

Many risk factors for the development of breast cancer are known but none of them has a character that at present makes general, primary preventive measures possible. Therefore, much interest during the past decades has focused on methods for early detection and treatment, with the aim of preventing metastatic, lethal cancer. This chapter discusses the three methods of mass breast cancer screening in widespread use at this time: breast self-examination (BSE), clinical breast examination (CBE), and mammography. Other available detection methods either are not sensitive or specific enough (e.g., thermography, diaphanoscopy, and ultrasonography) or are too complicated and expensive (e.g., computed tomography and magnetic resonance imaging) to be used for mass breast cancer screening,

even if they may have some potential as supplemental diagnostic tools in clinical situations.

Breast Self-Examination

In the absence of screening, more than 90% of breast cancers are detected by women themselves through the incidental finding of a lump or irregularity in the breast parenchyma. It is natural to assume that increased awareness among women may lead to earlier diagnosis and increased curability of breast cancer. Programs promoting BSE have been developed in many countries. The information on BSE is disseminated by cancer societies and health authorities. Written information is usually in the form of pamphlets. BSE campaigns will probably be most efficient if this written information is supplemented by practical training in BSE given during visits to physicians' offices, through courses at places of work, and so on.

Many studies on BSE have been reported (1). Most concern compliance rates in relation to mode of instruction, age, education, social and economic factors, and other variables. Even after intensive education, the general rate of compliance with regular monthly BSE seems to be rather low and is seldom higher than 50%.

Two studies deserve special comment as they tried to show whether screening with BSE really reduces the breast cancer mortality rate. The UK Trial of Early Detection of Breast Cancer, which was set up in 1979, used a semi-experimental approach by comparing breast cancer mortality in three regions: one where women were invited to undergo annual CBE and biannual mammography, one where women received intensive education in BSE, and one control region without a screening program. After a follow-up of about 10 years, no difference in the breast cancer mortality rate was found between the BSE and the control regions (2). In Finland, a very ambitious BSE education program was conducted between 1973 and 1975 (3). A cohort study was performed some years later of women who had returned self-administered calendars recording their practice of BSE over a 2-year period. Compared with the general Finnish population, the cohort had a 25% lower breast cancer mortality rate (3). However, because of possible selection bias (only women who returned calendars were included in the cohort), no definite conclusions could be drawn from this observation.

Even though there is at present no scientifically solid evidence that BSE reduces the breast cancer mortality rate, it seems very likely that BSE in some women prevents lethal disease. BSE is an inexpensive measure, and it can be repeated at short intervals; these are good reasons to promote the general use of BSE in women older than 40 years.

Clinical Breast Examination

Breast cancer is only rarely an incidental finding at routine clinical examination. Nevertheless, all clinicians should be well acquainted with the technique of CBE, and CBE should be included in routine physical examinations, especially of women older than 40. Including CBE in the physical examination also gives the physician an opportunity to instruct the patient in BSE.

During the 1950s and 1960s, some screening trials with CBE were performed. However, CBE is a very inefficient screening instrument. Even though the cumulative incidence of breast cancer over an extended period of time is quite high, the prevalence of palpable cancer at a given time is very low. In the middle of the 1960s, a population-based study of screening with CBE was performed in Malmö, Sweden (4). The results were disappointing. In women 40 to 70 years old, breast cancer was detected in only 2.1 per 1000 women at the first screening and 1.2 per 1000 women at rescreening

17 months later. The rate of benign lesions detected was more than 10 times as high, and a large number of diagnostic biopsies had to be performed. The conclusion was that screening with CBE was inefficient and would create huge practical problems.

In many screening programs, a combination of mammography and CBE is used as the primary screening instrument. This is discussed further in the next section on mammography. Neither BSE nor CBE can replace mammography in screening for breast cancer, but both can serve as supplements to mammography.

Mammography

The superiority of mammography among breast cancer screening methods lies in its ability to detect nonpalpable early cancer and precancerous lesions (cancer in situ). Mammography uses low-voltage x-rays, which in combination with compression of the breast makes it possible to image the soft tissues in great detail. Although mammography was developed already during the 1930s, it was not until the beginning of the 1960s that mammography's capacity to detect subclinical cancers—and thereby its potential for screening—was recognized (5). Once these benefits were recognized, some centers in the United States and Europe began to use mammography for screening. A large number of more or less systematic studies of screening mammography have been reported to date. Most interesting of these are the randomized trials that try to elucidate the effect of screening on breast cancer mortality rates. Both randomized and nonrandomized studies of mammography have also greatly contributed to the knowledge of the biology of early breast cancer.

To judge from the Swedish experience, the first screening (the "prevalence screening") of an unselected group of previously unscreened women aged 40 to 69, usually reveals four to six invasive cancers and one to two cancers in situ per 1000 women examined. About half of the cancers are subclinical, and the distribution of pathologic stages is clearly shifted toward more early stages compared with the stage distribution for spontaneously detected cancers (6). The cancer detection rate increases with age from about 1.5 per 10,000 women screened in the age group 40 to 44 years to about 10 per 10,000 women screened in the age group 65 to

69 years. At rescreening of the same population 2 years later, the breast cancer detection rate is usually about the same as at the prevalence screening; the majority of detected cancers are now subclinical, and the shift in the stage distribution toward early pathologic stages is even more pronounced than at the prevalence screening. A small number of cancers will always appear between screening rounds. These so-called interval cancers tend to have a stage distribution rather similar to that for spontaneously detected cancers.

Randomized Trials

Early cancers detected by screening seem to have a good prognosis, to judge from survival curves. However, this is not sufficient proof of a benefit from screening. One reason is *lead-time bias*, which refers to the fact that if detection by screening is pushed back in time, then measurement of survival can spuriously suggest a benefit. A second reason is *length-biased sampling*, which concerns the fact that screening preferably selects less malignant, slowly growing tumors that have a long preclinical stage.

To study whether screening really reduces breast cancer mortality rates, the Health Insurance Plan of Greater New York trial was started in 1963 (the "HIP trial"). From the insurance register, 31,000 women aged 40 to 64 were randomly selected and invited to undergo screening with mammography and CBE, repeated yearly for 4 consecutive years. This group was compared with a control group of similar size and composition. Only 65% of invited women participated. After 9 years of observation, the breast cancer mortality rate was about 30% lower in the invited group than in the control group, a statistically significant difference (7). The effect was confined to women 50 years or older; there was no benefit for women aged 40 to 49 years. However, results after 18 years of follow-up indicated a similar reduction in the breast cancer mortality rate of about 25% for women younger than as well as older than 50 (8).

In Europe, the development of screening mammography was influenced by studies conducted in Sweden during the 1970s. In 1977, after two pilot studies (9,10) had shown that mammography alone with one oblique projection could be used as an effective and inexpensive primary screening instrument,

Sweden's National Board of Health and Welfare initiated a population-based randomized study (the "two-county trial") of screening mammography. Women aged 40 or older were invited to undergo periodic screening with one-projection mammography repeated at 2- to 2.5-year intervals. After an observation time of 7 years, a significant reduction of about 30% in the breast cancer mortality rate was observed among women who were 40 to 74 years old at the time of randomization (11). Similar to the reports of the HIP trial, the early reports found no benefit in women aged 40 to 49 at the time of invitation, but prolonged observation revealed a small but not statistically significant mortality benefit in this age group (12). In addition to the two-county trial, three more randomized trials of screening mammography were started in Sweden between 1976 and 1981 in Malmö (13), Stockholm (14), and Gothenburg.

As the four Swedish randomized trials had a rather similar design, pooled analyses of these trials have been performed to obtain more precise risk estimates and allow statistically more meaningful stratification into age groups. These analyses included about 157,000 women in the invited group and about 126,000 in the control group, with attendance rates varying between 74% and 89% in the different trials. The first published results of this overview (15,16,17) showed that after an observation period of 6 to 12 years, among women in the invited group, there was a statistically significant reduction of approximately 30% in the breast cancer mortality rate in the 50 to 69 age group while the reduction in the breast cancer mortality rate in the 40 to 49 age group was small and statistically not significant. A further analysis after 4 more years of observation, however, showed an almost statistically significant reduction of approximately 20% in the breast cancer mortality rate in women who were 40 to 49 years old at the time of invitation (18,19).

Randomized trials of screening mammography have also been performed in the United Kingdom (Edinburgh) and Canada. The Edinburgh trial, started in 1978, recruited women 45 to 65 years old and included annual CBE plus biannual mammography. After 10 years of observation, a 14% to 21% statistically nonsignificant reduction in the breast cancer mortality rate was found independent of age at the time of invitation (20).

The Canadian National Breast Screening Study (NBSS) recruited participants between

1980 and 1985. It included two separate randomized studies. In one study, NBSS 1, women aged 40 to 49 were randomly assigned to undergo either annual mammography plus CBE or only initial CBE. In the other trial, NBSS 2, annual mammography plus CBE was compared with annual CBE alone in women aged 50 to 59. After an observation period of about 7 years, none of these trials showed a difference in breast cancer mortality between the two compared groups (21,22). For the 40- to 49-year age group, this result is not surprising as no trial so far had shown a clear benefit of screening after such a short follow-up. More puzzling is the result in the 50- to 59-year age group, in which one would expect an obvious benefit of mammography after 7 years. The selection caused by the design of the studies—actually only a minority of the invited women participated in the trials—may also have reduced the possibility of positive result (23–25). Results after longer follow-up will, however, be interesting to follow.

With regard to the collective evidence, there is little doubt at present that screening with mammography or mammography plus CBE in women aged 50 to 69 reduces the breast cancer mortality rate by about 30% within the first 7–10 years of observation (26). The results reported in the randomized trials are dominated by the prevalence screening and the first few rescreenings; the effect of periodic screening over a long time has been impossible to study. In the HIP trial, the systematic screening in the study group was limited to the first 4 years, and in the Swedish trials, the control groups were invited to undergo screening some years after the time of randomization. It seems likely, however, that the real, long-term reduction in the breast cancer mortality rate in women who start screening at age 50 is at least on the order of 30%.

Some Nonrandomized Studies

The largest systematic but not randomized study of screening mammography is the Breast Cancer Detection Demonstration Project (BCDDP) in the United States, which started in 1973 and recruited more than a quarter of a million women aged 35 to 74 years. The participants were screened on an annual basis using a combination of medical history, CBE, mammography, and until 1977, thermography. The participants were also taught BSE and advised to perform it monthly. Several reports from this project gave information on cancer detection

rates in women according to age, mode of detection, stage distribution of detected cancers, and survival according to stage (27,28). Survival curves from this study strongly support the concept that breast cancer detected early by screening mammography really is a curable disease even if the possibility of lead-time bias and length-biased sampling means that the studies cannot prove that screening really causes a reduction in breast cancer mortality.

Several nonrandomized, population-based studies have been reported from Europe. The most well known are the DOM (Diagnostisch Onderzoek Mammacarcinoom) and Nijmegen projects in the Netherlands (29,30) and the Florence project in Italy (31), which provided valuable information on interval cancers and early indicators of screening efficacy (32–34). The DOM and Florence projects also conducted case-control studies within the invited populations. These studies seemed to show that screening reduced the risk of dying of breast cancer by 50% to 70% (31,35). However, it has later been shown that this type of analysis has a serious bias, as women not complying with screening ("refusers") a priori represent a high-risk group.

Questions Related to Screening Mammography

In the following sections, some special questions related to screening mammography are discussed.

Mammography in Women Aged 40 to 49 Years

The great controversy at present concerns the age group 40 to 49. Early results from the randomized trials failed to show a reduction in the breast cancer mortality rate in this group. However, prolonged follow-up of the pooled data from the Swedish trials suggested a benefit on the order of 20%. Similar results were obtained by a meta-analysis of all randomized controlled trials of screening mammography (36). The present knowledge is summarized in Table 2-1. Some of the reported benefits have no doubt been caused by continued screening after age 50, but the magnitude of this influence is at present unknown (37–39).

None of the trials reported so far were specifically designed to answer the question of whether it is more beneficial to start screening

T A B L E 2-1

Relative Risks of Dying of Breast Cancer (Invited Group Versus Control Group) in the Age Group 40 to 49: Results of Randomized Trials

Trial	Relative Risk	95% Confidence Interval
Health Insurance Plan	0.77	0.55–1.11
Malmö	0.67	0.35–1.27
Kopparberg*	0.67	0.37–1.22
Ostergötland*	1.02	0.59–1.77
Stockholm	1.08	0.54–2.17
Gothenburg	0.59	0.33–1.06
Edinburgh	0.73	0.43–1.25
Canadian National Breast Screening Study (NBSS) 1	1.10	0.79–1.54
Pooled Swedish rials	0.77	0.59–1.01
Meta-analysis, all trials	0.85	0.71–1.01
Meta-analysis, all trials (except NBSS 1)	0.76	0.62–0.93

† Kopparberg and Ostergötland are the two counties in the "two-county trial."

Sources: Falun meeting on breast cancer screening with mammography in women aged 40–49 years: report of the organizing committee and collaborators. Int J Cancer 1996;64:693–699. Smart CR, Hendrick RE, Rutledge JH, Smith RA. Benefit of mammography screening in women aged 40–49 years—current evidence from randomized controlled trials. *Cancer* 1995;75:1619–26.

around age 40 than at age 50. Some years ago, a trial was started in the United Kingdom to compare women invited to undergo annual mammography screening at ages 40 to 41 with a control group not invited until age 50. Under the auspices of the International Union Against Cancer and with the support of the National Cancer Institute of the United States, an extended inter-European trial with similar design ["Eurotrial 40" (40)] is planned at present. If this trial is realized, the combined United Kingdom and European trials will contain 150,000 women in the invited group and 300,000 in the control group, and the first mortality analyses will be possible around the year 2010.

In Sweden, a huge amount of information on screening mammography has accumulated since the middle of the 1980s. At present, all Swedish counties actively invite women to periodic screening with mammography, and the compliance rate is high. As about half of the counties use 40 years as the lower age limit and the other half use 50 years, and as the counties started screening at different times, there are opportunities for retrospective comparative cohort studies that may elucidate the effect of different starting ages. Such studies are planned at present.

However, the problem with the age group 40 to 49 goes beyond demonstrating a significant reduction in breast cancer mortality rates. The low prevalence of mammographically detectable cancer in this age group makes the mortality gain in absolute terms small even if a relative benefit can be demonstrated. Mammography seems also to detect breast cancer less efficiently in the age group 40 to 49 than in older women. One would expect the ratio between the detection rate and the annual incidence rate registered in the region before screening began to be more or less constant regardless of age. However, this is not the case. At prevalence screenings in Sweden, this ratio has as a rule been 1 to 2 in the age group 40 to 49 compared with 3 or more in the older age groups. One reason for this trend is certainly that the dense parenchyma in the premenopausal breast makes the cancers less easy to detect. Another cause could be that breast cancers in women aged 40 to 49 on average grow more rapidly and therefore are more difficult to detect early by screening (41,42).

Another area of concern in the age group 40 to 49 is that the rate of mammographically uncertain findings requiring supplementary examinations and biopsies is rather high in relation to the cancer detection rate (6,43). In the Stockholm trial (43), which invited women aged 40 to 65, it was calculated that false-positive findings in the first screening round resulted in a cost of around $1 million per 100,000 women screened and that about 40% of this cost was associated with examinations performed in women younger than 50. Even more important is, of course, the anxiety caused among the women concerned, especially as it often took considerable time before cancer could be regarded as excluded. At present, many believe that screening before age 50 does more harm than good.

Mammography Alone Versus Mammography Plus Clinical Breast Examination

In the United States and Canada, screening consists of mammography plus CBE, while in Sweden and some other European countries, mammography alone is used as the primary screening instrument. An argument for CBE is that some palpable cancers (~5%) are not detected by mammography. This is especially common for lobular carcinomas. The advantages of using mammography alone as the primary screening instrument are the considerably lower costs and the sharp demarcation obtained between the screening procedure and the clinical situation. The results can be illustrated by a screening program in a Swedish county (6) of women aged 40 to 69. The attendance rate was 87% at the first screening and 78% at the second screening. Of 1000 women at the first screening, 46 were recalled for supplementary mammography; only 9 of these were referred for clinical examination and biopsy. Five of these women had cancer as demonstrated by histologic examination. The figures found at rescreening 2 years later were very similar.

Active Invitation Versus General Recommendations

In many countries, including the United States, the impetus for screening comes mainly from general recommendations issued by health authorities, cancer societies, and specialist organizations; women are not actively invited to undergo mammography. Whether a woman undergoes screening then becomes largely dependent on her own initiative and responsibility. The problem with this approach is the generally low attendance rate, usually below 50%, and the great dependence on factors such as education, social class, income, and geographic location. Active invitation of women in concerned age groups is much more effective, producing attendance rates usually on the order of 70% to 90%.

Interval Between Screening Rounds

All screening is based on periodic examinations; this is necessary for a quantitative effect. The optimal interval between consecutive screenings is not known but ongoing randomized studies in the United Kingdom and Finland are comparing different screening intervals. Current recommendations are mainly based on the experience with so-called interval cancers. There is general agreement that the interval between consecutive screening rounds should not be shorter than 1 year and not longer than 3 years. Indications that breast cancers in younger women (40–49 years) may grow more rapidly (41,42) speak in favor of annual screening in this age group.

Type of Mammography

Since the 1960s, when the HIP trial was started, considerable technical developments in mammography have led to reductions in the radiation dose and improvements in the quality of the image. This progress has been made possible by the development of special machines that generate optimal low-energy x-rays, special devices for compression of the breast, more sensitive films, and intensifying screens and grids. The importance of mammography quality assurance programs has been recognized in all countries with screening programs, and in addition to monitoring the quality of mammography equipment, countries can monitor medical parameters such as cancer detection rates and rates of recall for supplementary mammography, CBE, or biopsy to determine the efficacy of screening programs. Mammography has essentially become a subspecialty of radiology, and radiologists who practice mammography are usually required to complete special training programs and courses.

Unlike clinical mammography, which is done using three projections (mediolateral, craniocaudal, and mediolateral oblique), screening mammography uses one projection (mediolateral oblique) or two projections (mediolateral oblique and craniocaudal). There seem to be negligible differences between one- and two-projection screening mammography with regard to the cancer detection rate, but two-projection mammography reduces the rate of recall for supplementary mammography (44) and is therefore now generally preferred, especially in younger women. Independent reading of the mammograms by two radiologists has often been recommended and in one systematic study increased the cancer detection rate by 15% (45).

Radiation Risks

The radiation risks of mammography have been much discussed. That ionizing radiation can cause breast cancer is well known from epidemiologic analyses of atomic bomb survivors and cohorts of women exposed to ionizing radiation for medical reasons (46). As a rule, the doses that have induced breast cancer have been higher than 0.5 Gy, but theoretical risks of lower doses can be calculated by linear extrapolation. During the 1960s, when mammography was first used for screening, the doses were relatively high (50 mGy or more) and even though the theoretical risk of breast cancer induction was low, this theoretical risk caused concern about mass screening with mammography and frightened many women away from participation in screening programs. Owing to technical developments, radiation doses have decreased dramatically and at present are ideally about 4 mGy for two-projection mammography. In practice, a dose of 5 to 10 mGy per screening seems more realistic as the conditions are not always ideal and as some women are recalled for supplementary mammography. The theoretical risk of radiation-induced breast cancer after such low doses is very low in absolute terms. However, because mammography is an intervention performed in a population without known disease, the risk must be weighed against the assumed benefit. The benefit-risk ratio can be expressed as "years of life saved by screening detection of breast cancer"/"years of life lost because of radiation-induced breast cancer." Estimates of this ratio are complicated by the fact that different epidemiologic materials lead to rather different risk assumptions. Other complications for the theoretical risk calculations are the accumulation of the radiation dose over time and the latency time for radiation-induced cancer. Even with the most pessimistic risk assumptions it is, however, obvious that the benefit to risk ratio is very high for women who start screening at age 50 or later. Due to the still somewhat uncertain benefit of screening in women between 40 and 50 the radiation risk may still be an argument, but probably not a very strong one, against mammography screening in this age group.

Specific High-Risk Groups

Some groups of women have an exceptionally high risk of breast cancer. One group is, of course, women operated on for breast cancer. Such women have a high risk of developing a new cancer in the contralateral breast and, after breast-conserving treatment, a new cancer or recurrence in the ipsilateral breast. Another group consists of women operated on for benign breast lesions with proliferative, atypical epithelial changes or cancer in situ. The mentioned groups are usually followed with CBE two to three times per year and mammography annually regardless of age.

Women with a genetic predisposition to breast cancer constitute another high-risk group. During recent years, mutations in specific genes (*BRCA1*, *BRCA2*, and others) were found in women with hereditary breast cancer and also in healthy women from families with high rates of breast cancer (47). The latter women have an exceptionally high risk of developing breast cancer, often at a remarkably young age. If bilateral mastectomy is not performed, these women may require close surveillance with mammography, CBE, and other screening methods such as ultrasonography and magnetic resonance imaging. However, little is known at present about the effectiveness of such surveillance.

Older Women

Mammographic screening in women older than 70 is so far insufficiently studied. Of the randomized studies to date, only the two-county trial had no upper age limit for invited women and because of a low compliance rate among the oldest women, only the age group 70 to 74 has been included in the mortality analyses. The reduction in the breast cancer mortality rate in this age group seemed to be insignificant, but these results have little relevance because the group was small and screening in women older than 70 was terminated after the second screening round (15). In a separate report from the two-county trial (48), a significant reduction in the breast cancer mortality rate of 32% was found in women who were 65 to 74 years old at the time of randomization. However, it is not known to what degree this benefit derived from women older than 70. Several studies have shown that the cancer detection rate is high and the rate of false-positive findings is low in old women; the fatty, unstructured breast in these women seems to be an ideal object for mammography (6,10,48).

Some have argued against screening in older women, citing the opinion that breast cancer is not as lethal in older women as in younger women and also referring to the relatively short normal life expectancy in the elderly. The first assumption does not seem to be true: Several studies showed that the relative survival for elderly breast cancer patients is worse than that for younger ones (49,50). Concerning the second argument, women between 70 and 80 years old without breast cancer now have an expected survival of 15 to 10 years. There are certainly good reasons to focus more interest on screening in elderly women—perhaps especially those between 70 and 75 years old.

Cost-Benefit Considerations

Several cost-benefit calculations have been reported on the basis of experience from the randomized trials. For the age group 50 to 69, the cost per year of life saved has been calculated to be $3000 to $5000 in Europe (51); similar calculations in the United States (52) revealed costs on the order of $15,000 to $30,000. The higher calculated costs in the United States are due to annual instead of biannual screening, more expensive mammography, compulsory CBE, and a higher biopsy rate. For the age group 40 to 49, all calculations are very uncertain because the reduction in the mortality rate is still unclear. Assuming, however, a reduction in the breast cancer mortality rate of 20%, the cost in the United States has been calculated to be $40,000 to $50,000 per year of life saved (53).

On the whole, the cost-benefit analyses suggest that the costs of breast cancer screening are reasonable compared with costs of other life-saving measures such as kidney and heart transplantations and some radical treatment for symptomatic cancer.

Screening Guidelines in Different Countries

Most developed countries with a high incidence of breast cancer have issued more or less official guidelines on screening for breast cancer. In 1983, the American Cancer Society (ACS) in cooperation with the National Cancer Institute (NCI) presented such guidelines. They recommended monthly BSE for all women older than 20, CBE every 3 years between ages 20 and 40, annual CBE after age 40, and mammography every 1 to 2 years between ages 40 and 50 and annually after age 50. In 1993, after an international workshop (54), NCI omitted the recommendations for screening with CBE and mammography in women younger than 50. However, as a result of a new conference in January 1997 (55) both NCI and ACS now recommend annual mammography starting at age 40.

In Sweden, the National Board of Health and Welfare in 1986 issued recommendations to the county councils (which are responsible for the health service) on active invitation to screening mammography. The Board recommended that counties use a lower age limit not below 40 and not over 50 and an upper age limit of 75. For women younger than 55, screening every 18 months was recommended; for women older than 55, biannual screening was recommended. In 1989, the Board recommended that in case of scarce resources, women aged 50 to 69 should be given priority. As a result, the whole country is at present covered by screening programs with 40 as the lower age limit in about half of the counties. At present, a revision of the 1986 guidelines is being prepared within the National Board of Health and Welfare.

Systems similar to the Swedish one, which is based on active invitation, have been introduced in the United Kingdom, Finland, the Netherlands, and Iceland, but with 50 years as the lower age limit. In the cancer control program of the European Union, mammographic screening is given high priority and strongly recommended for all women aged 50 to 69.

Some Concluding Remarks

At present, there is almost universal consensus concerning the value of mammographic screening in women aged 50 to 69. Besides reducing the breast cancer mortality rate, screening also increases the possibility of breast-conserving treatment and reduces the need for adjuvant endocrine or cytotoxic treatment.

Screening in women younger than 50 is still controversial, even if there are some indications that screening in the age group 40 to 49 reduces the relative breast cancer mortality rate. The evidence, however, is not too convincing, especially as some part of the registered benefit certainly derives from continued screening after age 50. On the debit side is a high rate of uncertain findings in relation to the rate of detected cancers. More knowledge of the effect of screening on breast cancer mortality rates in this age group can probably be obtained by retrospective epidemiologic analyses of the large body of data from the Swedish service screening. The ongoing UK trial and the planned Eurotrial (40) may ultimately answer the question of whether it is beneficial to start screening at age 40 instead of age 50, but answers will not be available until around the year 2010.

A reasonable compromise at present could be to start screening at age 45. The prevalence of detectable cancer before this age is very low, and the benefit, if any, of screening in age 40–44 must be marginal and can hardly outweigh the negative side effects. More attention should be focused on women older than 70, especially those aged 70 to 74, in whom considerable benefit can be expected. In countries without active invitation to screening, much could be gained by efforts to increase the compliance rate in screening programs, which at present is low among some categories of women.

A woman attending screening usually regards it as a means of either excluding breast cancer or detecting a cancer that can be easily cured but that if not detected by screening might have killed her. This is of course a great simplification of the reality. All women who participate in screening should be informed about some simple principles of the procedure. They should thus know that an essential benefit can be obtained only by repeated screenings at regular intervals. They should also know that screening can never detect all breast cancers and, of course, not prevent the development of cancer later on. Finally, they should be aware of the considerable probability of uncertain results, which may cause anxiety and inconvenience in the form of supplemental examinations and biopsies.

In a way, screening for early detection of breast cancer is a medical anomaly that converts many perfectly healthy women into patients. However, until acceptable primary preventive methods are found, screening will probably continue to be the most effective way to reduce the consequences of breast cancer.

REFERENCES

1. Baines CJ. Breast self-examination. *Cancer* 1992;69(suppl 7):1942–1946.

2. UK Trial of Early Detection of Breast Cancer Group. Breast cancer mortality after 10 years in the UK trial of early detection of breast cancer. *Breast* 1993;2:13–20.

3. Gastrin G, Miller AB, To T, et al. Incidence and mortality from breast cancer in the Mama program for breast screening in Finland, 1973–1986. *Cancer* 1994;73:2168–2174.

4. Langeland P. Population screening for female breast tumours. A clinical investigation. *Acta Radiol Suppl* 297;1970.

5. Egan RL. Experience with mammography in a tumor institution. Evaluation of 1000 studies. *Radiology* 1960;75:894–900.

6. Thurfjell EL, Lindgren JA. Population-based mammography screening in Swedish clinical practice: prevalence and incidence screening in Uppsala county. *Radiology* 1994;193:351–357.

7. Shapiro S. Evidence on screening for breast cancer from a randomized trial. *Cancer* 1977;39:2772–2782.

8. Shapiro S. Determining the efficacy of breast cancer screening. In: Fortner JG, Rhoads JE, eds. *Accomplishments in cancer research.* Philadelphia: JB Lippincott, 1989:61–74.

9. Jakobsson S, Lundgren B, Melander O, Norin T. Mass-screening of a female population for detection of early carcinoma of the breast. *Acta Radiol* 1975;14:424–432.

10. Lundgren B, Jakobsson S. Single view mammography. A simple and efficient approach to breast cancer screening. *Cancer* 1976;38:1124–1129.

11. Tabar L, Fagerberg CJG, Gad A, et al. Reduction in mortality from breast cancer after mass screening with mammography. *Lancet* 1985;1:829–832.

12. Tabar L, Fagerbert G, Chen HH, et al. Screening for breast cancer in women aged under 50: mode of detection, incidence, fatality and histology. *J Med Screen* 1995;2:94–98.

13. Andersson J, Aspegren K, Janzon L, et al. Mammographic screening and mortality from

breast cancer: the Malmö mammographic screening trial. *BMJ* 1988;297:943–948.

14. Frisell J, Lidbrink E, Hellström L, Rutqvist LE. Follow-up after 11 years. Update of mortality results in the Stockholm mammographic screening trial. In: Lidbrink E. Mammographic screening for breast cancer. Aspects on benefit and risks (dissertation). Stockholm: Karolinska Institute, 1995.

15. Nyström L, Rutqvist LE, Wall S, et al. Breast cancer screening with mammography: overview of Swedish randomised trials. *Lancet* 1993;341: 973–978.

16. Nyström L, Larsson LG, Rutqvist LE, et al. Determination of cause of death among breast cancer cases in the Swedish randomized mammography screening trials. A comparison between official statistics and validation by an endpoint committee. *Acta Oncol* 1995;34:145–152.

17. Larsson LG, Nyström L, Wall S, et al. The Swedish randomised mammography screening trials: analysis of their effect on the breast cancer related excess mortality. *J Med Screen* 1996;3: 129–132.

18. Falun meeting on breast cancer screening with mammography in women aged 40–49 years: report of the organising committee and collaborators. *Int J Cancer* 1996;64:693–699.

19. Larsson LG, Andersson I, Bjurstam N, et al. Updated overview of the Swedish randomized trials on breast cancer screening with mammography: age group 40–49 at randomization. *JNCI* 1997; monograph No. 22:57–61.

20. Alexander FE, Anderson TJ, Brown HK, et al. The Edinburgh randomised trial of breast cancer screening: results of 10 years of follow-up. *Br J Cancer* 1994;70:542–548.

21. Miller AB, Baines CJ, To T, Wall C. Canadian National Breast Screening Study #1. Breast cancer detection and death rates among women aged 40 to 49 years. *Can Med Assoc J* 1992;147: 1459–1476.

22. Miller AB, Baines CJ, To T, Wall C. Canadian National Breast Screening Study #2. Breast cancer detection and death rates among women aged 50 to 59 years. *Can Med Assoc J* 1992; 147:1477–1488.

23. Boyd NF, Jong RA, Yaffe MJ, et al. A critical appraisal of the Canadian National Breast Cancer Screening Study. *Radiology* 1993;189:661–663.

24. Tarone RE. The excess of patients with advanced breast cancer in young women screened with mammography in the Canadian National Breast Screening Study. *Cancer* 1995;75:997–1003.

25. Baines CJ. The Canadian National Breast Screening Study. *Ann Intern Med* 1994;120: 326–334.

26. Shapiro S. Screening: assessment of current studies. *Cancer* 1994;74:231–238.

27. Baker LH. Breast Cancer Detection Demonstration Project: five-year summary report. *CA Cancer J Clin* 1982;32:194–225.

28. Smart CR, Hartmann WH, Beahrs OH, Garfinkel L. Insights into breast cancer screening of younger women. *Cancer* 1993;72:1449–1456.

29. de Waard F, Collette HJA, Romback JJ, et al. The DOM project for the early detection of breast cancer, Utrecht, the Netherlands. *J Chronic Dis* 1984;37:1–44.

30. Peeters PHM, Verbeek ALM, Hendriks JHCL, van Bon MJH. Screening for breast cancer in Nijmegen. Report of 6 screening rounds, 1975–1986. *Int J Cancer* 1989;43:226–230.

31. Palli D, Del Turco MR, Buitti E, et al. A case-control study of the efficacy of a non-randomized breast cancer screening program in Florence (Italy). *Int J Cancer* 1986;38:501–504.

32. Peeters PHM, Verbeek ALM, Hendriks JHCL, et al. The occurrence of interval cancers in the Nijmegen screening programme. *Br J Cancer* 1989;59:929–932.

33. Paci E, Ciatto S, Buiatti E, et al. Early indicators of efficacy of breast cancer screening programmes. Results of the Florence district programme. *Int J Cancer* 1990;46:198–202.

34. Peer P, Holland R, Hendriks J, et al. Age-specific effectiveness of the Nijmegen population-based breast cancer-screening program: assessment of early indicators of screening effectiveness. *J Natl Cancer Inst* 1994;86:436–441.

35. Collette HJA, Day NE, Rombach JJ, de Waard F. Evaluation of screening for breast cancer in a non-randomised study (the DOM project) by means of a case-control study. *Lancet* 1984;1 2:1224–1226.

36. Smart CR, Hendrick RE, Rutledge JH, Smith RA. Benefit of mammography screening in women aged 40–49 years—current evidence from randomized controlled trials. *Cancer* 1995;75:1619–1626.

37. Shapiro S, Venet W, Strax P, et al. Ten- to fourteen-year effect of screening on breast cancer mortality. *J Natl Cancer Inst* 1982;60:349–355.

38. de Koning HJ, Boer R, Warmerdam PG, et al. Quantitative interpretation of age-specific mortality reductions from the Swedish breast cancer-screening trials. *J Natl Cancer Inst* 1995;87:1217–1223.

39. Tabar L, Duffy SW, Chen HH. Re: Quantitative interpretation of age-specific mortality reductions from the Swedish breast cancer-screening trials. *J Natl Cancer Inst* 1996;88:52–53.

40. *Eurotrial 40. A randomized population-based trial on the efficacy of screening mammography in women under 50. Study protocol.* Geneva, International Union Against Cancer, September 1995.

41. Peer P, van Dijck J, Hendriks J, et al. Age-dependent growth rate of primary breast cancer. *Cancer* 1993;71:3547–3551.

42. Tabar L, Fagerberg G, Chen HH, et al. Tumour development, histology and grade of breast cancers: prognosis and progression. *Int J Cancer* 1996;66:413–419.

43. Lidbrink E, Elfving J, Frisell J, Jonsson E. Neglected aspects of false positive findings of mammography in breast cancer screening: analyses of false positive cases from the Stockholm trial. *BMJ* 1996;312:273–312.

44. Thurfjell E, Taube A, Tabar L. One- versus two-view mammography screening. A prospective population-based study. *Acta Radiol* 1994;35:340–344.

45. Thurfjell E, Lernevall A, Taube A. Benefit of independent double reading in a population-based mammography screening program. *Radiology* 1994;191:241–244.

46. United Nations Scientific Committee on the Effects of Atomic Radiation. *1994 Report.* New York: United Nations, 1994.

47. Olsson H, Borg Å. Genetic pre-disposition to breast cancer. *Acta Oncol* 1996;35:1–8.

48. Chen HH, Tabar L, Fagerberg G, Duffy SW. Effect of breast cancer screening after age 65. *J Med Screen* 1995;2:10–14.

49. Adami HC, Malker B, Holmberg L, et al. The relationship between survival and age at diagnosis in breast cancer. *N Engl J Med* 1986;14:559–563.

50. Constanza ME. Breast cancer screening in older women. Synopsis of a forum. *Cancer* 1992;69 (suppl):1925–1931.

51. de Koning H, van Ineveld M, van Oortmarssen G, et al. Breast cancer screening and cost-effectiveness: policy alternatives, quality of life considerations and the possible impact of uncertain factors. *Int J Cancer* 1991;49:531–537.

52. Elixhauser A. Costs of breast cancer and the cost-effectiveness of breast cancer screening. *Int J Techol Assess Health Care* 1991;7:604–615.

53. Rosenquist CJ, Lindfors KK. Screening mammography in women aged 40–49 years: analysis of cost-effectiveness. *Radiology* 1994;191:647–650.

54. Fletcher SW, Black W, Harris R, et al. Report of the International Workshop on Screening for Breast Cancer. *J Natl Cancer Inst* 1993;85:1644–1656.

55. NIH consensus development conference on breast cancer screening for women ages 40–49. Jan 21–23, 1997. Program and abstracts. National Inst. Health, 1997.

Indications and Techniques for Breast Biopsy

MONICA MORROW

The most common clinical indications for breast biopsy are a dominant breast mass, pathologic nipple discharge, or an abnormal-appearing mammogram. The determination of what constitutes a dominant mass is frequently difficult, particularly in the premenopausal woman. The normal glandular tissue of the breast is nodular, and this nodularity is usually most pronounced in the upper outer quadrant of the breast and the inframammary ridge area. Such nodularity, particularly when it waxes and wanes during the menstrual cycle, is a physiologic process and is not an indication for breast biopsy. Breast nodularity is often accompanied by breast pain. Breast pain is an uncommon presenting symptom of breast carcinoma; fewer than 10% of patients with cancer have pain as an associated symptom. In the absence of clinical or mammographic evidence of a breast mass, breast pain should be managed nonoperatively. This is true even when the pain appears to be localized, because surgery, including radical surgical approaches such as mastectomy, is rarely successful in eradicating breast pain.

Dominant Masses

Dominant masses are characterized by their persistence throughout the menstrual cycle. They may be discrete or poorly defined, but differ in character from the surrounding breast tissue and the corresponding area in the contralateral breast. The differential diagnosis of dominant breast masses includes macrocysts, fibroadenoma, prominent areas of fibrocystic change, fat necrosis, and carcinoma. A dominant breast mass palpated in a premenopausal woman should be aspirated to determine if it is a cyst. Cysts are usually well demarcated from the surrounding breast tissue, and are somewhat mobile and firm. Cysts that are very full are often quite hard, and may be difficult to distinguish from solid masses by physical examination. Cysts require biopsy only if the aspirated fluid is bloody, the palpable abnormality does not resolve completely after the aspiration of fluid, or the same cyst recurs multiple times in a short time interval. The routine cytologic examination of cyst fluid is not indicated because of the low likelihood of carcinoma in the absence of the clinical findings just noted. In addition, the cytologic identification of atypical cells in cyst fluid is not uncommon, resulting in the clinical dilemma of a patient whose cyst resolves with aspiration, whose mammogram appears normal, and who has a cytology indicating the need for a biopsy. Ciatto et al (1) performed cytology on 6782 cyst fluid aspirates. Atypical cells were identified in 1677 and no cancers were identified. Five intracystic papillomas were found, but bloody fluid was present in all of these aspirates.

Cysts can occur at any age, but are particularly common in women in their 40s and those who are perimenopausal. In postmenopausal women who are not taking exogenous estrogen, cysts are uncommon and should be regarded with a higher degree of suspicion than in the premenopausal years. Aspiration is still an

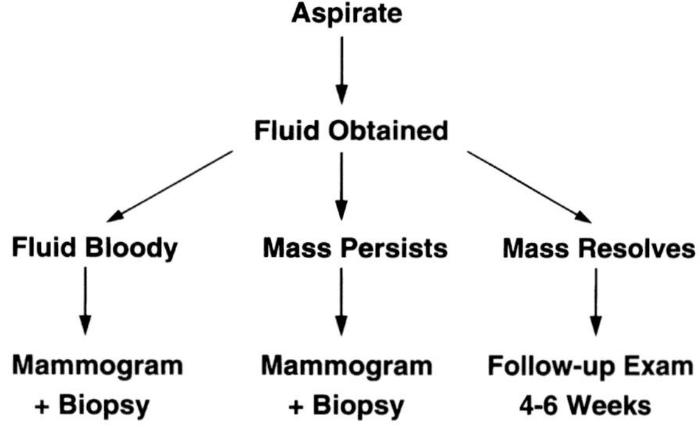

FIGURE 3-1

Algorithm for the evaluation and management of breast cysts.

appropriate first step, but a repeat examination 4 to 6 weeks after aspiration to check for recurrence of the cyst is essential. The algorithm for cyst management is summarized in Figure 3-1.

Noncystic masses in premenopausal women that are clearly different from the surrounding breast tissue should be evaluated by biopsy using one of the techniques described later in the chapter. Observation for one or two menstrual cycles is only appropriate for vague asymmetry or nodularity, when it is unclear that a dominant mass is present. A dominant breast mass should not be dismissed as a cyst unless the diagnosis is documented by sonography or aspiration.

In postmenopausal women, clinical examination of the breasts is frequently easier owing to atrophy of the nodular glandular elements. Benign breast problems causing palpable masses are less frequent in this age group, and carcinoma is more common; therefore, small areas of nodularity that might be observed in a premenopausal woman should be considered for prompt biopsy in a postmenopausal woman.

Nipple Discharge

Nipple discharge is a common complaint, but an uncommon sign of breast carcinoma. Three percent to 11% of women with carcinoma have an associated nipple discharge. The likelihood of a nipple discharge being secondary to malignancy increases with age. In one study, 32% of women over age 60 presenting with nipple discharge and no mass had carcinoma, compared

to 7% of women under age 60 with the same presentation (2). The initial step in the evaluation of nipple discharge is to determine whether it is physiologic or pathologic. Discharges are classified as pathologic if they are spontaneous, and localized to one duct. Pathologic discharges may be bloody or serous, and are almost always unilateral. In contrast, physiologic discharges occur only with nipple compression, frequently originate from multiple ducts, and are often bilateral. The clinical evaluation of a pathologic discharge should include testing the fluid for occult blood and identifying the quadrant of the breast from which the discharge originates. Although 70% to 85% of the discharges due to carcinoma contain blood (3), a nonbloody discharge that meets the other criteria of a pathologic discharge is an indication for a breast biopsy. Cytology is not usually useful in the evaluation of nipple discharge because the absence of malignant cells does not reliably exclude carcinoma, and positive cytologic findings will not differentiate between intraductal and invasive carcinoma.

As part of the evaluation of a pathologic discharge, a mammogram should be obtained to look for nonpalpable masses, calcifications, or dilated ducts. When a discharge occurs in association with a mass, the mass should be evaluated by biopsy. In the absence of a mass, a terminal duct excision should be performed. The role of galactography in the management of nipple discharge is controversial. Tabar et al (4) studied 116 women undergoing galactography for pathologic discharge. Ductal lesions were visualized in all women, but how this altered the surgical approach or avoided surgery is not clear. Galactography may be useful in identifying lesions in the periphery of the breast that would not be removed with a standard terminal duct excision, or in minimizing the amount of the ductal system that is removed in women of childbearing age. However, galactography does not provide a definitive diagnosis for intraductal lesions and does not obviate the need for histologic sampling in women with pathologic discharges.

Mammographic Abnormalities

In many surgical practices, a mammographic abnormality is one of the most frequent indications for breast biopsy. The initial clinical step in the evaluation of a mammographic abnormality is a careful physical examination. If there is any question about whether a palpable finding corresponds to a mammographically identified mass, a radiopaque marker should be placed on the abnormality and repeat mammographic views obtained. If the clinical and mammographic lesions correspond, the lesion can be approached as a palpable abnormality. If there is any doubt about this correspondence, a needle localization biopsy is the most prudent course.

The classic mammographic signs of clinically occult malignancy are clustered microcalcifications and small masses. A review of 5500 mammographically generated biopsies identified microcalcifications as the indication for biopsy in 45% of patients, masses in 43%, masses containing microcalcifications in 6%, and asymmetric density in 5% (5). The positive predictive value of most mammographic findings is low and cancer is identified in only 20% to 35% of biopsy specimens in most series (6–9). Special mammographic views are frequently helpful in the evaluation of equivocal findings on two-view mammography, and these views should be obtained prior to making a final determination of the need for biopsy. Morrow et al (9) studied 267 consecutive patients referred to a surgeon because of an abnormal-appearing mammogram. Sixty-seven percent of the group had an incomplete radiologic workup, and spot compression and magnification views were obtained before the need for biopsy was determined. After the additional evaluation, only 150 of the 267 abnormalities were found to be suspicious enough to warrant biopsy. Even when biopsy is clearly indicated on the basis of the initial mammogram, magnification views are useful in delineating the extent of the lesion.

Techniques of Breast Biopsy

Palpable Masses

Palpable breast masses can be diagnosed with fine-needle aspiration (FNA) biopsy, core cutting needle biopsy, excisional biopsy, or incisional biopsy. The accuracy, techniques, and advantages of each of these approaches are discussed.

Fine-Needle Aspiration

FNA is becoming increasingly popular for the diagnosis of dominant breast masses. Accuracy rates for FNA are high. A review of seven published reports of 4943 FNA procedures noted a sensitivity of 87%, and the incidence of insufficient specimens varied from 4% to 13% (10). Kline et al (11) reviewed 3545 breast aspirates and reported a 9.6% rate of false-negative results. In half of the false-negative cases the needle tract did not extend into the tumor. Other factors reported to be associated with false-negative aspirates include small tumor size, fibrotic tumors, and infiltrating lobular, tubular, and cribriform histologies (11–13). False-positive aspirates are extremely uncommon, being reported in fewer than 1% of cases in most large series (10–14).

FNA has the advantage of being quick, relatively painless, and inexpensive to perform. Results are available within 24 hours, and immediate interpretation of smears is often feasible. Since the diagnosis of malignancy by FNA is quite reliable, treatment options can be discussed with the patient and definitive surgery performed without the need for a biopsy. This approach avoids the problem of incorporating the biopsy incision in the definitive surgical resection. Aspirates that are interpreted as suspicious or atypical are an indication for a surgical biopsy. Insufficient specimens provide no useful information and are an indication for a repeat FNA or another type of biopsy. In one series (14), physician experience was the factor that correlated best with a low rate of insufficient specimens.

The major drawback to the use of FNA in many institutions is the lack of an experienced cytopathologist. In addition, FNA will not reliably distinguish invasive from intraductal carcinoma, potentially leading to the overtreatment of gross ductal carcinoma in situ, and FNA provides no histologic detail such as the presence of an extensive intraductal component associated with the invasive cancer, which might influence the extent of a lumpectomy.

The major controversy surrounding the use of FNA is the management of the dominant mass with a benign aspirate. The so-called triple test uses physical examination, mammography, and FNA in an attempt to avoid surgical biopsy of benign breast lesions. When all three of these modalities indicate benign disease, the chance of carcinoma being present is 0.6% according to one review (15). However, Bell et al (16) noted a 3.4% incidence of carcinoma in 285 women for whom the results of the triple test were negative. When one considers observation of a dominant mass in the setting of negative triple test results, all elements of the triple test must be evaluable. The extremely low incidence of malignancy cited above does not apply in patients in whom the mass is not visible on the mammogram, or those with an insufficient cytologic aspirate. In addition, the accuracy of a clinical or mammographic diagnosis of a benign lesion is lowest in young women, the group in whom biopsy is most likely to be omitted. If a dominant mass is to be observed, a defined follow-up plan must be established to allow for the early detection of missed cancers. The use of FNA in the evaluation of solid masses is summarized in Figure 3-2.

Technique The breast mass is fixed in the operator's nondominant hand and the skin is cleansed with antiseptic. A small amount of 1% lidocaine is used to anesthetize the skin at the puncture site. Needles varying in size from 21 to 27 gauge have been used for FNA. The use of a syringe holder, which aids in creating a vacuum for aspiration, is preferred although a standard syringe can also be used. The needle is inserted into the mass, and when firm tissue is encountered, suction is applied from the syringe. The needle is moved back and forth within the tumor to facilitate dislodging cells. When aspirated material is visible in the hub of the needle, a satisfactory specimen has usually been obtained. In order to minimize the number of insufficient specimens, a second aspirate is

obtained through the same skin puncture site. Depending on the preference of the cytologist, the aspirated material is smeared onto microscope slides or placed into a fixative for cell block preparation.

There are no real contraindications to aspiration cytology. The procedure may be done in anticoagulated patients as long as firm pressure is applied to the site at the completion of the aspiration. Mammography done within 2 weeks of an FNA may result in false-positive readings due to hematoma obscuring the regular contours of benign breast masses (17). The most common complication of FNA is bruising. Pneumothorax has been reported after the procedure, but is very rare. This complication can be prevented by avoiding a direct perpendicular approach to lesions deep within the breast.

Core Cutting Needle Biopsy

Core cutting needle biopsies have many of the advantages of FNA, but because a core of tissue is obtained for histologic examination, more details of tumor structure are available and ductal carcinoma in situ can be identified. The adequacy of the specimen can be evaluated at the time of the biopsy, allowing additional tissue to be removed when the specimen appears to be nothing but fat, and the material is suitable for interpretation by any pathologist. Fentiman et al (18) performed core biopsy on 135 patients with breast cancer and 107 (79%) were successfully diagnosed. In a similar study of 150 core biopsies, Minkowitz et al (19) determined an 89% sensitivity and a 100% specificity for the core technique. In both series, a higher incidence of false-negative results was reported

Algorithm for the management of solid breast masses using fine-needle aspiration (FNA) cytology. The decision to follow a solid mass on the basis of benign findings by physical examination, mammography, and FNA should be made after a consideration of the patient's age and other recognized breast cancer risk factors.

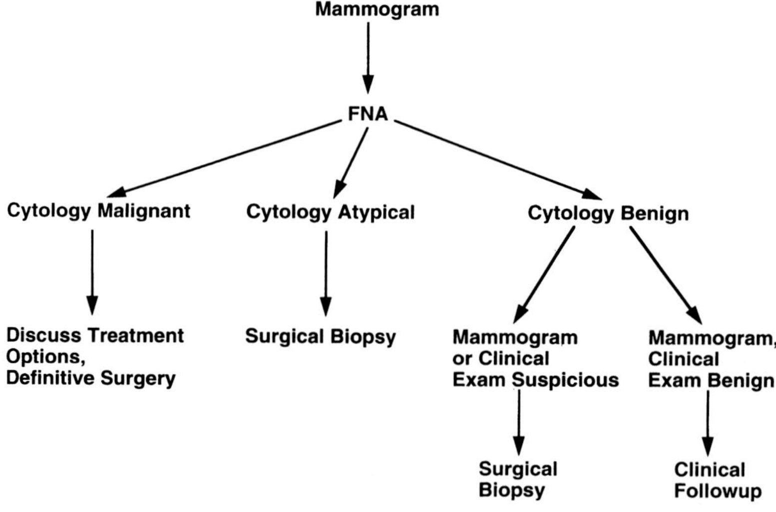

for small tumors. Shabot et al (20) prospectively compared the diagnostic accuracy of aspiration cytology and core needle biopsy in 81 patients with breast masses. Aspiration cytology was diagnostic in 95% of patients, compared to a 70% diagnostic rate for core biopsy ($p = 0.008$). False-positive diagnoses are rare with the core biopsy technique, but could occur with lesions such as radial scars. False-negative results may occur with extremely hard tumors, because the sampling needle is deflected into the surrounding fat. The choice between core biopsy and FNA is often dependent on the availability of a cytopathologist.

Technique Core needle biopsies can be performed with Tru-Cut needles or the spring-loaded Bioptycut device. The Bioptycut needle has a higher diagnostic sensitivity than the Tru-Cut needle (21), but it is also more expensive. Seeding of core needle tracts with tumor cells has been reported, so it is prudent to place the biopsy tract so that it will be excised during definitive therapy. This is probably a theoretical concern in patients undergoing breast-conserving surgery who will receive irradiation, but in patients undergoing mastectomy, excision of the puncture site is desirable. Complications of core biopsy are uncommon and include hematoma, infection, and pneumothorax.

Excisional Biopsy

Excisional biopsy is the complete removal of a breast abnormality. When the excisional biopsy of a cancer includes a margin of normal breast tissue, it will often serve as the definitive lumpectomy. Excisional biopsy is an outpatient procedure that can almost always be performed using local anesthesia supplemented with intravenous sedation as necessary. In the past, patients undergoing a breast biopsy were often admitted to the hospital and given general anesthesia, with a plan to proceed directly to a mastectomy if a frozen section revealed carcinoma. There is little rationale for such an approach today. Data from retrospective and prospective trials demonstrate no survival advantage for patients undergoing biopsy followed immediately by definitive surgery when compared to patients undergoing two separate operative procedures (22,23). The performance of a separate biopsy (two-step procedure) allows the clinician to review the pathology of the entire malignancy before discussing treatment options, and

allows the patient to seek consultation with a radiation oncologist or a reconstructive surgeon prior to making a treatment choice. For many women, the time for consultation with other members of the breast cancer care team and the option of a second opinion are critical to the decision-making process. Delays of up to 1 month from the time of diagnosis to definitive therapy have not been shown to alter prognosis (22,23), so performing definitive surgery is not an emergency.

Prior to an excisional biopsy, high-quality diagnostic mammography that includes magnification views of the site of the palpable abnormality should be performed. The purpose of this is to assess the extent of the palpable mass and any associated nonpalpable component, and to ensure that no nonpalpable abnormali-

A mammogram obtained following a breast biopsy that demonstrated a 1-cm carcinoma. The large postbiopsy hematoma affects the surrounding breast parenchyma, and limits the assessment of the patient's suitability for breast-conserving therapy.

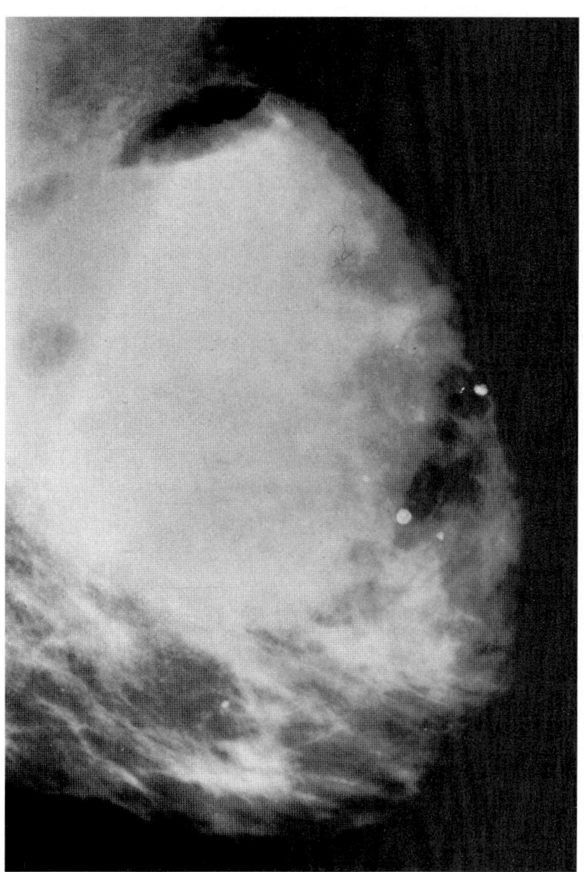

ties are present elsewhere in either breast. This information is essential to evaluate the patient's suitability for breast-conserving therapy if a diagnosis of cancer is made. Adequate mammograms in the immediate postbiopsy period are often difficult to obtain, owing to pain on compressing the breast or hematoma and post-biopsy inflammation obscuring the breast parenchyma (Fig. 3-3). Using information obtained from magnification mammography of the primary tumor site, Kearney and Morrow (24) obtained histologically negative margins with a single conservative diagnostic biopsy in 227 (95%) of 239 patients. Magnification mammography also readily identifies patients requiring wider excisions for complete tumor removal (25).

Technique Cosmetic outcome and the possible need for definitive cancer surgery must be balanced when one considers the site of incision. Incisions in Langer's lines usually produce the best cosmetic result for lesions in the upper half of the breast. In the lower half of the breast the choice between a radial incision and an incision in Langer's lines will depend on the contour of the breast and the amount of tissue to be excised (Fig. 3-4).

When malignancy is suspected, the incision should be placed over the mass to allow its removal as a single specimen, and to provide adequate visualization to achieve hemostasis. This approach will also facilitate re-excision of the cavity when necessary to obtain cancer-negative margins. Tunneling for small distances to improve cosmesis is appropriate, but the use of circumareolar incisions to remove lesions in the periphery of the breast should be avoided.

Skin removal is neither necessary nor desirable unless the lesion is adherent to the dermis. An important step in avoiding visible depressions in the breast contour is preservation of the subcutaneous fat. Once the skin is incised, the breast tissue should be divided to a point 0.5 to 1.0 cm superficial to the breast mass and then excision is carried out (Fig. 3-5). Lesions that appear to be fibroadenomas can be shelled out at the level of the capsule as long as care is taken to remove the entire lesion. Other masses should be removed with a small margin (5–10 mm) of normal breast tissue. Electrocautery should be used with care until the lesion has been removed, because thermal injury makes evaluation of margins difficult and may interfere with the histologic diagnosis of small tumors.

Proper specimen management is critical to the success of an excisional biopsy. If a margin of normal tissue has been removed as part of the biopsy, orienting sutures should be placed. The use of two sutures will allow orientation of the specimen by the pathologist. The intact specimen should be examined to confirm that the lesion in question has been removed. When there is suspicion of malignancy, the adequacy of the margins can be grossly assessed. The

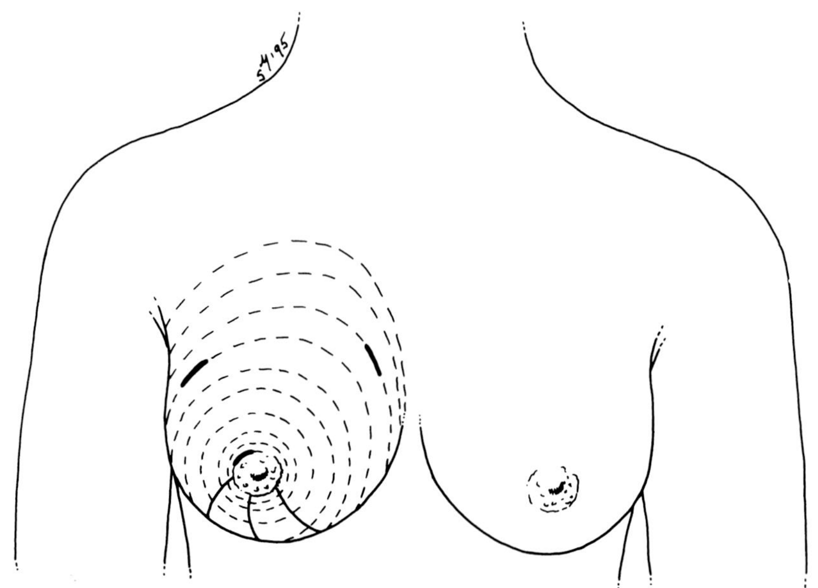

F I G U R E 3-4

Incision placement for breast biopsy. The dotted lines indicate Langer's lines and solid lines illustrate the site of incision placement in different parts of the breast.

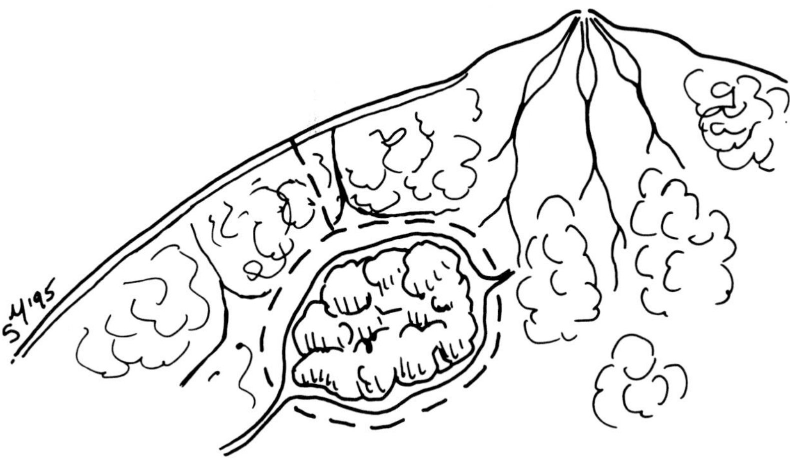

FIGURE **3-5**

Approach to lesions within the substance of the breast by incising the subcutaneous tissue and overlying parenchyma (dotted line) to a point approximately 1 cm superficial to the lesion.

specimen is sent fresh to pathology and margins are inked to allow identification of patients who require re-excision.

Prior to closure, careful palpation of the biopsy site should be carried out to confirm removal of the lesion in its entirety. Meticulous hemostasis is important, and use of drains should be avoided. Reapproximation of the breast parenchyma should also be avoided because this often distorts the contour of the breast and worsens the cosmetic result. This distortion is often not evident when the patient is supine with her arms relaxed. The deep dermis is reapproximated with several interrupted sutures and a subcuticular skin closure is utilized. Complications of excisional biopsy are uncommon and include infection, hematoma, and failure to remove the palpable mass.

Incisional Biopsy

The use of incisional biopsy is reserved for masses too large to be excised as a diagnostic procedure, most commonly locally advanced breast cancer. Today there are few indications for incisional biopsy. Diagnostic material can be obtained using FNA or core needle biopsy with lower morbidity and lower cost, and immunohistochemical techniques allow the determination of hormone receptor status and the study of tumor markers from small specimens. Incisional biopsy is appropriate when it becomes apparent intraoperatively that what appeared to be a dominant mass is a diffuse process within the breast. This situation usually occurs with benign fibrocystic changes, and rather than remove an entire quadrant of the breast, an inci-

sional biopsy of the clinical abnormality should be performed.

Nipple Discharge

Terminal Duct Excision

The standard method for the diagnosis of pathologic nipple discharge is a terminal duct excision. Terminal duct excision, like other excisional breast biopsies, is an outpatient procedure that is readily performed under local anesthesia, usually with supplemental sedation. Patients should be advised preoperatively that there may be some permanent numbness of the nipple-areolar complex following the biopsy, and women of childbearing age will be unable to lactate. In the patient who has had preoperative galactography demonstrating a localized ductal abnormality, a needle localization of the abnormality may be performed. This approach may be advantageous in the young patient who wishes to maintain the ability to lactate in the future.

Technique A circumareolar incision is placed over the quadrant of the breast where the discharge originates (Fig. 3-6A). The incision may involve up to one half of the circumference of the areola if necessary for exposure. Incisions of more than half of the areolar circumference risk devascularization of the nipple-areolar complex. With the knife, the nipple is dissected free from the underlying breast tissue as a full-thickness dermal flap (Fig. 3-6B). Dissection deep to the level of the dermis runs the risk that the ductal pathology, which is usually proximal

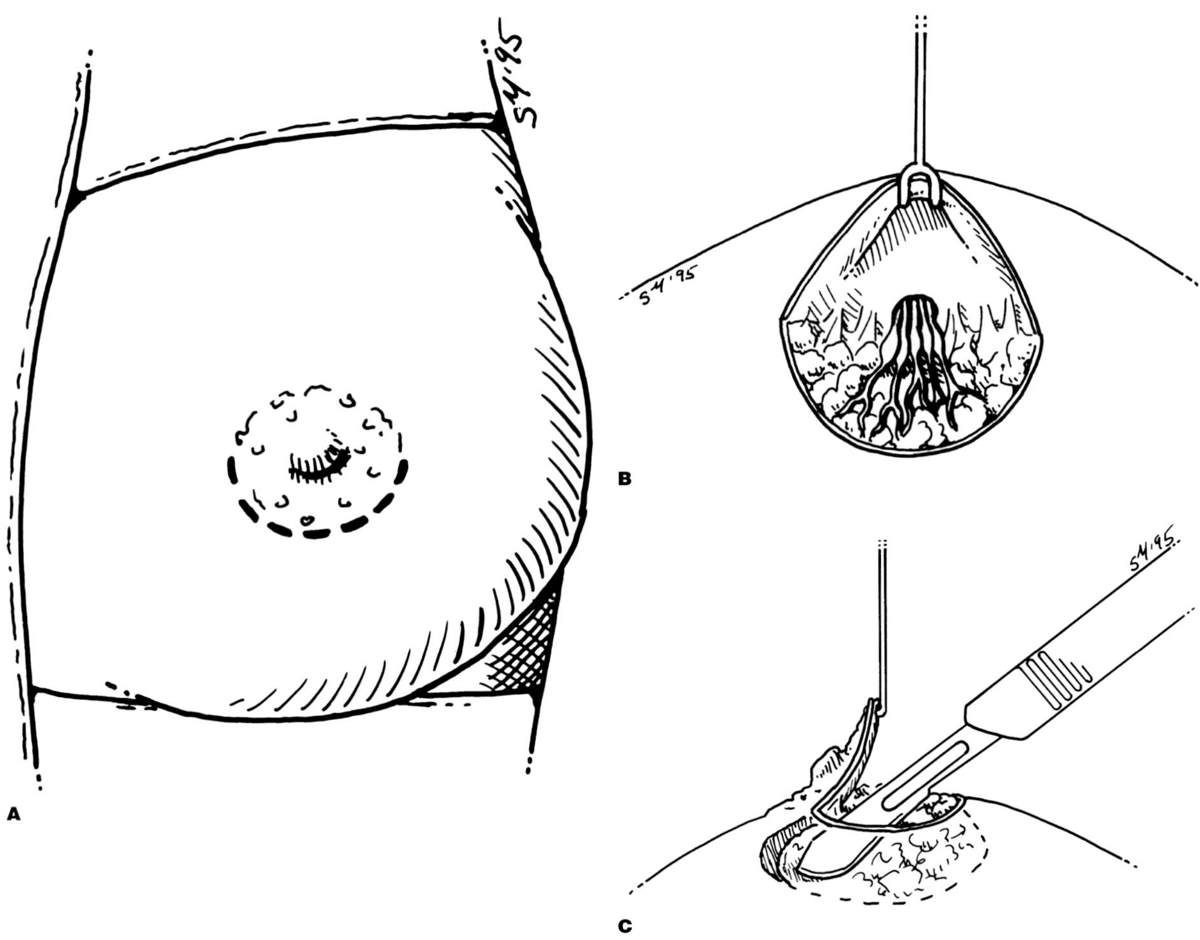

FIGURE 3-6

A. A circumareolar incision centered over the discharging duct is used for terminal duct excision. B. The nipple-areolar complex is dissected free from the underlying breast tissue as a full-thickness dermal flap. C. If a single abnormal duct is not identified intraoperatively, the entire central core of ductal tissue is excised.

in the duct, will not be removed. As the nipple is dissected free and the proximal ducts are divided, the abnormal duct can usually be identified visually or by the presence of discharge. Some surgeons prefer to cannulate the discharging duct with a fine probe prior to making the incision. If a single abnormal duct is identified, it is followed distally in the breast for a distance of 2 to 3cm and then transected. The point of transection should be observed for discharge, which would indicate that the pathology was more peripheral in the duct. Ligation of the transected duct is unnecessary. If an abnormal duct is not identified intraoperatively, the entire central core of ductal tissue is excised to a depth of 2 to 3cm (Fig. 3-6C). Attempts

to reapproximate the breast tissue should be avoided. An excellent cosmetic result is obtained with careful approximation of the dermis and subcuticular closure of the skin.

Mammographic Abnormalities

Needle Localization Biopsy

The most important factors in the success of a needle localization biopsy are accurate placement of the guide, a thorough understanding by the surgeon of the relationship between the guide and the mammographic abnormality, and communication between the surgeon and the radiologist. Gallagher et al (26) reviewed 100 consecutive needle localization biopsies performed by a single surgeon in a 1-year period. In 96 procedures the wire was within 5 mm of the abnormality. The median specimen volume was 6.0 cm^3, and one patient required a second biopsy because of failure to excise the lesion. Other series reported that 59% to 78% of localizations are within 1 cm of the target (27–29). Whether a guidewire, dye, or a combination of the two is used appears to be primarily a matter of preference. Failure rates of needle localization biopsy vary widely, ranging from less than 1% to 18% (30,31), but most modern series reported failure to excise the mammographic lesion in 1% to 2% (32–34) of patients.

The majority of needle localization biopsies can be done under local anesthesia, with supplemental sedation as necessary. As discussed previously, most mammographically identified breast abnormalities are benign, and the routine removal of very large amounts of breast tissue should be avoided.

Technique Prior to beginning the procedure, the surgeon must carefully review the mammograms to understand the relationship between the localizing wire and the mammographic abnormality. Marking the point where the wire enters the skin with a radiopaque marker makes it easy to determine how much of the wire is within the breast. The ideal localization is one in which the wire passes through the abnormality. Wire placement more than 1 cm from the target is not particularly helpful to the surgeon, and repositioning should be considered. Measurements of the distance from the localizing wire to the lesion, taken with the patient erect and the breast compressed, are of little use to the surgeon in the operating room.

Incision placement is critical to the success of needle localization biopsy. The incision should be placed at the point of entry of the wire into the breast only when the wire has a short course within the breast. When the wire traverses a large amount of the breast, the incision should be made just proximal to the area of the pathology and the wire identified within the breast parenchyma (Fig. 3-7). The appropriate location for the incision can be determined by noting the relationship between the nipple, the entry point of the wire in the skin, and the lesion on both mammographic views. Incision over the area of the pathology allows the use of a smaller incision, facilitates hemostasis, and allows the removal of a single specimen. In addition, if a carcinoma requiring re-excision lumpectomy is identified, the re-excision is readily accomplished.

After the breast tissue is entered, the localizing wire is identified within the breast parenchyma. When this is accomplished, the distal portion of the wire is stabilized with a clamp and the remainder of the wire is brought into the incision. Caution should be used when dividing breast tissue with the cautery prior to the identification of the wire, because the wire can be readily transected with the cautery. Care should be taken at all times to avoid pulling on the wire, grasping it with clamps, or moving it to determine its course within the breast. These maneuvers, particularly in women with fatty breasts, run the risk of dislodging the wire from the area of the target.

The breast tissue over the proximal portion of the wire is incised until the area of the pathology is approached. This approach is facilitated by the use of a guidewire with a thickened distal segment, with the thickened segment positioned in the lesion. When the

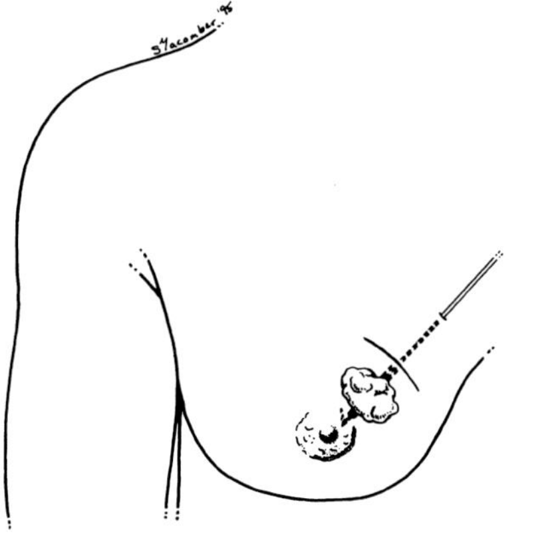
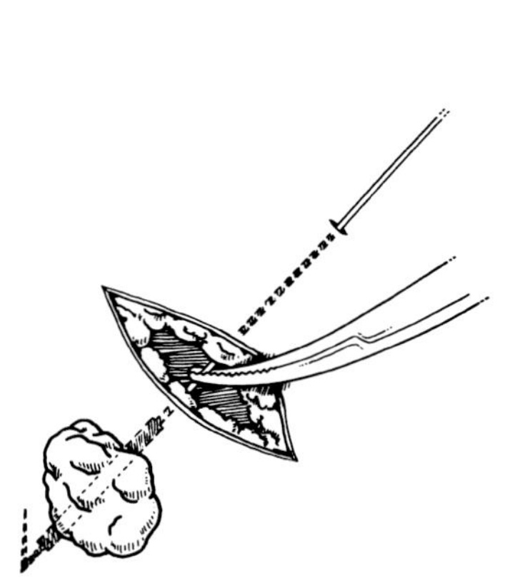

F I G U R E **3-7**

Incisions for needle localization breast biopsy should be placed adjacent to the area of pathology, not at the entry point of the wire into the breast. The wire is then identified in the breast parenchyma and brought into the wound.

change in the caliber of the wire is identified, the dissection is moved away from the wire to allow removal of the entire lesion with a small margin of normal breast tissue. Cautery should be avoided in the area of the lesion, because cautery artifact can make both the diagnosis of small lesions and an assessment of margin status difficult.

Specimen radiography is a mandatory part of needle localization biopsy. It is the only way to determine whether calcifications have been removed, and although many mammographically identified masses are palpable intraoperatively, a specimen radiograph ensures that the palpable abnormality corresponds to the mammographic lesion being sought, and serves as a record that the lesion has been removed. The specimen is marked with orienting sutures and the pathologist is provided with a copy of the specimen radiograph. As with other breast biopsies, inking of the specimen to determine margin status should be routine. Frozen section has little role in the management of nonpalpable abnormalities. Sacchini et al (35) reported a 12% discordance rate between frozen section and permanent section results in a series of 403 nonpalpable abnormalities. Problems were primarily due to the inability to reliably distinguish atypical hyperplasia from intraductal carcinoma, and difficulties in identifying a small area of invasion in large areas of intraductal carcinoma. Frozen section of small lesions runs the risk of distorting all of the available diagnostic material with frozen section artifact. The widespread availability of immunohistochemical hormone receptor determination, and the fact that a diagnostic needle localization is rarely undertaken with a plan to proceed to definitive surgery, make frozen section unnecessary in the management of nonpalpable abnormalities.

When the specimen radiograph fails to confirm the presence of the lesion, both the surgeon and the radiologist should review the localization films to determine whether the lesion was truly localized. If, in retrospect, the lesion was not localized, further excision of breast tissue at the site of the wire is of little merit and the procedure should be terminated. Failure to localize the lesion is a relatively uncommon cause of failure to excise a mammographic abnormality. More commonly, limited exposure from a poorly placed incision and traction on the localizing wire are the causes of failure. If the localization appears to be on target, the removal of additional breast tissue from the distal portion of the biopsy cavity will usually result in excision of the mammographic abnormality. If the lesion is not visualized in the second specimen, the procedure should be terminated. When the patient can comfortably tolerate compression, a mammogram should be obtained to confirm persistence of the lesion and a repeat biopsy undertaken.

In addition to failure to remove the mammographic abnormality, complications of needle localization biopsy include retention of a portion of the wire in the breast, infection, and hematoma.

Image-Guided Core Needle Biopsy

An alternative to excisional biopsy in the management of mammographic abnormalities is stereotactic core needle biopsy. Nonpalpable masses can also be sampled using ultrasound guidance. The potential advantages of a core biopsy include less pain, the absence of surgical scars, and lower cost compared to open surgical biopsy. A review of seven series comparing stereotactic core biopsies to surgical excision demonstrated sensitivities ranging from 71% to 100% for core biopsy when the technique was used in selected patients (36). The sensitivity of the procedure varies with the type of lesion being targeted, and is lower for microcalcifications than mass lesions (36,37). The routine use of specimen radiography with core biopsies done for calcifications will allow a determination that the appropriate area has been sampled. As experience has been gained with the core biopsy technique, a number of core diagnoses that are indications for surgical biopsy have been identified. The most frequently encountered of these is atypical ductal hyperplasia, which is associated with carcinoma in 30% to 50% of cases (38,39). A core diagnosis of radial scar is also an indication for a surgical biopsy to exclude coexistent carcinoma. Another indication for a repeat biopsy is lack of concordance between the core biopsy findings and the appearance of the mammographic target. Prior to core biopsy, a differential diagnosis for the mammographic abnormality should be developed. Lack of concordance between the histologic diagnosis and the mammographic diagnosis suggests that the lesion may not have been sampled, and is an indication for a repeat biopsy. Dershaw et al (38) observed this problem in 15 of 314 women undergoing core biopsy. A diagnosis of lobular carcinoma in situ should not be accepted as a cause for a mammographic abnormality, and is an indication for repeat biopsy.

One limitation of core biopsy is that it does not always provide the accurate characterization of an entire malignant lesion, which is essential for treatment planning. Jackman et al (39) observed that of 43 lesions diagnosed by core biopsy as intraductal carcinoma, 8 (19%) contained invasive carcinoma. Similar results were reported by Parker et al (37) in their large multi-institutional series. The clinical implications of an incomplete diagnosis are reflected in the series of Evans (40), in which 12% of patients diagnosed with carcinoma by core biopsy required more than one surgical procedure.

Contraindications to core biopsy include very-low-suspicion mammographic abnormalities that can be safely followed, patients with lesions that cannot be accurately targeted such as lesions immediately beneath the skin or those that are diffuse, and patients who are unable to cooperate with the procedure. Breast implants and extremely small lesions that would be completely removed with the procedure are also contraindications. The cost-effectiveness of core biopsy varies with the degree of suspicion of the lesion being sampled and the type of local therapy selected after cancer is diagnosed (36,40).

REFERENCES

1. Ciatto S, Cariaggi P, Bulgaresi P. The value of routine cytologic examination of cyst fluids. *Acta Cytol* 1987;31:301–304.

2. Seltzer M, Perloff L, Kellye R, Fitts W. The significance of age in patients with nipple discharge. *Surg Gynecol Obstet* 1979;131:519–522.

3. Murad T, Contesso G, Mouriesse H. Nipple discharge from the breast. *Ann Surg* 1989;195:250–264.

4. Tabar L, Dean PB, Pentek Z. Galactography: the diagnostic procedure of choice for nipple discharge. *Radiology* 1983;149:31–38.

5. Talamonti M, Morrow M. The abnormal mammogram. In: Harris JR, Lippman M, Morrow M, Hellman S, eds. *Diseases of the breast.* New York: Lippincott-Raven, 1996:114–121.

6. Silverstein M, Gamagami P, Colburn W, et al. Nonpalpable breast lesions: diagnosis with slightly overpenetrated screen-film mammogra-phy and hook wire directed biopsy in 1014 cases. *Radiology* 1989;171:633–638.

7. Wilhelm MC, Edge S, Cole D, et al. Nonpalpable invasive breast cancer. *Ann Surg* 1991;213:600–605.

8. Knutzen A, Gisvold J. Likelihood of malignant disease for various categories of mammographically detected, nonpalpable breast lesions. *Mayo Clin Proc* 1993;68:454–460.

9. Morrow M, Schmidt R, Cregger B, et al. Preoperative evaluation of abnormal mammographic findings to avoid unnecessary breast biopsies. *Arch Surg* 1994;129:1090–1096.

10. Hamond S, Keyhani-Rafagha S, O'Toole RV. Statistical analysis of fine needle aspiration of the breast. A review of 678 cases plus 4265 cases from the literature. *Acta Cytol* 1987;31:276–280.

11. Kline TS, Joshi LP, Neal HS. Fine needle aspiration of the breasts: diagnoses and pitfalls. *Cancer* 1979;44:1458–1464.

12. Lamb J, Anderson TJ. Influence of cancer histology on the success of fine needle aspiration of the breast. *J Clin Pathol* 1989;42:733–735.

13. Patel JJ, Gartell PC, Smallwood JA, et al. Fine needle aspiration cytology of breast masses; an evaluation of its accuracy and reasons for diagnostic failure. *Ann R Coll Surg Engl* 1987;69:156–159.

14. Barrows GH, Anderson TJ, Lamb JL, Dixon JM. Fine needle aspiration of breast cancer. Relationship of clinical factors to cytology results in 689 primary malignancies. *Cancer* 1986;58:1493–1498.

15. Donegan WL. Evaluation of a palpable breast mass. *N Engl J Med* 1992;327:937–942.

16. Bell DA, Hajdu SI, Urban JA, Gaston JP. Role of aspiration cytology in the diagnosis and management of mammary lesions in office practice. *Cancer* 1983;51:1182–1189.

17. Sickles EA, Klein DL, Goodson WH, Hunt TIC. Mammography after needle aspiration of palpable breast masses. *Am J Surg* 1983;145:395–397.

18. Fentiman IS, Millis RR, Hayward JL. Value of needle biopsy in the outpatient diagnosis of breast cancer. *Arch Surg* 1989;115:652–654.

19. Minkowitz S, Moskowitz R, Khafuf R, Alderete MN. Tru-Cut needle biopsy of the breast. An analysis of its specificity and sensitivity. *Cancer* 1985;57:320–323.

20. Shabot MM, Goldberg IM, Schick P, et al. Aspiration cytology is superior to TruCutR needle biopsy in establishing the diagnosis of clinically

suspicious breast masses. *Ann Surg* 1982; 196:122–126.

21. McMahon AJ, Lutfy AM, Matthew A, et al. Needle core biopsy of the breast with a spring-loaded device. *Br J Surg* 1992;79:1042–1045.

22. Fisher ER, Sass R, Fisher B. Biologic considerations regarding the one and two step procedures in the management of patients with invasive carcinoma of the breast. *Surg Gynecol Obstet* 1985;161:245–249.

23. Bertario L, Reduzzi D, Piromalli D, et al. Outpatient biopsy of breast cancer: influence on survival. *Ann Surg* 1985;201:64–67.

24. Kearney T, Morrow M. Effect of re-excision on the success of breast conserving surgery. *Ann Surg Oncol* 1995;2:303–307.

25. Morrow M, Schmidt R, Hassett C. Patient selection for breast conservation therapy with magnification mammography. *Surgery* 1995;118: 621–626.

26. Gallagher WJ, Cardenosa G, Rubens JR, et al. Minimal-volume excision of nonpalpable breast lesions. *Am J Radiol* 1989;153:957–961.

27. Gisvold JJ, Martin JK. Pre-biopsy localization of nonpalpable breast masses. *Am J Radiol* 1984;143:477–481.

28. Tinnemans JGM, Wobbes TH, Hendricks KJC, et al. Localization and excision of nonpalpable breast lesions: a surgical evaluation of three methods. *Arch Surg* 1987;122:802–806.

29. Bigelow R, Smith R, Goodman PA, Wilson GS. Needle localization of nonpalpable breast masses. *Arch Surg* 1985;129:565–569.

30. Roses DF, Mitnick J, Harris MN, et al. The risk of carcinoma in wire localization biopsies for mammographically detected clustered calcifications. *Surgery* 1991;110:877–886.

31. Norton LW, Zeligman BE, Pearlman NW. Accuracy and cost of needle localization breast biopsy. *Arch Surg* 1988;123:947–950.

32. Meyer JE, Eberlein TJ, Stomper PC, Sonnenfeld MR. Biopsy of occult breast lesions. Analysis of 1261 abnormalities. *JAMA* 1990;263:2341–2343.

33. Thompson WR, Bowen JR, Dorman BA, et al. Mammographic localization and biopsy of non-palpable breast lesions. *Arch Surg* 1991; 126:730–734.

34. Alexander HR, Candela FC, Dershaw DD, Kinne DW. Needle localized mammographic lesions. Results and evolving treatment strategy. *Arch Surg* 1990;125:1441–1444.

35. Sacchini V, Luini A, Agristi R, et al. Nonpalpable breast lesions. Analysis of 952 operated cases. *Breast Cancer Res Treat* 1995;36:32–59.

36. Morrow M. When can stereotactic core biopsy replace excisional biopsy? A clinical perspective. *Breast Cancer Res Treat* 1995;36:1–9.

37. Parker SH, Burbank F, Jackman RJ, et al. Percutaneous large core breast biopsy: a multi-institutional study. *Radiology* 1994;193:359–364.

38. Dershaw DD, Liberman L, Abramson AF. Nondiagnostic stereotaxic core breast biopsy: results of re-biopsy. *Radiology* 1996;198:323–325.

39. Jackman RJ, Nowels KW, Shepard MJ, et al. Stereotaxic large-core needle biopsy of 450 non-palpable breast lesions with surgical correlation in lesions with cancer or atypical hyperplasia. *Radiology* 1994;193:91–95.

40. Evans WP. Stereotactic core biopsy. In: Harris JR, Lippman ME, Morrow M, Hellman S, eds. *Diseases of the breast.* Philadelphia: Lippincott-Raven, 1996:144–152.

Breast-Conserving Therapy for Early-Stage Breast Cancer

UMBERTO VERONESI

History of Breast-Conserving Therapy

The treatment of breast cancer remained substantially unchanged for some 80 years after the publication by Halsted in 1892 of the first report of radical mastectomy. Some variations in surgical technique were introduced during the first half of this century, either to reduce the extent of surgical ablation (for instance, conservation of the pectoralis major muscle) or to enlarge the extent of the tissues removed (for instance, removal of the internal mammary nodes). The need for extirpation of the entire breast was, however, never put under discussion. A handful of pioneers challenged the necessity of radical mastectomy, but they never received attention or recognition. Among them, one should mention the German gynecologist Hirsch (1), the French radiotherapist Baclesse (2), the English surgeon Keynes (3), and the American surgeon Crile (4).

Some 30 years ago, the issue of breast conservation was introduced with force in many cancer centers, for the following reasons: 1) All controlled studies comparing highly aggressive local-regional treatments with less aggressive ones showed no differences in survival. 2) The new concept of the natural history of breast cancer included the principle that prognosis depended chiefly on the presence or absence of occult metastatic foci in distant organs. 3) The introduction of mammography made it possible to identify nonpalpable, clinically silent lesions. All these events, which occurred in the 1960s, laid the groundwork for a more scientific approach to breast preservation.

Unfortunately, the first randomized trial comparing breast-conserving therapy with mastectomy (5), conducted in the 1960s at Guy's Hospital in London, showed a worrying increase in mortality rates among women treated with a breast-conserving procedure. It is now recognized that the failure of the London trial was due to the inadequate radiotherapeutic and surgical approaches (axillary dissection was not performed in node-positive patients, and insufficient doses of radiotherapy were delivered to the breast and axilla). However, the results from the Guy's Hospital study, published in 1972 (5), made it ethically difficult for institutional review boards to accept further proposals for randomized trials comparing radical mastectomy with less radical surgical procedures. Fortunately, in 1969, at a meeting of breast cancer experts called by the World Health Organization in Geneva (6), a proposal for such a trial presented by the Milan Cancer Institute won approval despite considerable opposition. The Milan trial was designed to compare the Halsted mastectomy with extensive breast resection and complete axillary dissection followed by radiotherapy to the ipsilateral breast with a dose of 50 Gy plus a boost dose to the scar of an additional 10 Gy. This trial was completed by the end of the 1970s, and the results were published in 1981 (7). The results showed similar rates of local recurrence and identical long-term survival rates with both treatments, indicating that appropriate breast-conserving therapy is as safe as the Halsted mastectomy. The results of the Milan trial were confirmed by subsequent trials in various countries.

Results of Randomized Trials

Only the most important randomized trials with at least 300 patients are considered in this review.

Trials Comparing Conservative Treatment with Mastectomy

As previously mentioned, the first trial comparing conservative treatment with mastectomy was conducted at Guy's Hospital in London (5). The study was conducted between 1961 and 1970 and involved a total of 370 patients. The patients were randomly assigned to one of two groups. The first group was treated with radical mastectomy plus radiotherapy to the axilla, supraclavicular triangle, and internal mammary chain (25–27 Gy). The second group was treated with breast resection plus radiotherapy to the breast (35–38 Gy) and regional nodes (25–27 Gy) similar to the mastectomy group. The early results of this trial, published in 1972 (5), showed that among stage II patients treated conservatively, there was a significant increase in the local-regional recurrent rate and a reduced survival rate. A more recent report of this trial showed that even in stage I patients, mastectomy was superior to conservative treatment (8).

The Milan trial conducted between 1973 and 1980 was the first to show that breast-conserving therapy is a safe method of treatment in patients with small cancers of the breast. This trial randomly assigned 701 patients with T1N0 breast carcinoma to undergo either Halsted mastectomy or quadrantectomy, axillary dissection, and radiotherapy of 60 Gy to the breast only (QUART). Early data were published in 1977 (9,10), and more complete results were published in 1981 (7). The results showed identical disease-free and overall survival rates in both groups. The results were confirmed in more recent publications (11) after 16 years of follow-up.

Data from the National Surgical Adjuvant Breast and Bowel Project (NSABP) B-06 trial were first published in 1985 (12) and were updated in 1989 (13) and 1995 (14). This trial was started in 1976 and accrued a total of 1855 patients who were randomly assigned to undergo total mastectomy, lumpectomy, or lumpectomy plus radiotherapy (50 Gy). In addition, all patients were treated with a subtotal axillary dissection. Patient accrual into this trial stopped in 1984. Although the survival rates did not differ between the three groups, patients treated conservatively had a considerably higher rate of local recurrence (39% for patients treated with lumpectomy and 10% for patients treated with lumpectomy plus radiotherapy) than did patients treated with mastectomy. In the lumpectomy-plus-radiotherapy group, patients who had positive lymph nodes and were treated with adjuvant chemotherapy had a reduced rate of local recurrence, while in the lumpectomy-only group, the use of adjuvant chemotherapy did not affect the local recurrence rate.

Between 1980 and 1986, the European Organization for Research and Treatment of Cancer (EORTC) carried out an extensive trial in Europe (15). A total of 903 patients with stage I or II disease were randomly assigned to undergo breast resection, axillary dissection, and radiotherapy to the breast (50 Gy plus 25 Gy with an iridium implant) or modified radical mastectomy. The interesting aspect of the EORTC trial was the inclusion of patients with large tumors ($\leq$5 cm). The data obtained from the trial helped to confirm previous results. The survival curves of the two groups were superimposable even though the rate of local recurrence was higher in the group treated with breast conservation (15).

Between 1983 and 1989, the Danish Breast Cooperative Group conducted a randomized trial comparing breast-conserving therapy with mastectomy in 905 patients. Breast-conserving therapy consisted of wide breast resection plus axillary dissection and radiotherapy to the ipsilateral breast (50 Gy plus 10–25 Gy). A total of 450 patients were assigned to receive breast-conserving therapy, whereas 455 were assigned to undergo mastectomy. The survival and local-regional recurrence rates were equal in the two groups (16).

Trials Comparing Two Different Conservative Procedures

As previously mentioned, the NSABP B-06 trial (14) compared two different conservative treatments (lumpectomy and lumpectomy plus radiotherapy) and showed similar survival rates with both treatments but a fourfold increase

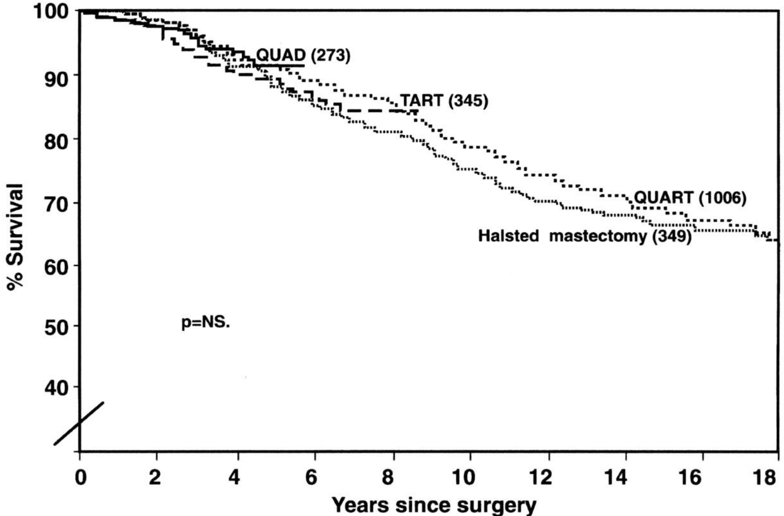

Cumulative incidence of local recurrence according to treatment in the first, second, and third Milan trials. NS = not significant; QUAD = quadrantectomy plus axillary dissection; QUART = quadrantectomy and axillary dissection plus radiotherapy; TART = lumpectomy and axillary dissection plus radiotherapy. (Reproduced by permission from Veronesi U, Salvadori B, Luini A, et al. Breast conservation is a safe method in patients with small cancer of the breast. Long-term results of three randomized trials on 1,973 patients. *Eur J Cancer* 1995;31: 1574–1579.)

Overall survival according to treatment in the first, second, and third Milan trials. NS = not significant; QUAD = quadrantectomy plus axillary dissection; QUART = quadrantectomy and axillary dissection plus radiotherapy; TART = lumpectomy and axillary dissection plus radiotherapy. (Reproduced by permission from Veronesi U, Salvadori B, Luini A, et al. Breast conservation is a safe method in patients with small cancer of the breast. Long-term results of three randomized trials on 1,973 patients. *Eur J Cancer* 1995;31:1574–1579.)

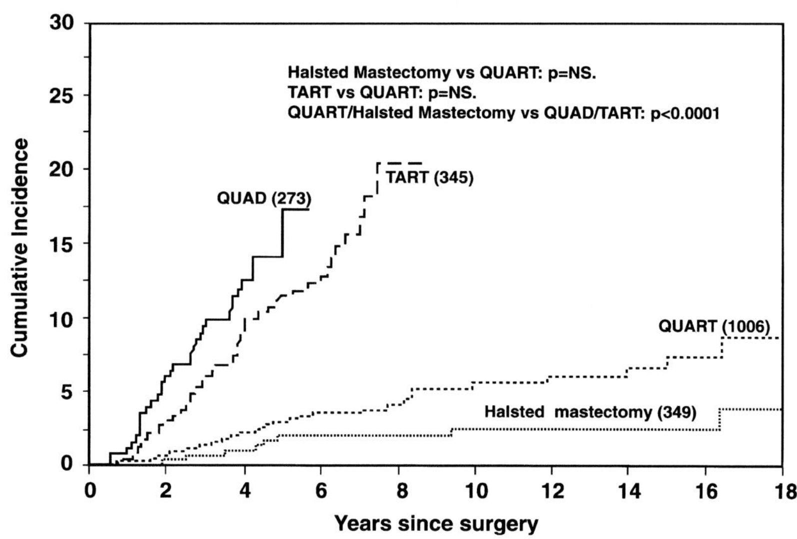

in local recurrences in patients not receiving radiotherapy.

Between 1981 and 1988, the Uppsala-Orebro Breast Cancer Study Group randomly assigned 381 patients to receive either sector resection plus axillary dissection (194 patients) or sector resection plus axillary dissection followed by radiotherapy (54 Gy; 187 patients) (17). Local recurrences were two times more frequent in patients treated with resection without radiotherapy than they were in patients who received resection plus radiotherapy. Survival curves were similar in the two groups (17,18).

In the second Milan trial, conducted between 1985 and 1987, a total of 705 patients were randomly assigned to undergo either QUART (50 plus 10 Gy) or lumpectomy and axillary dissection plus radiotherapy (45 plus 15 Gy by interstitial radioactive iridium). The results showed similar survival curves but a threefold increase in local recurrences in the lumpectomy group (19).

A third clinical trial was conducted in Milan between 1988 and 1989. A total of 567 women with early breast cancer (tumor diameter <2.5 cm) were randomly assigned to undergo QUART or quadrantectomy and axillary dissection but no radiotherapy (QUAD). The local recurrence rate was considerably higher in patients treated with QUAD than it was in patients treated with QUART (20). The annual rate of recurrence was 3.3% in the QUAD group and 0.46% in the QUART group. However, in women older than 55 years, the recurrence rate was low even in the QUAD group (annual rate of 1.5%) (Figs. 4-1 and 4-2).

Issues in Breast-Conserving Therapy

The introduction of breast-conserving therapy raised a series of issues, some of which have not yet been resolved. These issues are discussed in this section. In the case of controversial issues, the available data are reviewed, and recommendations for treatment are given.

Significance of Size of Primary Tumor

One of the most important issues in breast-conserving therapy is the indication for breast-conserving therapy in relation to the size of the primary carcinoma. The first Milan trial accrued patients with tumors less than 2 cm in maximum diameter (7). The two major subsequent trials of the NSABP (14) and EORTC (15) explored the possibility of expanding the indications for breast-conserving therapy to include treatment of tumors up to 4 cm (NSABP) or 5 cm (EORTC) in diameter.

The results of these trials showed that size of the primary carcinoma is not a limiting factor for breast conservation. In addition, the long-term results of the NSABP and EORTC studies showed no survival differences when breast-conserving therapy was compared with mastectomy. However, the size of the tumor is an important factor in breast conservation from the standpoint of quality of results. If the size of the breast is small, breast conservation is unsatisfactory even for small tumors and is impractical for large tumors.

Another important issue in breast-conserving therapy is the presence of tumor cells at the resection margins. In the NSABP trial (12,13), margin positivity was a criterion for exclusion from the breast conservation group and assignment to treatment with mastectomy. Other studies provided evidence that even when margins are positive, a re-resection will, in the majority of patients, result in clear margins and maintain the patient as a candidate for breast conservation (21). In this context, the NSABP trial clearly showed that margin negativity does not indicate the absence of residual cancer cells: In some 40% of patients with negative margins treated with lumpectomy, a local relapse occurred, showing that in spite of margin negativity, cancer cells were in fact present in the residual mammary tissue (13). These data have strongly called in question the reliability of the status of resection margins as a predictor of local recurrence. It must be added that in the second Milan trial, in the lumpectomy-plus-radiotherapy group, patients with positive resection margins had a limited increase in local recurrences compared with patients with negative margins (19,22). In the Milan trials, the status of the resection margins of the quadrantectomy specimen was not considered important because with this quadrantectomy, positive margins are exceptionally rare.

Proper Extent of Local Excision

The proper extent of local resection is one of the crucial problems of breast conservation. How large must the resection margins be to avoid an excess risk of local recurrence? The final answer should result from the judgment of the surgeon once he or she has discussed with the patient the various options and the cosmetic expectations. What is certain is that the wider the excision, the lower the risk for local recurrences; the survival duration is not affected by the extent of resection. What should be avoided is the sharp and sometimes brutal request of the surgeon that a woman choose between "lumpectomy" (with a high risk of local relapses) and "mastectomy." The surgeon must inform the patient that many intermediate options, among them wide tylectomy, sector resection, and quadrantectomy, are also available and result in very low rates of local recurrence and acceptable cosmetic outcomes. Otherwise, under the pressure of their anxiety, most patients will choose mastectomy, which can be avoided in most patients. This rudimental way of approaching the patient with incomplete information has most likely resulted in increased rates of unnecessarily mutilated women in many countries.

On the other hand, the surgeon must know that a wide excision of normal breast tissue around the primary carcinoma will create a large defect in the breast that will require remodeling of the breast shape.

With the techniques available today, it is possible to achieve better aesthetic results than were previously possible with breast-conserving therapy. Even when the cosmetic result of the treated breast is good, this breast is often smaller than the opposite breast. If the difference is minimal, surgical correction of the contralateral breast is not needed, and the edema resulting from subsequent radiotherapy to the treated breast will help to restore the symmetry between the two sides. If the difference is considerable, the opposite breast should be remodeled as well.

Role of Axillary Dissection

The need for axillary dissection as part of breast-conserving therapy is a subject of debate. Axillary dissection has been a constant component of breast cancer surgery since the first Halsted mastectomy. Axillary dissection was originally considered an important therapeutic procedure because gross axillary involvement was very common in patients treated during the first half of the century. However, the role of this procedure has slowly changed over the past 20 years. Axillary dissection has become an "informational" procedure in women with a clinically uninvolved axilla, with the aim of discovering occult lymph node metastases.

In the case of axillary involvement, an indicator of poor prognosis, adjuvant systemic treatment needs to be considered. In very small early breast carcinomas (<1 cm), the risk of occult axillary involvement is on the order of 5% to 10%. The morbidity associated with dissecting axillary nodes, which are normal in 90% to 95% of these women with tumors smaller than 1 cm, is a heavy price to pay for obtaining, in only a minority of women, information that may be helpful in the planning of subsequent therapeutic programs. Moreover, many recent studies showed that useful prognostic information can be obtained with accurate pathologic, biologic, and molecular biologic examination of the primary carcinoma (23,24). It appears, therefore, that axillary dissection in patients with small carcinomas of the breast and with clinically negative nodes may represent overtreatment (25). In women with carcinomas smaller than 1 cm, axillary dissection will probably soon be abandoned. In exceptional cases where a tumor of such small size shows unfavorable prognostic characteristics (histopathologic grade 3, high proliferative index, absence of estrogen receptors, etc), adjuvant treatment may be applied. An alternative treatment of the clinically negative axilla may be the administration of radiotherapy, which if strictly limited to the axillary field should not create any risk of damage to the brachial plexus. A trial designed to evaluate the ability of radiotherapy to destroy occult cancer foci in clinically negative patients is in progress in Milan. A new solution to the problem of the axillary dissections in axillary negative patients is the "sentinel node" technique, recently proposed. With this method, which employs either a blue dye or a radioactive colloid albumin, the first axillary node draining the mammary lymph from the area where the tumor is located is isolated, removed, and histologically examined. If negative, the remaining nodes will be negative, with an accuracy around 95%, and axillary dissection may be avoided (26).

Role of Radiotherapy

The importance of radiotherapy in breast-conserving therapy is well established. There is no doubt that the administration of radiotherapy after surgical treatment for breast carcinoma considerably reduces the risk of local recurrence.

In the NSABP experience, among women treated with lumpectomy with free resection margins, the risk of local recurrences was 40% without the use of adjuvant radiotherapy but only 10% with the use of radiotherapy. Similar results were observed in two other clinical trials of lumpectomy with or without radiotherapy: the Uppsala trial (18) and the Milan 3 trial (20).

Nonetheless, some aspects of the role of radiotherapy need further discussion. The first is the fact that although radiotherapy reduces the risk of local recurrence, it does not influence the overall survival of the patient. Therefore, the patient must be aware that choosing not to undergo radiotherapy will increase the risk of local relapse (which may be quantified) but will not increase the risk of dying of breast cancer.

The second aspect is the effectiveness of radiotherapy in different age groups. According to the Milan experience, radiotherapy is essential in young women and important in middle-aged women but considerably less important in women older than 55. Among patients who undergo adequate local treatment such as quadrantectomy but who do not receive radiotherapy, the annual rate of local recurrence is 1.53% among women older than 55 years, compared with 2.99% in women between 45 and 55 years old and 6.93% in women younger than 45 (11). Women older than 55, when informed about the low annual rate of local relapse with surgery alone, may decide not to undergo radiotherapy.

Biologic Significance of Local Recurrence

The biologic significance of locally recurrent disease after breast-conserving therapy is an area of controversy. Two recent articles (27,28) were devoted to clarifying whether local recurrences represent the expression of a particularly aggressive tumor type or simply reflect the result of incomplete removal of the primary carcinoma.

Several studies were conducted to identify risk factors for the development of local recurrences. Among these risk factors are the histologic type, pathologic grade, proliferative rate, the presence of an extensive intraductal component (EIC), resection margin status, peritu-

moral lymphatic spread, and other biologic and biomolecular markers (29–32). It would be useful to be able to distinguish markers for increased risk of local recurrence from markers that may also indicate an increased risk for the development of distant disease.

With this objective, an extensive study was recently conducted in Milan. A review of 2233 patients treated with quadrantectomy and radiotherapy showed that a number of biologic and pathologic factors influence the local spread of disease, the development of distant metastases, or both.

Patient age and peritumoral vascular invasion were found to be predictors of both local and distant recurrences, while tumor size and axillary lymph node involvement appeared to be associated only with an increased risk of distant disease. The presence of an EIC appeared to be an important predictor of local recurrence but not distant metastases. This specific risk appears to be inversely proportional to the extent of resection of normal breast tissue around the primary carcinoma: In patients treated with quadrantectomy, the presence of an EIC has limited prognostic value for local recurrences, while in patients treated with lumpectomy, the presence of an EIC has much greater prognostic significance (11).

The data from the Milan study showed a probability of recurrence, starting from the second year after surgery, of about 1% per year. In patients who had a local recurrence, the potential for distant metastases varied greatly according to the time elapsed between the surgical removal of the primary tumor and the appearance of the local recurrence. The risk of developing a distant metastasis was more than six times greater in patients who had a local recurrence in the first year after primary surgery than it was in patients who had a local recurrence more than 3 years after the primary procedure. The relative risk decreased to 2.2 in patients with a local recurrence in the second year after surgery and to 1.2 in patients with a local recurrence in the third year. The 5-year survival rate for patients who experienced local recurrences was approximately 70% (28).

How, then, should local relapse be managed in terms of both local and systemic treatment? If the local recurrence is a small (<1 cm) single mass and is strictly limited to the scar of the previous resection, a re-resection of the breast may be indicated. If the recurrences are multiple, of large size, or not strictly limited to the site of the previously resected primary carcinoma, a mastectomy should be performed. For local recurrences occurring during the first 2 years after surgery, in young patients (<35 years old), or in patients with evidence of peritumoral lymphatic invasion, systemic therapy should be recommended. On the other hand, for local relapses occurring more than 2 years after surgery, in patients whose primary carcinoma contained an EIC, or in patients who were treated with inadequate surgery, additional systemic therapy may be avoided.

Role of Plastic Surgery in Breast-Conserving Therapy

The cosmetic requirements of breast surgery create a role for the plastic surgeon in the treatment of primary breast cancer. As the surgical reshaping of the contralateral breast to achieve a symmetric result becomes increasingly common, the role of the plastic surgeon in breast-conserving therapy is becoming more important. A team that includes the leading breast surgeon, the plastic surgeon, and a pathologist and a radiologist (for intraoperative pathologic and radiologic verifications) appears to provide the ideal cooperative approach to effectively treating primary breast carcinoma. We are facing a period during which, owing to extensive detection campaigns, most breast carcinomas are discovered at a very early phase of development, when the disease is local and the risk of dissemination is very low. Under these conditions, the greatest efforts must be concentrated on appropriate local-regional treatment to maximize local control of the disease and to minimize cosmetic defects.

Preoperative Chemotherapy To Enable Breast-Conserving Therapy

Many patients with medium or large tumors (>3 cm) who, because of the dimensions of their tumors, are not candidates for conservative surgery may be treated with breast-conserving therapy after the administration of preoperative chemotherapy for a short period. Generally, three or four courses of combination chemotherapy can reduce the size of the tumor enough to allow a conservative breast resection. In a significant percentage of patients, the mass will disappear clinically, while the complete pathologic disappearance of the carcinoma is a rare event (33,34). In one of the main studies of preoperative chemotherapy (33), no significant differences were seen in the response rates of primary carcinomas to the various combinations of chemotherapeutic agents utilized (Table 4-1).

Recommendations for the surgical approach after preoperative chemotherapy were recently set forth. First, the extent of tumor regression must be evaluated not only by careful and frequent physical examination, but also by strict mammographic monitoring. Tumor measurements should be recorded after each physical examination. Second, when choosing the type of operation, the surgeon should consider not only the size of the tumor but also the volume of the breast and the possible cosmetic

T A B L E   **4-1**

Local (LR) and Distant Recurrences (DR) as First Event According to Axillary Nodal Status and Type of Chemotherapy (Milan Study)

Drug Regimen (No. of Cycles)	N	Positive Nodes (%)	LR	DR	Negative Nodes (%)	LR	DR
CMF (3)	32	23 (71.9)	3	9	9 (28.1)	2	—
CMF (4)	33	19 (57.6)	2	6	14 (42.4)	—	2
FAC (3)	30	19 (63.3)	1	6	11 (36.7)	1	—
FAC (4)	32	11 (34.3)	1	1	21 (65.6)	1	2
FEC (3)	33	24 (72.7)	1	10	9 (27.3)	—	2
FNC (3)	33	15 (45.5)	—	4	8 (54.5)	—	3
ADM (3)	33	25 (75.8)	4	4	8 (24.2)	1	1
Total	226	136 (60.1)	12	45	90 (39.9)	5	10

CMF = cyclophosphamide, methotrexate, fluorouracil; FAC = fluorouracil, doxorubicin, cyclophosphamide; FEC = fluorouracil, etoposide, cisplatin; FNC = fluorouracil hitoxantrone cyclophosphamide; ADM = doxorubicin.

Source: Veronesi U, Bonadonna G, Zurrida S. Conservation surgery after primary chemotherapy in large carcinomas of the breast. *Ann Surg* 1995; 222:612–618.

outcome. Third, while at the operating table, the surgeon must be assisted by an experienced pathologist who will carefully examine the specimen and perform multiple biopsies to obtain samples for frozen-section evaluation when necessary to quantify the extent of tumor regression. Fourth, microcalcifications must always be considered carefully, because they are unlikely to disappear after chemotherapy, and the re-excised specimen must contain all of them. Fifth, the placement of tattoo marks on the skin to guide the surgeon must be done prior to the institution of chemotherapy. Sixth, when breast remodeling is performed hastily or without sufficient care, the poor cosmetic result abrogates the raison d'être of the whole approach.

The main problem associated with preoperative chemotherapy is patients' fear of such treatment. Very often women are frightened by the idea of starting treatment with chemotherapy instead of surgery. Because chemotherapy is considered by many patients to be a sign of utmost gravity of disease, serious depression may ensue. Moreover, unpleasant side effects, particularly alopecia, are a deterrent to this approach. Therefore, the task of future research should be the identification of a combination of drugs that will minimize side effects but maintain good efficacy in the control of the primary carcinoma.

Conclusions

Breast-conserving therapy is becoming increasingly common in breast cancer treatment. Further improvements in the early diagnosis of breast cancer will emphasize this trend in the future. Survival rates after conservative surgery are equal to those obtained with radical mastectomy. However, excessively conservative surgery or the withholding of radiotherapy will increase the risk of local recurrence, leading to a high rate of salvage mastectomies. Finally, the possibility of saving the breast when a tumor is discovered while still small is an important motivation for the participation of women in screening and early detection programs.

REFERENCES

1. Hirsch J. Radiumchirurgia des brust Krebses. *Dtsch Med Wochenschr* 1927;43:1419–1421.

2. Baclesse F. Roentgen therapy as the sole method of treatment of cancer of the breast. *Am J Roent Radium Ther Nucl Med* 1949;62:311–313.

3. Keynes G. Conservative treatment of cancer of the breast. *BMJ* 1937;2:643–647.

4. Crile G Jr. Results of simplified treatment of breast cancer. *Surg Gynecol Obstet* 1964;118:517–523.

5. Atkins H, Hayward JL, Klugman DJ, Wayte AB. Treatment of early breast cancer: a report after 10 years of clinical trial. *BMJ* 1972;2:423–429.

6. *Meeting of investigators for evaluation of methods and diagnosis and treatment of breast cancer. Final report.* World Health Organization, Geneva, December 8–12, 1969.

7. Veronesi U, Saccozzi R, Del Vecchio M, et al. Comparing radical mastectomy with quadrantectomy, axillary dissection, and radiotherapy in patients with small cancers of the breast. *N Engl J Med* 1981;305:6–11.

8. Hayward JL. The Guy's trial of treatment of early breast cancer. *World J Surg* 1988;1:314–316.

9. Veronesi U. New trends in the treatment of breast cancer at the Cancer Institute of Milan. *AJR Am J Roentgenol* 1977;128:287–289.

10. Veronesi U, Banfi A, Saccozzi R, et al. Conservative treatment of breast cancer. *Cancer* 1977; 39:2822–2826.

11. Veronesi U, Salvadori B, Luini A, et al. Breast conservation is a safe method in patients with small cancer of the breast. Long-term results of three randomized trials on 1,973 patients. *Eur J Cancer* 1995;31:1574–1579.

12. Fisher B, Bauer M, Margolese R, et al. Five-year results of a randomized clinical trial comparing total mastectomy and segmental mastectomy with or without radiation in the treatment of breast cancer. *N Engl J Med* 1985;312:665–673.

13. Fisher B, Redmond C, Poisson R, et al. Eight-year results of a randomized clinical trial comparing total mastectomy and lumpectomy with or without irradiation in the treatment of breast cancer. *N Engl J Med* 1989;320:822–828.

14. Fisher B, Anderson S, Redmond CK, et al. Reanalysis and results after 12 years of follow-up in a randomized clinical trial comparing total mastectomy with lumpectomy with or without irradiation in the treatment of breast cancer. *N Engl J Med* 1995;333:1496–1498.

15. van Dongen JA, Bartelink H, Fentiman IS. Randomized clinical trial to assess the value of breast-conserving therapy in stage I and II breast

cancer, EORTC 10801 Trial. National Institutes of Health Consensus Development Conference on the Treatment of Early-Stage Breast Cancer. *Monogr Natl Cancer Inst* 1992;11:15–18.

16. Blichert-Toft M, Rose C, Andersen JA, et al. Danish randomized trial comparing breast conservation therapy with mastectomy: six years of life-table analysis. National Institutes of Health Consensus Development Conference on the Treatment of Early-Stage Breast Cancer. *Monogr Natl Cancer Inst* 1992;11:19–25.

17. The Uppsala-Orebro Breast Cancer Study Group. Sector resection with or without postoperative radiotherapy for stage I breast cancer: a randomized trial. *J Natl Cancer Inst* 1990;31:277–280.

18. Liljegren G, Holmberg L, Adami HO, et al. Sector resection with or without postoperative radiotherapy for stage I breast cancer: five-year results of a randomized trial. Uppsala-Orebro Breast Cancer Study Group. *J Natl Cancer Inst* 1994;86:652–654.

19. Veronesi U, Volterrani F, Luini A, et al. Quadrantectomy versus lumpectomy for small size breast cancer. *Eur J Cancer* 1990;26:671–673.

20. Veronesi U, Luini A, Del Vecchio M, et al. Radiotherapy after breast-preserving surgery in women with localized cancer of the breast. *N Engl J Med* 1993;328:1587–1591.

21. Schmitt SY, Abner A, Gelman R, et al. The relationship between microscopic margins of resection and the risk of local recurrence in patients treated with breast conserving surgery and radiation therapy. *Cancer* 1994;74:1746–1751.

22. Veronesi U, Andreola S, Agresti R, et al. The examination of resection margins with conservative surgery: what is the value? In: Wise L, Johnson H Jr, eds. *Controversies in management*. New York: Futura, 1994:165–168.

23. Silvestrini R, Daidone MG, Luisi A, et al. Biologic and clinicopathologic factors as indicators of specific relapse types in node-negative breast cancer. *J Clin Oncol* 1995;13:697–704.

24. Silvestrini R, Daidone MG, Benini E. Validation of p53 accumulation as a predictor of distant metastasis at 10 years of follow-up in 1400 node-negative breast cancers. *Clin Cancer Res* 1996;2:2007–2013.

25. Greco M, Agresti R, Raselli R, et al. Axillary dissection can be avoided in selected breast cancer patients: analysis of 401 cases. *Anticancer Res* 1996;16:3913–3918.

26. Veronesi U, Paganelli G, Galimberti V, et al. Sentinel-node biopsy to avoid axillary dissection in breast cancer with clinically negative lymph-nodes. *Lancet* 1997;349:1864–1867.

27. Fisher B, Anderson S, Fisher ER, et al. Significance of ipsilateral breast tumor recurrent after lumpectomy. *Lancet* 1991;338:327–331.

28. Veronesi U, Marubini E, Del Vecchio M, et al. Local recurrences and distant metastases after conservative breast cancer treatment: partly independent events. *J Natl Cancer Inst* 1995;87:19–27.

29. Schnitt SJ, Connolly JL, Harris JR, et al. Pathologic predictors of early local recurrence in stage I and II breast cancer treated by primary radiation therapy. *Cancer* 1984;53:1049–1057.

30. Stotter AT, McNeese MD, Ames FC, et al. Predicting the rate and extent of locoregional failure after breast cancer. *Cancer* 1989;64:2217–2225.

31. Recht A, Schnitt SJ, Connolly JL, et al. Prognosis following local or regional recurrence after conservative surgery and radiotherapy for early stage breast carcinoma. *Int J Radiat Oncol Biol Phys* 1989;16:3–9.

32. Holland R, Veling SH, Mravunac M, et al. Histologic multifocality of Tis, T1–2 breast carcinomas. Implications for clinical trials of breast conserving surgery. *Cancer* 1985;56:979–990.

33. Bonadonna G, Veronesi U, Brambilla C, et al. Primary chemotherapy to avoid mastectomy in tumors with diameters of three centimeters or more. *J Natl Cancer Inst* 1990;82:1539–1545.

34. Veronesi U, Bonadonna G, Zurrida S. Conservation surgery after primary chemotherapy in large carcinomas of the breast. *Ann Surg* 1995;222:612–618.

Overview of Breast Reconstruction

STEPHEN S. KROLL
SIRPA ASKO-SELJAVAARA

Growing Interest in Breast Reconstruction

Twenty-five years ago, postmastectomy breast reconstruction was rare, even in the United States. The results were inconsistent and, more often than not, unsatisfying. Today breast reconstruction is common, particularly in cancer centers in the United States but also increasingly in medical centers throughout the world (1–4). At the University of Texas M. D. Anderson Cancer Center in Houston, Texas, for example, breast reconstruction is now the most commonly performed major reconstructive operation. The reasons for this increase include better reconstructive techniques with improved results, increasing awareness on the part of women about the availability of breast reconstruction, an improved climate of cooperation between oncologic and reconstructive surgeons, and increased availability of plastic surgeons capable of performing breast reconstruction. These changes have resulted in fewer limitations, lowered psychological stress, and a more complete rehabilitation for breast cancer patients.

Rationale for Breast Reconstruction

Mastectomy, in the eyes of a woman who is compelled to submit to it for treatment of breast cancer, is often considered a deforming operation. Some women are able to cope with the deformity with ease, but many (if not most) others are not (5). Especially in the woman with large breasts, unilateral mastectomy causes an asymmetry that must be corrected by wearing an external breast prosthesis. Although the prosthesis is concealed by clothing, many women complain that it is uncomfortable, limits the type of clothing that they can wear, and can become dislodged during strenuous activities like swimming and dancing. Moreover, each morning when the prosthesis is applied, the patient is reminded of her deformity. Breast reconstruction serves to correct many of these problems, allowing women who are psychologically or physically uncomfortable with their deformity to regard themselves once again as completely feminine, attractive, and normal.

The goal of breast reconstruction is to restore symmetry and a normal female contour so that the patient will appear normal in her clothing without having to wear a prosthesis. Patients should be warned not to expect the breasts to look normal in the unclothed state. A normal clothed appearance, however, is a realistic goal that can almost always be met so that the patient's expectations will rarely be disappointed. The surgeon may well strive to accomplish something better and not infrequently may achieve a result that does appear nearly normal without clothing (Fig. 5-1). Nevertheless, it is unwise to promise that quality of result to a patient. It is better to promise less than can be delivered, because the vagaries of blood supply and scar behavior make the results of even the best surgeons' work impossible to predict accurately. Patients are never unhappy when the results exceed their expectations.

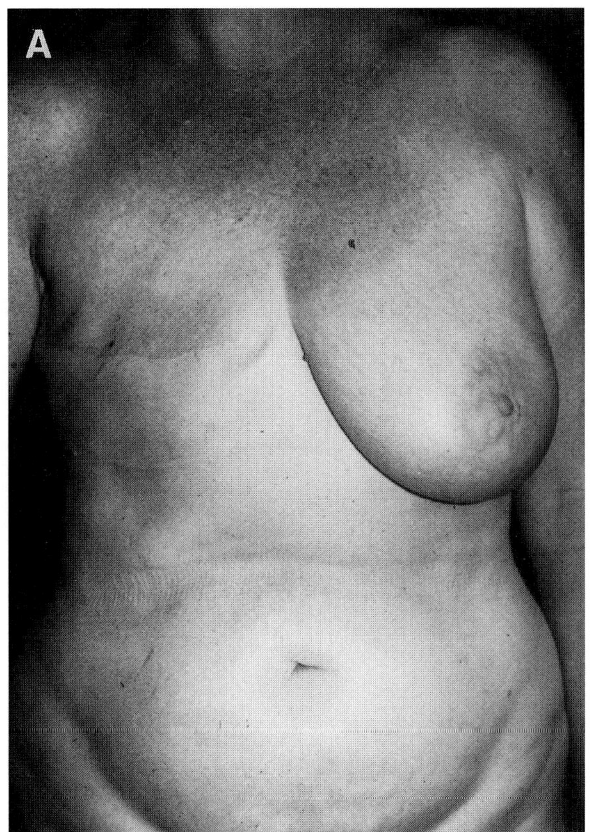
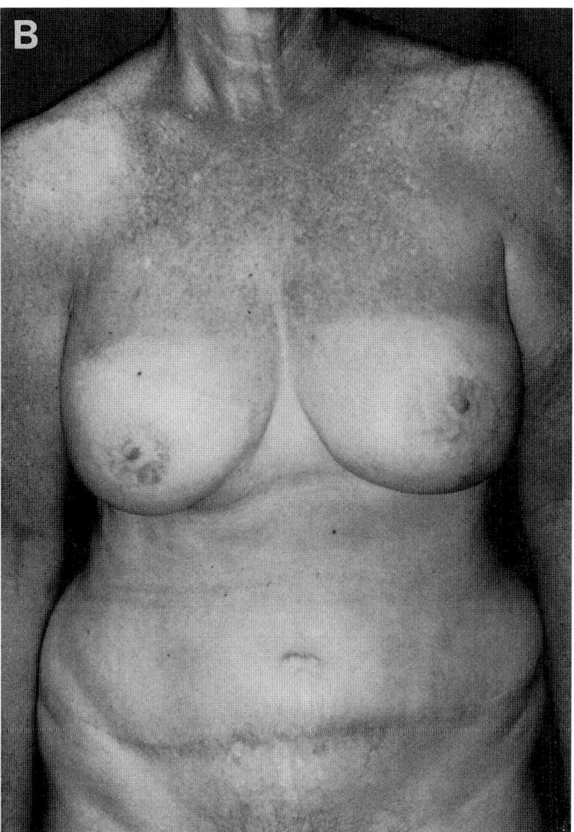

F I G U R E **5-1**

A. A 49-year-old woman after right modified radical mastectomy. [Reproduced by permission from Kroll SS. Breast reconstruction with the transverse rectus abdominis myocutaneous (TRAM) flap. In: Kroll SS, ed. *Reconstructive plastic surgery for cancer.* Philadelphia: Mosby, 1996:276–285.] *B.* The patient 6 years after right TRAM flap breast reconstruction and left mastopexy. (Reproduced by permission from Kroll SS, Miller MJ, Schusterman MA, et al. Rationale for elective contralateral mastectomy with immediate bilateral reconstruction. *Ann Surg Oncol* 1994;1:457–461.)

Available Methods

Reconstructive surgeons and their patients have a wide variety of methods of breast reconstruction available to them. These methods can be divided into two general categories: those based on implants and those based on autogenous tissues. Implant-based methods include simple implant insertion (6–8), tissue expansion with subsequent implant placement (9,10), and the latissimus dorsi myocutaneous flap used over an implant (11,12). Autogenous tissue methods involve the use of flaps including the transverse rectus abdominis myocutaneous (TRAM) flap (13–15), the gluteal free flaps (16–19),and other less commonly used free flaps such as the

lateral thigh flap (20) and the extended latissimus dorsi flap (21). All the autogenous methods create a breast mound without using an alloplastic implant. As such, they tend to be more complex than those methods that utilize an implant but generally lead to better and more consistently successful results.

Implant-Based Reconstructions

The simplest method of breast mound reconstruction is just to replace the breast tissue with an implant and then cover it with locally available skin. This is most often possible when the original breast is very ptotic and when much of the breast skin has been preserved in the mas-

F I G U R E 5-2

A 48-year-old woman 1 year after left breast reconstruction with a silicone gel implant and right mastopexy.

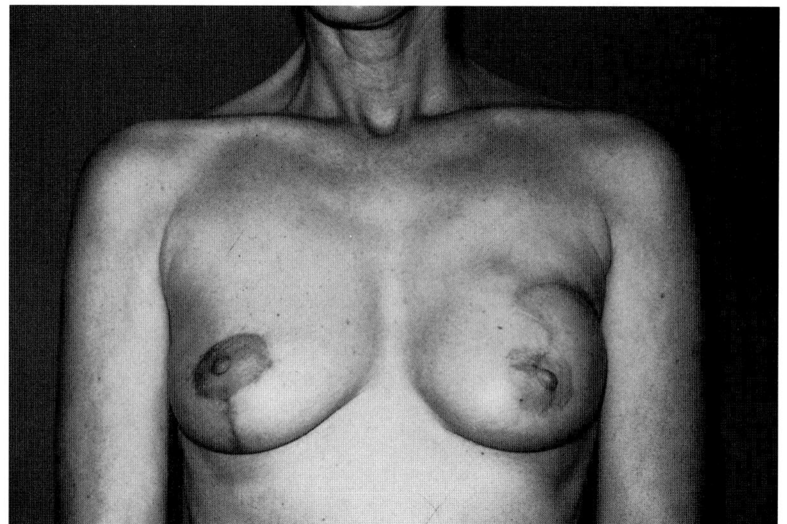

F I G U R E 5-3

A. The latissimus dorsi flap plan. (Reproduced by permission from Singletary SE, Hortobagyi GN, Kroll SS. Surgical and medical management of local-regional treatment failures in advanced primary breast CA. *Surg Oncol Clin North Am* 1995;4:671–684.) *B*. A 60-year-old woman after right modified radical mastectomy. *C*. The result of reconstruction with a latissimus dorsi flap overlying a silicone gel implant. *D*. The donor site.

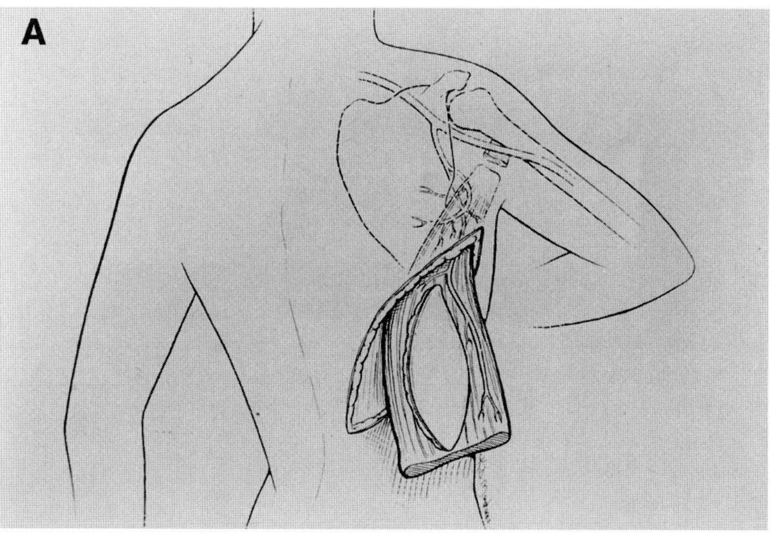

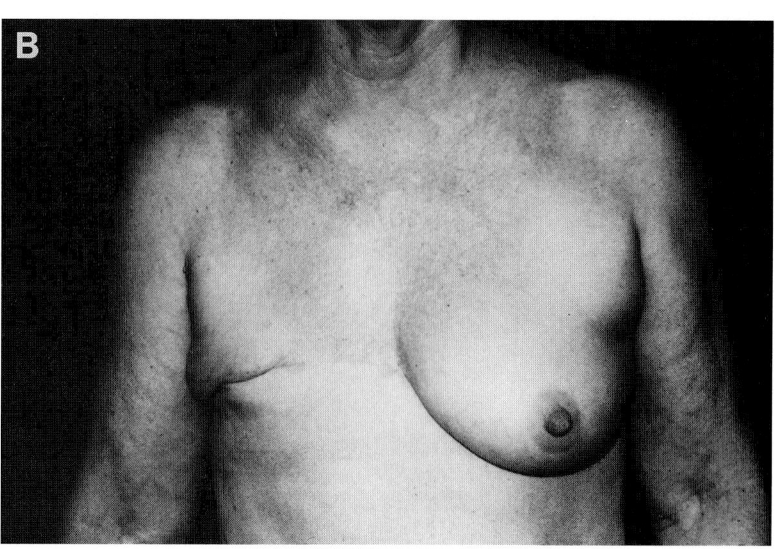

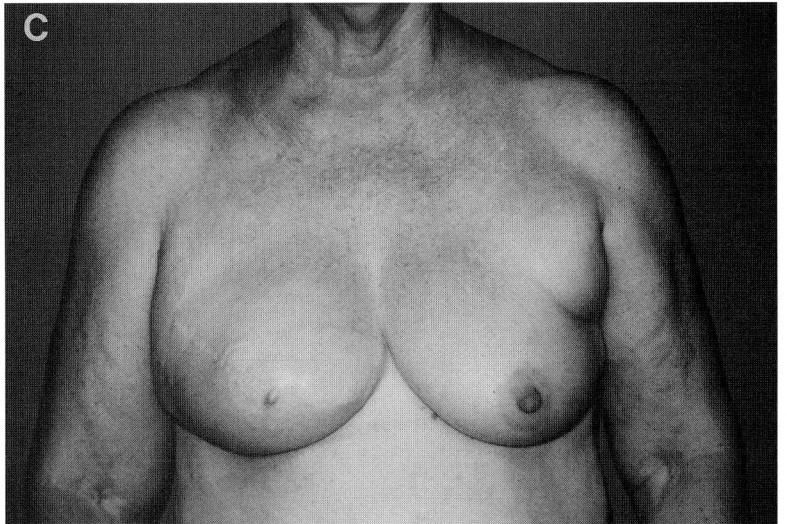

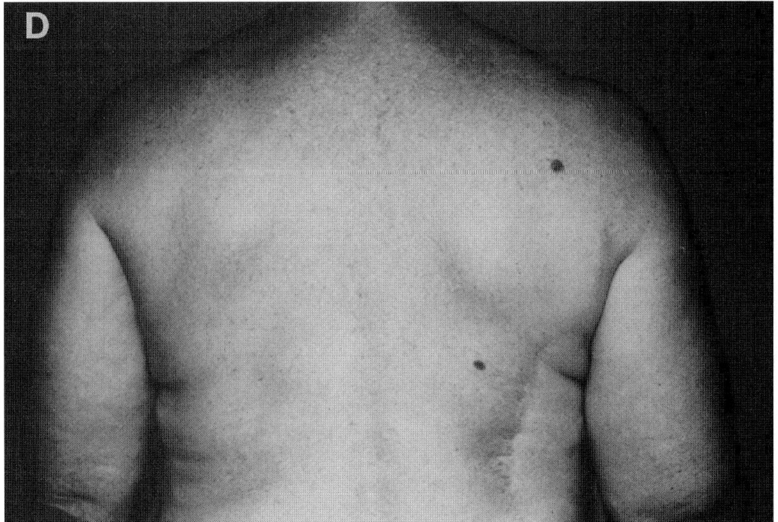

F I G U R E   **5-3**
Continued

tectomy. Generally the preference is to place the implant beneath the pectoralis major muscle, at least in the upper pole of the breast, to reduce the risk of capsular contracture (22). Combined with an opposite mastopexy to provide symmetry, simple implant insertion in this situation can lead to a very acceptable result with a minimum of additional surgery.

If there is insufficient local skin to provide coverage of the implant and permit adequate breast ptosis, tissue expansion can be used to overcome the skin deficiency and allow successful breast mound reconstruction without importing distant skin and creating additional scarring (Fig. 5-2). The textured expanders have been more successful than the smooth-walled ones (23–25); the former allow more rapid expansion with less capsular contracture. Expansion should begin within 2 weeks after

surgery, before a rigid scar capsule has had a chance to form. The expander should ultimately be overfilled so that the reconstructed breast is larger than the opposite normal one. This overexpanded state should be maintained for at least 4 months so that the skin expansion becomes relatively permanent. The device is then replaced by a permanent implant of the proper size to match the opposite breast.

Tissue expansion and simple implant placement appeal to many women because these techniques do not require extensive surgery and no visible scars are created other than those required by the mastectomy. Unfortunately, the long-term results with implant-based methods have not equaled those obtained with autogenous tissue. Capsular contracture (26) occurs in virtually all patients with implants, and in breast reconstruction, unlike breast augmentation, the prosthesis is close to the skin so the contracture is readily apparent. We found that within 5 years, two thirds of our patients who had breast reconstruction with smooth-walled silicone gel implants developed a noticeable capsular contracture, and at least one third required a surgical correction (27). Although capsular contracture rates using polyurethane foam–covered implants were lower, those devices are no longer available. Newer textured saline implants are advertised as having a lower contracture rate than the smooth-walled implants, but it is unclear whether this is really true. The M. D. Anderson experience to date suggests that the risk of capsular contracture using the newest textured implants probably is lower than that with smooth-walled implants, but the risk, along with that of deflation, infection, and rippling, is still significant enough to make implant-based reconstruction unpredictable.

The use of the latissimus dorsi myocutaneous flap over an implant is a time-tested technique that is capable of achieving quite good results (Fig. 5-3). By bringing new skin from the back to replace the skin removed in the mastectomy, the vagaries of tissue expansion are avoided, and re-establishment of breast shape and ptosis is predictably achieved. Unfortunately, capsular contracture is not prevented. For this reason, we have become less enthusiastic about the standard latissimus dorsi flap (used with an implant) than we were in years past.

Implant-based reconstruction has several other risks in addition to capsular contracture. Periprosthetic infection occurs in approximately 1% of patients, and requires removal of the implant. Implant shell failure with leakage of the contents is common in implants that have been in place for many years, and requires implant replacement. Some patients have had to have their implants removed because of chronic unexplained pain, even when capsular contracture was absent. If the patient gains weight, the normal breast gets larger while the implant-based one does not. Finally, there are questions about silicone's relationship with autoimmune diseases (28–32). We are not convinced, at the time of this writing, that a causative relationship exists. Nevertheless, we cannot dismiss the possibility entirely. Moreover, even if there is no causative relationship, the anxiety about the risks of silicone implants has been a serious problem for women with implant-based reconstruction and for their surgeons. For all these reasons, the alternative of reconstruction with only autogenous tissue has become increasingly popular.

Autogenous Tissue Reconstruction

Autogenous tissue breast reconstruction is more complex than reconstruction with implants, but it confers many long-term advantages. First, all the risks and anxieties associated with silicone implants are eliminated. Second, because the mature normal breast is largely composed of fat, reconstruction with subcutaneous fatty tissues creates a breast mound that looks and feels much like a real breast. The reconstructed breast also physically mimics a real breast, exhibiting ptosis and falling off to the side naturally when the patient is supine. Third, if the patient gains weight, the reconstructed breast (containing fatty tissues) will get larger just like a real breast. Finally, because the breast mound is entirely autogenous tissue, severed nerve endings can grow into it, and some degree of normal sensation is usually restored.

TRAM Flap

The most commonly used technique for autogenous tissue breast reconstruction, both in our institution and elsewhere, is that involving the TRAM flap (13–15,33). The TRAM flap combines the transfer of enough tissue to easily reconstruct one breast (and often two breasts) with a donor site that is easily hidden by clothing (Fig. 5-4). In some patients, the removal of redundant tissue on the lower abdomen improves the appearance of the donor site, although this does not invariably occur. The TRAM flap procedure is technically not overly difficult, and failures in experienced hands (although not necessarily in inexperienced ones) are uncommon. For these reasons, use of the TRAM flap has become the most popular and commonly used method of breast reconstruction in our institution.

There are several variations of the TRAM flap, but they can be divided into two categories: the conventional TRAM flap and the free TRAM flap (3,33–35). The conventional TRAM flap gets its blood supply from the superior epigastric vessels (36,37) via the full length of the rectus abdominis muscle between the xiphoid and the lower edge of the flap (Fig. 5-5). In healthy nonsmoking patients, the blood supply from one muscle alone is usually adequate; in patients who smoke and in others at higher risk of complications, the use of two pedicles is

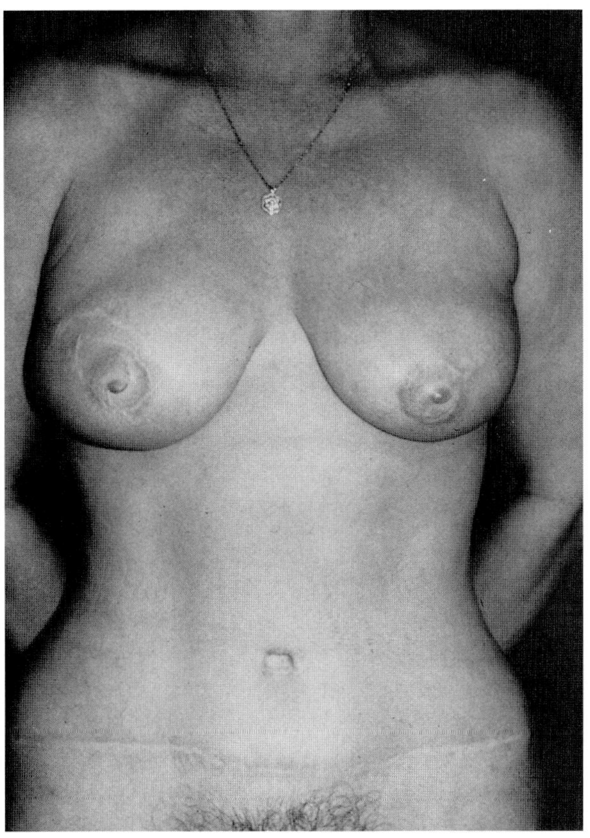

FIGURE 5-4

A 43-year-old woman 2 years after bilateral immediate free TRAM flap breast reconstruction. (Reproduced by permission from Kroll SS, Miller MJ, Schusterman MA, et al. Rationale for elective contralateral mastectomy with immediate bilateral reconstruction. *Ann Surg Oncol* 1994;1:457–461.)

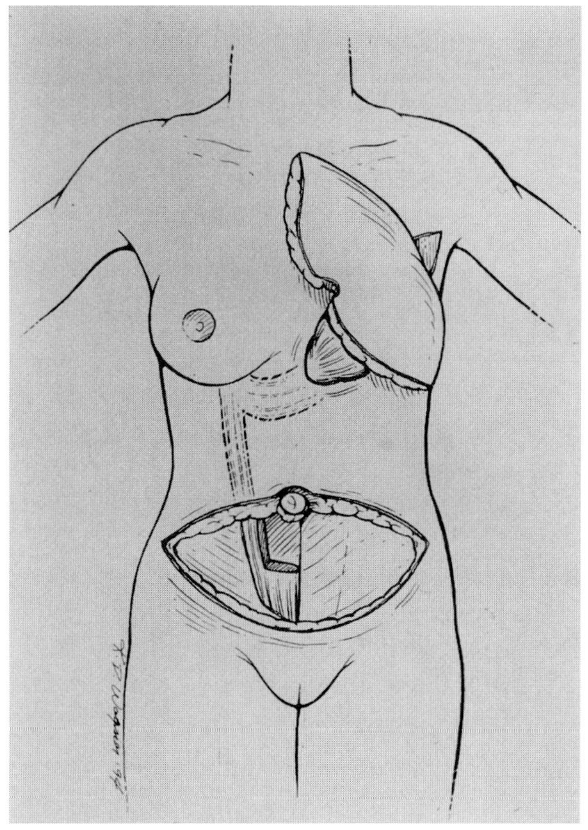

FIGURE 5-5

The conventional TRAM flap. The flap is left attached to the muscle pedicle and transferred through a subcutaneous tunnel to the chest wall. (Reproduced by permission from Singletary SE, Hortobagyi GN, Kroll SS. Surgical and medical management of local-regional treatment failures in advanced primary breast CA. *Surg Oncol Clin North Am* 1995;4:671–684.)

TABLE 5-1

Incidence of Ischemic Necrosis in 331 TRAM Flaps

		Percentage of Flaps			
TRAM Type	**n**	**Total Loss**	**Major Loss**	**Minor Loss**	**Fat Necrosis**
Free	136	0.7	0.7	2.9	11.0
Conventional	195	0.0	2.1	21.0	25.6

TRAM = transverse rectus abdominis myocutaneous.

better and will reduce the incidence of flap necrosis. The conventional TRAM flap is capable of achieving excellent results (Fig. 5-6). It has the advantage of not requiring microvascular equipment or expertise, but it has two disadvantages compared to the free TRAM flap: It requires the sacrifice of more muscle and has a less robust blood supply.

The free TRAM flap is more technically complex in that it requires specialized equipment and surgeons who are trained in microvascular free tissue transfer. It does, however, have several important advantages. First, the blood supply to the flap is more direct and therefore more effective (Table 5-1) (37). Partial flap loss is much less common in patients who have

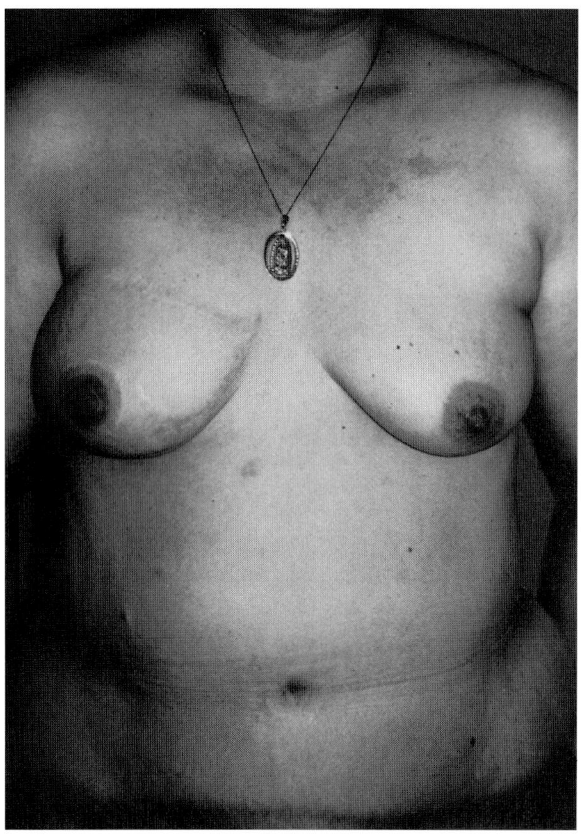

A 43-year-old woman 8 years after reconstruction of the right breast with a conventional TRAM flap.

reconstruction with the free TRAM flap, and when it does occur, it tends to be minor in degree (38). In addition, because of the more robust blood supply, the surgeon has more freedom to bend and twist the flap into whatever shape is required to create an aesthetically successful breast. For these reasons, the average aesthetic results of free TRAM flap reconstruction tend to be slightly better than those achieved with conventional flaps (38).

Second, the amount of muscle sacrificed in performing a free TRAM flap is much less than that required using a conventional flap. This leads to a stronger postoperative abdominal wall, at least as measured by the ability to perform sit-ups (39). Moreover, the upper part of the abdominal wall is not disturbed at all. This is especially important because the epigastric region can be a frequent source of prolonged pain in conventional TRAM flap patients, especially in older women. With the free flap, epigastric abdominal wall disruption is completely eliminated. Consequently, the free

TRAM flap patients have less postoperative pain and a faster recovery.

The most significant long-term risk of any type of TRAM flap breast reconstruction is development of a postoperative abdominal bulge or hernia. When severe, this complication can be devastating and must be prevented at all cost. We found that if the abdominal wall is securely repaired by approximating the internal oblique fascia to the midline fascia deep to the linea alba with heavy suture material (such as No. 1 Prolene or Novafil), postoperative bulges and hernias are extremely rare (40). The weak fascia of the anterior rectus sheath lateral to the midline should not be relied on. On rare occasions, if the closure is unusually tight or if the fascia is of poor quality and does not hold the suture well, synthetic mesh is used to reinforce the abdominal wall further. In most cases, however, even after bilateral reconstruction, mesh is not necessary.

Gluteal Flaps

The superior and inferior gluteal free flaps are good autogenous tissue sources that can be used as an alternative to the TRAM flap or in patients in whom a TRAM flap cannot be used because of a previous abdominoplasty or other surgery. The gluteal flap reconstruction is technically more difficult to perform than the TRAM flap procedure, however, often requiring a vein graft and more time to perform. They also cause donor site changes that can be visible even through clothing when the patient is wearing pants. Consequently, they have not become as popular as the TRAM flap for general breast reconstruction. Both flaps are useful, however, in patients who have had a previous unilateral TRAM flap reconstruction and who subsequently develop a new contralateral breast cancer. In such patients, a gluteal free flap can be a good alternative capable of matching the existing TRAM flap reconstruction fairly well.

Extended Latissimus Dorsi Flap

The second most commonly used autogenous tissue breast reconstruction technique in our institution, after the TRAM flap procedure, is the extended latissimus dorsi flap method (21). This is a technically simple method that has a high success rate and is capable of achieving excellent results (Fig. 5-7). The method is identical to the standard latissimus dorsi flap procedure except that additional subcutaneous fat and skin are transferred with the flap so that an implant is not required. Operative time is less than that for any of the other autogenous tissue techniques. Failure is rare, unless the thoracodorsal vessels have previously been injured. Shaping of the breast is somewhat more difficult than with the TRAM flap, but the ultimate result is usually similar. The main disadvantage of the extended latissimus dorsi flap is the donor site scarring (Fig. 5-8). Many women do not seem to mind these scars, possibly in part because they do not usually look at them. The donor deformity is noticeable and can be visible when the patient is wearing a bathing suit. In spite of this, however, the method has become quite popular.

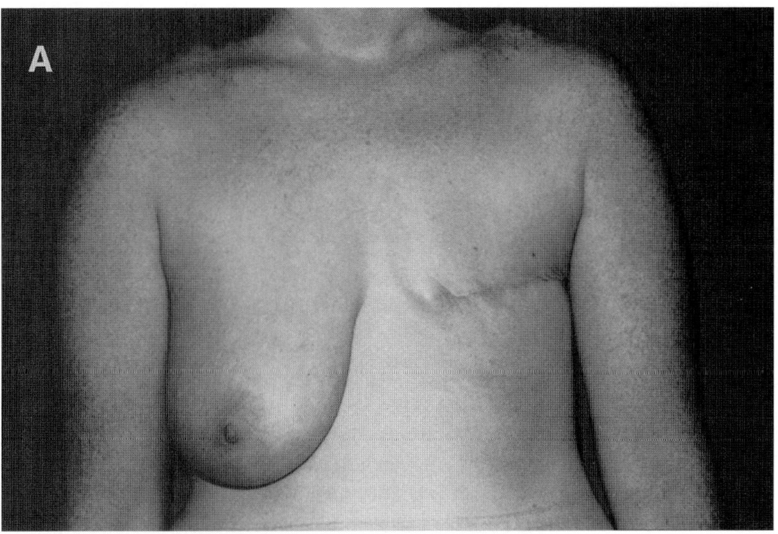

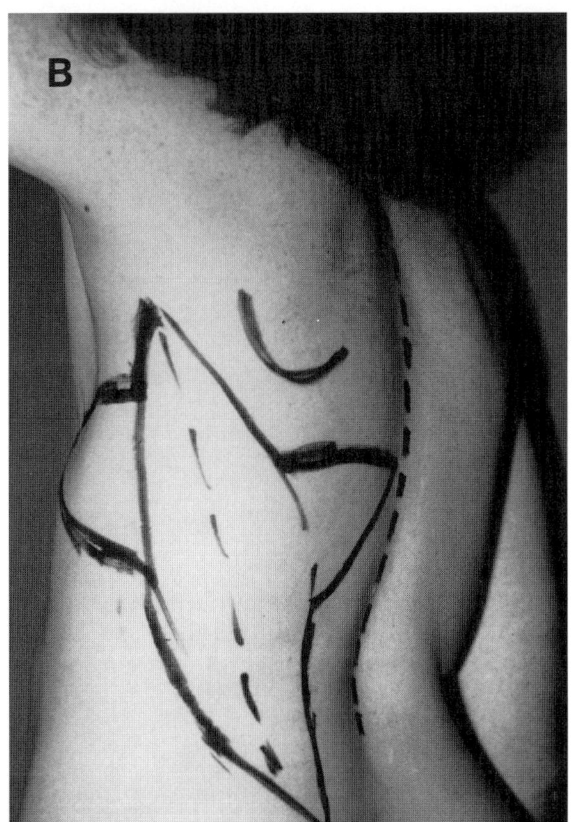

F I G U R E   **5-7**

A. A 31-year-old woman after a left modified radical mastectomy. *B.* A "fleur-de-lis" pattern for an extended latissimus dorsi flap. *C.* The patient 2 years after reconstruction.

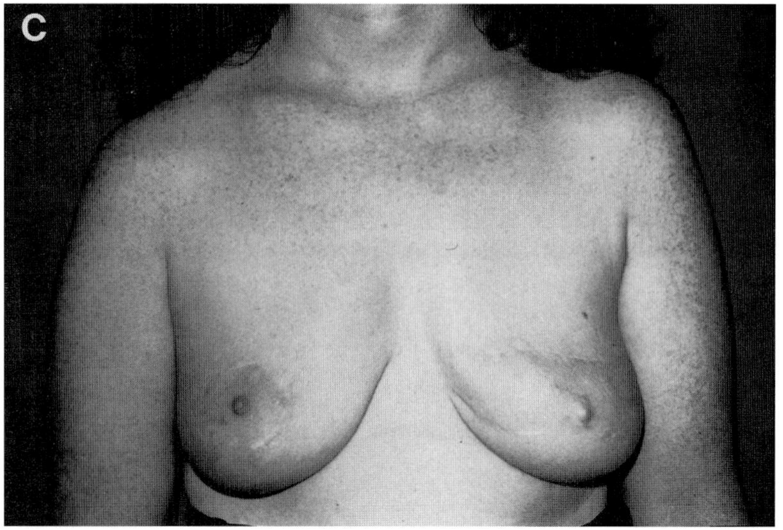

FIGURE 5-7
Continued

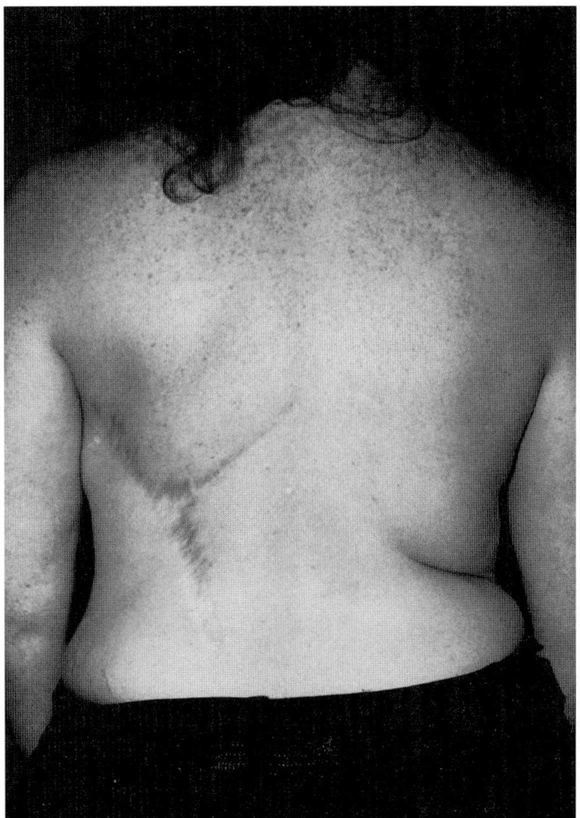

FIGURE 5-8
The donor site scarring from the "fleur-de-lis" type of extended latissimus dorsi flap.

"Ruben's Fat Pad" Flap

"Ruben's fat pad" flap technique (41) uses fatty tissue in the flank overlying the iliac crest. This free flap procedure is more technically difficult than the TRAM flap one, but has a relatively well-hidden donor site scar and the advantage of being available for use even for the patient who has had a previous TRAM flap or abdominoplasty. Usage of Ruben's flap is relatively new, and not enough of these procedures have been done to fairly assess its reliability or place in breast reconstruction. Nevertheless, this promising method is being used increasingly when a TRAM flap is not possible, and it deserves further study.

Immediate Versus Delayed Breast Reconstruction

Delayed breast reconstruction, performed months or years after the mastectomy, has stood the test of time and has several advantages. Women who have lived with their mastectomy scars for some time are usually sure of their motivations and tend to be satisfied with the results, even when less than perfect. Any required adjuvant chemotherapy or radiation will have been completed and will not interfere with the reconstruction. If they have survived many years without cancer, these women are usually oncologically stable and not likely to develop unexpected tumor recurrence. Nevertheless, immediate reconstruction has grown in popularity and is the preferred approach for most patients with early breast cancer (1,2,42,43).

Immediate reconstruction has a number of significant advantages. It is more convenient for patients, accomplishing most of their reconstructive needs simultaneously with the removal of their malignancy. Immediate reconstruction is psychologically easier because the patient is not confronted with the deformity of mastectomy. It is also less expensive than delayed reconstruction because one less hospitalization is required (44). With one less anesthetic induction, the patient is exposed to less anesthesia risk. Finally, the aesthetic results of immediate reconstruction tend to be better than those of delayed reconstruction because of the ability to preserve and use uninvolved breast skin (38).

Immediate reconstruction is especially advantageous to patients undergoing breast reconstruction with a free flap. After axillary dissection, the thoracodorsal artery and vein are usually exposed and available for use as recipient vessels. This recipient vessel exposure shortens the operating time for the reconstructive surgeon and eliminates the possibility of vascular injury when the vessels have to be dissected out of scar tissue in a delayed reconstruction.

Immediate reconstruction, especially when combined with a skin-preserving mastectomy, requires teamwork and coordination between the plastic and general surgical teams. The quality of the result depends not only on the work of the reconstructive surgeon but also on that of the general surgeon. He or she must be capable of working with limited skin incisions and yet maintaining sufficient blood supply to the mastectomy flaps that they remain viable. If use of a free flap is planned, the thoracodorsal vessels must be properly exposed and uninjured. The general surgeon is therefore an important member of the team.

Immediate breast reconstruction does not increase the likelihood of cancer recurrence, either locally or systemically (2,45). At the University of Texas M. D. Anderson Cancer Center, immediate reconstruction has been combined with skin-preserving mastectomy in more than 550 patients. Although local recurrences have occurred, the incidence of such events is similar to that found in patients in other comparable series treated without either immediate reconstruction or skin-preserving mastectomy (Table 5-2). We therefore see no reason why this reconstructive option should be denied to patients with early (T1 and T2) breast cancer who desire it. For patients with more advanced (T3) malignancies, immediate reconstruction is more controversial. Some surgeons prefer to avoid immediate reconstruction for such patients because they will often require urgent postoperative adjuvant radiotherapy or chemotherapy, or both, and the surgeon does not want to subject the flap to radiotherapy or run the risk that a surgical complication of the reconstruction might delay adjuvant treatment. Our own opinion at this time is that immediate reconstruction can be indicated for selected patients with T3 tumors but that because postoperative radiotherapy is more difficult after reconstruction, the radiation therapist should be consulted and the situation discussed prior to the surgery.

Role of Nipple and Areolar Reconstruction

Nipple reconstruction is technically simple and can generally be accomplished in an office or clinic setting using local anesthesia. Not all patients request reconstruction of the nipple, but for those who accept it, nipple reconstruction can add a significant degree of realism to the reconstructed breast. Because nipple reconstruction adds so much to breast reconstruction with so little risk, we believe that surgeons should encourage their patients to undergo it

T A B L E   **5-2**

Local Tumor Recurrence, Metastasis, and Mortality in Patients with T1 and T2 Breast Cancer Undergoing Skin-Preserving Mastectomy with Immediate Reconstruction

| | | **Percentage of Patients** | | |
	n	**Recurrence**	**Metastasis**	**Death**
All patients	545	2.6	5.1	2.2
Length (yr) of follow-up				
>1	394	3.6	6.9	3.0
>2	278	4.0	7.9	3.6
>3	176	5.1	9.7	4.0
>4	95	4.2	6.3	1.1
>5	39	7.8	10.3	2.6

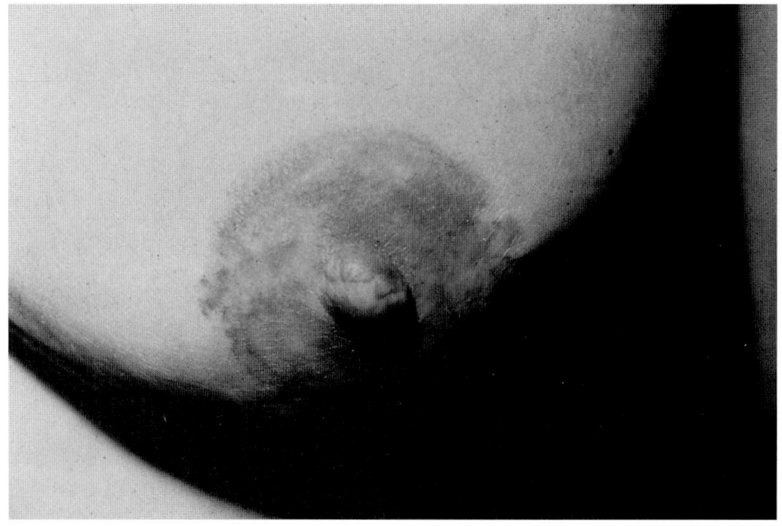

A reconstructed nipple-areolar complex. The use of medical-grade tattooing to simulate an areola not only is relatively painless, but also provides color to the nipple, reconstructed with small local flaps, as well. (Reproduced by permission from Kroll SS. Nipple and areolar reconstruction. In: Kroll SS, ed. *Reconstructive plastic surgery for cancer.* Philadelphia: Mosby, 1996: 314–318.)

by making it as painless, convenient, and inexpensive as possible. This is facilitated by reconstructing the areola with tattooing rather than a skin graft (46,47), because tattooing can be performed in the office or clinic with minimal anesthesia. It is possible to perform the areolar tattooing immediately following the nipple reconstruction, but the results seem to be better if the tattooing is delayed for a few weeks. Tattooing also permits coloration of the nipple itself, something a skin graft cannot accomplish (Fig. 5-9). For these reasons, nipple reconstruction methods that require skin grafting are best avoided.

Complications

Complications of implant-based reconstruction include capsular contracture, periprosthetic infection, leakage, and breast asymmetry, as discussed earlier. Infection requires that the implant be removed and not replaced (except by autogenous tissue). Leaking or deflated implants, and those that are rendered severely asymmetric by changes in the patient's weight, are ordinarily replaced with new ones in a relatively simple surgical procedure. Treatment of capsular contracture, if it causes severe disfigurement or pain, is more difficult. Release of the capsule relieves the symptoms, but the problem usually recurs quickly unless the implant is replaced with something different (such as autogenous tissue). Capsular contracture is especially likely in patients treated with radiotherapy (48), so implants should be avoided if irradiation is planned (49). Should a patient with an implant subsequently need radiotherapy, however, the implant is not ordinarily removed until the capsular contracture becomes symptomatic.

Complications are not rare after autogenous tissue reconstruction, but they are usually self-limited and do not lead to failure of the reconstruction. Most of them, in fact, will resolve without further surgery. Partial loss of a TRAM flap may require early surgical revision (50). Extensive flap loss may require augmentation or replacement with another flap (51). If such additional surgery is necessary, we prefer to do it early so that delays in the administration of adjuvant treatment are minimized.

Hernias and abdominal bulges occur in between 1% and 4% of TRAM flap patients and usually appear a few months after the reconstruction. Most such abdominal wall problems can be repaired successfully, and virtually all of them can be if the TRAM flap was unilateral (52). Synthetic mesh may be necessary to reinforce the abdominal wall in this situation. Because an abdominal bulge or hernia does not interfere with adjuvant treatment, its repair is generally deferred until all such treatment is completed.

Integration of Multimodality Therapy

Immediate reconstruction does not hinder administration of postoperative adjuvant chemotherapy or irradiation unless healing of the reconstructed breast is significantly delayed. Such delays in wound healing are usually caused by flap ischemia and partial necrosis, especially if the necrosis is not corrected by early debridement and surgical revision. Partial flap necrosis is much less common after reconstruction with free TRAM flaps than with conventional TRAM flaps (53); this is one reason why we prefer free TRAM flaps and use them regularly.

Similarly, the late appearance of fat necrosis (which can cause one or more firm nodules of scar tissue in the periphery of the reconstructed breast) is related to flap blood supply and is much less common with free TRAM flaps than conventional ones. Fat necrosis can be confused with tumor recurrence and for this reason often causes concern in the patient and oncologist. If the mass suspected of being fat necrosis is in a typical location (usually the point in the reconstructed breast most distant from its blood supply) and if it appears to be softening and decreasing in size with time, it can probably be treated with observation and benign neglect. If there is doubt about the diagnosis, needle biopsy can be used for confirmation. If the mass is getting larger, however, biopsy should be performed immediately. If the nodule is attached to the skin, it is probably not fat necrosis and biopsy is required.

Conclusions

Breast reconstruction is of great assistance to women who have difficulty coping with the deformity caused by mastectomy. Many methods of breast reconstruction are available, and all have advantages and devotees. Our own preference, for patients who are suitable candidates, is to use only autologous tissues. Our first choice for most patients is the free TRAM flap. We find this technique, especially when combined with a skin-preserving mastectomy and used for immediate reconstruction, to be exceedingly reliable and effective. Other effective but less frequently used methods of breast reconstruction are the extended latissimus dorsi flap, the gluteal free flaps, and the "Ruben's fat pad" flap techniques. For patients who are not appropriate candidates for autologous tissue reconstruction, or for those who for their own reasons prefer the use of breast implants, implant-based reconstruction can also be effective. Provided that patients have reasonable expectations, breast reconstruction usually succeeds in achieving its goals, and most patients are highly satisfied with the outcome.

REFERENCES

1. Noone RB, Murphy JB, Spear SL, Little JW. A 6-year experience with immediate reconstruction after mastectomy for cancer. *Plast Reconstr Surg* 1985;76:258–269.

2. Noone RB, Frazier TG, Noone GC, et al. Recurrence of breast carcinoma following immediate reconstruction: a 13-year review. *Plast Reconstr Surg* 1994;93:96–106.

3. Suominen E, Asko-Seljavaara S, Tuominen H, Tukainen E. Free microvascular TRAM flaps for breast reconstruction: the first 50 patients. *Eur J Plast Surg* 1995;18:1–6.

4. DeMay M, Lejour M, Declety A, Meythiaz A. Late results and current indications of latissimus dorsi breast reconstructions. *Br J Plast Surg* 1991;44:1–4.

5. Schain WS, Wellisch DK, Pasnau RO. The sooner the better: a study of psychological factors in women undergoing immediate versus delayed breast reconstruction. *Am J Psychiatry* 1985;142:40–46.

6. Little JW, Golembe EV, Fisher JB. The "living bra" in immediate and delayed reconstruction of the breast following mastectomy for malignant and nonmalignant disease. *Plast Reconstr Surg* 1981;68:392.

7. Woods JE. Breast reconstruction: current state of the art. *Mayo Clin Proc* 1986;61:579–585.

8. Jarrett JR, Cutler RG, Teal DF. Subcutaneous mastectomy in small, large, or ptotic breasts with immediate placement of implants. *Plast Reconstr Surg* 1978;62:702.

9. Gibney J. Use of a permanent tissue expander for breast reconstruction. *Plast Reconstr Surg* 1989;84:607–617.

10. Becker H. Breast reconstruction using an inflatable breast implant with detachable reservoir. *Plast Reconstr Surg* 1984;73:678–683.

11. Bostwick J, Vasconez LO, Jurkiewicz MJ. Breast reconstruction after a radical mastectomy. *Plast Reconstr Surg* 1978;61:682.

12. Biggs TM, Cronin ED. Technical aspects of the latissimus dorsi myocutaneous flap in breast reconstruction. *Ann Plast Surg* 1981;6:381.

13. Hartrampf CR Jr, Scheflan M, Black PW. Breast reconstruction with a transverse abdominal island flap. *Plast Reconstr Surg* 1982;69:216–224.

14. Hartrampf CR Jr, Bennett GK. Autogenous tissue reconstruction in the mastectomy patient:

a critical review of 300 patients. *Ann Surg* 1987;205:508–518.

15. Elliott LF, Hartrampf CR Jr. Tailoring of the new breast using the transverse abdominal island flap. *Plast Reconstr Surg* 1983;72:887–893.

16. Shaw WW. Breast reconstruction by superior gluteal microvascular free flaps without silicone implants. *Plast Reconstr Surg* 1983;72:490–499.

17. Nahai F. Inferior gluteus maximus musculocutaneous flap for breast reconstruction. *Perspect Plast Surg* 1992;6:65.

18. Codner MA, Nahai F. The gluteal free flap breast reconstruction: making it work. *Clin Plast Surg* 1994;21:289–296.

19. Shaw WW. Microvascular free flaps: the first decade. *Clin Plast Surg* 1983;10:3–20.

20. Elliott LF, Beegle PH, Hartrampf CR Jr. The lateral transverse thigh free flap: an alternative for autogenous-tissue breast reconstruction. *Plast Reconstr Surg* 1990;85:169–181.

21. McCraw JB, Papp C, Edwards A, McMellin A. The autogenous latissimus breast reconstruction. *Clin Plast Surg* 1994;21:279–288.

22. Woods JE, Irons GB, Arnold PG. The case for submuscular implantation of prostheses in reconstructive surgery. *Ann Plast Surg* 1980;5: 115.

23. Spear SL, Stefan MM, Travaglino-Parda R. Breast reconstruction with expanders and implants. In: Kroll SS, ed. *Oncologic plastic surgery: reconstructive surgery for cancer patients*. Philadelphia: Mosby, 1996:305–313.

24. Ohlsen HL. A clinical comparison of the tendency to capsular contracture between smooth and textured gel-filled silicone mammary implants. *Plast Reconstr Surg* 1992;90:247–254.

25. Pollack H. Breast capsular contracture: a retrospective study of textured versus smooth silicone implants. *Plast Reconstr Surg* 1993;91: 404–407.

26. McCraw JB, Maxwell GP. Early and late capsular "deformation" as a cause of unsatisfactory results in the latissimus dorsi breast reconstruction. *Clin Plast Surg* 1988;15:717–726.

27. Kroll SS, Baldwin BJ. A comparison of outcomes using three different methods of breast reconstruction. *Plast Reconstr Surg* 1992;90:455–462.

28. Heggers JP, Kossovsky N, Parsons RW, et al. Biocompatibility of silicone implants. *Ann Plast Surg* 1983;11:38–45.

29. McGrath MH, Burkhardt BR. The safety and efficacy of breast implants for augmentation mammaplasty. *Plast Reconstr Surg* 1984;74:550–560.

30. Kossovsky N, Heggers JP, Robson MC. The bioreactivity of silicone. In: Williams DF, ed. *CRC critical reviews in biocompatibility*. Boca Raton: CRC Press, 1987:53–85.

31. Brody GS, Conway DP, Deapen DM, et al. Consensus statement on the relationship of breast implants to connective-tissue disorders. *Plast Reconstr Surg* 1992;90:1102–1105.

32. Fisher JC. The silicone controversy—when will science prevail? *N Engl J Med* 1992;326:1696–1698.

33. Schusterman MA, Kroll SS, Miller MJ, et al. The free TRAM flap for breast reconstruction: a single center's experience with 211 consecutive cases. *Ann Plast Surg* 1994;32:234–242.

34. Holmstrom H. The free abdominoplasty flap and its use in breast reconstruction. *Scand J Plast Reconstr Surg* 1979;13:423.

35. Grotting JC, Urist MM, Maddox WA, Vasconez LO. Conventional TRAM flap versus free microsurgical TRAM flap for immediate breast reconstruction. *Plast Reconstr Surg* 1989;83:842–844.

36. Moon HK, Taylor GI. The vascular anatomy of rectus abdominis musculocutaneous flaps based on the deep superior epigastric system. *Plast Reconstr Surg* 1988;82:815–829.

37. Boyd JB, Taylor GI, Corlett R. The vascular territories of the superior epigastric and the deep inferior epigastric systems. *Plast Reconstr Surg* 1984;73:1–14.

38. Kroll SS, Coffey JA Jr, Winn RJ, Schusterman MA. A comparison of factors affecting aesthetic outcomes of TRAM flap breast reconstruction. *Plast Reconstr Surg* 1995;96:860–864.

39. Kroll SS, Schusterman MA, Reece GP, et al. Abdominal wall strength, bulging, and hernia after TRAM flap breast reconstruction. *Plast Reconstr Surg* 1995;96:616–619.

40. Kroll SS, Marchi M. Comparison of strategies for preventing abdominal-wall weakness after TRAM flap breast reconstruction. *Plast Reconstr Surg* 1992;89:1045–1053.

41. Hartrampf CR Jr, Noel RT, Drazan L, et al. Ruben's fat pad for breast reconstruction: a peri-iliac soft-tissue free flap. *Plast Reconstr Surg* 1994;93:402–407.

42. Beasley ME. The pedicled TRAM as preference for immediate autogenous tissue breast reconstruction. *Clin Plast Surg* 1994;21:191–205.

43. Vinton AL, Traverso LW, Zehring RD. Immediate breast reconstruction following mastectomy is as safe as mastectomy alone. *Arch Surg* 1990;125:1303–1308.

44. Elkowitz A, Colen S, Slavin S, et al. Various methods of breast reconstruction after mastectomy: an economic comparison. *Plast Reconstr Surg* 1993;92:77–83.

45. Kroll SS, Ames F, Singletary SE, Schusterman MA. The oncologic risks of skin preservation at mastectomy with immediate breast reconstruction. *Surg Gynecol Obstet* 1991;172:17–20.

46. Spear SL, Convit R, Little JW. Intradermal tattoo as an adjunct to nipple-areolar reconstruction. *Plast Reconstr Surg* 1989;83:907–911.

47. Kroll SS. Nipple and areolar reconstruction. In: Kroll SS, ed. *Oncologic plastic surgery: reconstructive surgery for cancer patients.* Philadelphia: Mosby, 1996:314–318.

48. Schuster RH, Kuske RR, Young VL, Fineberg B. Breast reconstruction in women treated with radiation therapy for breast cancer: cosmesis, complications, and tumor control. *Plast Reconstr Surg* 1992;90:445–454.

49. Kroll SS, Schusterman MA, Reece GP, et al. Breast reconstruction with myocutaneous flaps in previously irradiated patients. *Plast Reconstr Surg* 1994;93:460–469.

50. Kroll SS. The early management of flap necrosis in breast reconstruction. *Plast Reconstr Surg* 1991;87:893–901.

51. Kroll SS, Freeman P. Striving for excellence in breast reconstruction: the salvage of poor results. *Ann Plast Surg* 1989;22:58–64.

52. Kroll SS, Schusterman MA, Mistry D. The internal oblique repair of abdominal bulges secondary to TRAM flap breast reconstruction. *Plast Reconstr Surg* 1995;96:100–104.

53. Schusterman MA, Kroll SS, Weldon ME. Immediate breast reconstruction: why the free TRAM over the conventional TRAM flap? *Plast Reconstr Surg* 1992;90:255–262.

CHAPTER 6

Adjuvant Therapy for Breast Cancer

AHMAD AWADA
JOSEPH KERGER
JOSÉE-ANNE ROY
MARTINE J. PICCART-GEBHART

*B*reast cancer, once it has recurred at distant sites, is a lethal disease. This rule, which has very few exceptions, highlights the crucial role of adjuvant therapy in the treatment of early breast cancer. The major end point of adjuvant therapy is cure for a larger and larger proportion of patients.

Slow but constant progress is being made in the identification of effective adjuvant therapy regimens; however, there is increasing awareness that these treatments may not be devoid of serious side effects in the long run. This chapter summarizes the current knowledge in the changing field of adjuvant therapy as well as the most promising new approaches in the early stages of clinical development.

Adjuvant Therapy for Node-Positive Breast Cancer

Hormonal Therapy

Hormonal manipulation has been used for the treatment of breast cancer for a century (1). However, the effectiveness of hormonal agents as adjuvant therapy was not widely appreciated until the publication in 1988 of an overview of randomized trials (2), the first update of which was published in 1992 (3). The roles of tamoxifen and ovarian ablation as adjuvant therapy for breast cancer were closely examined in these reports.

Tamoxifen

In the 1992 overview (3), data on 30,000 women enrolled in randomized trials of adjuvant tamoxifen were analyzed. These trials included not only trials of tamoxifen versus no tamoxifen but also trials of tamoxifen plus chemotherapy versus the same chemotherapy alone (Table 6-1). Data on recurrence and mortality at 10 years were analyzed for the entire cohort and for particular subsets, such as node-negative and node-positive patients.

Tamoxifen was found to produce a significant reduction in the annual odds of recurrence and death. Indirect comparisons strongly suggested that women 50 years or older, those with estrogen receptor–positive tumors, and those who took tamoxifen for at least 2 years had a greater benefit with therapy. However, the reductions in the annual odds of mortality for tamoxifen given for an average of 2 years or for an average of more than 2 years were comparable, with overlapping confidence intervals, leaving uncertainty about the optimal duration of treatment. Results recently issued by three cooperative groups shed light on this important question (4–6). More than 3500 postmenopausal patients with operable node-positive or node-negative invasive breast cancer were randomized in the Swedish trial to receive tamoxifen for 2 or 5 years (4). At a median follow-up of $5^{1}/_{2}$ years, there was a significant improvement in event-free survival and overall survival rates for the patients receiving tamoxifen for 5 years.

T A B L E   **6-1**

Overview of Findings from Early Breast Cancer Trialists' Collaborative Group 1992[a]

Treatment	Reduction in Annual Odds of		Absolute Difference at 10 Years in	
	Recurrence (%)	Mortality (%)	Recurrence-Free Survival (%)	Survival (%)
Ovarian ablation in patients <50 yr old	26 ± 6	25 ± 7	10.2 ± 2.7	10.6 ± 2.7
Tamoxifen[b]	25 ± 2	17 ± 2	6.6 ± 0.9	6.2 ± 0.9
Node-negative patients	28 ± 4	17 ± 5	5.1 ± 1.4	3.5 ± 1.4
Node-positive patients	33 ± 2	18 ± 2	8.8 ± 1.1	8.2 ± 1.1
Polychemotherapy[b]	28 ± 3	16 ± 3	8.4 ± 1.3	6.3 ± 1.4
Node-negative patients	26 ± 7	18 ± 8	7.1 ± 2.7	4.0 ± 2.8
Node-positive patients	30 ± 3	18 ± 3	8.7 ± 1.5	6.8 ± 1.6

[a] Based on 133 randomized trials conducted between 1957 and 1985 involving 75,000 women (3).

[b] Overall analysis.

In the National Surgical Adjuvant Breast and Bowel Project (NSABP) trial B-14 (5), 1172 breast cancer patients with node-negative and estrogen receptor–positive tumors were randomized to stop tamoxifen treatment after 5 years or to pursue the drug for an additional 5 years. Preliminary results indicate no further benefit from use of tamoxifen for more than 5 years.

The results of a small Scottish trial were similar: No additional benefit was observed in patients randomized to continue tamoxifen indefinitely as compared to patients receiving treatment for 5 years, and there was a suggestion that treatment for longer than 5 years may increase the risk of endometrial carcinoma (6).

While we wait for the results of other important clinical trials addressing the issue of the optimal duration of tamoxifen therapy, it seems reasonable to adopt 5-year tamoxifen therapy in daily clinical practice.

In addition to a significant reduction in the annual odds of recurrence and death, adjuvant tamoxifen confers additional advantages, such as a reduction in the incidence of contralateral breast cancer and potential protection from cardiovascular events and physiologic bone loss.

A reduction in the incidence of contralateral breast cancer in patients receiving adjuvant tamoxifen was observed in several trials (7,8). Similarly, the 1992 overview (3) reported that contralateral breast cancer developed in 2% (184/9135) of the control patients, in contrast with 1.3% (122/9128) of the tamoxifen-treated patients (3).

Both the Stockholm trial (9) and the Scottish trial (10) showed a decreased number of cardiac events in women receiving adjuvant tamoxifen. In the 1992 overview analysis (3), tamoxifen was associated with a reduction of 12% [standard deviation (SD) = 6, $p = 0.05$] in non-breast-cancer deaths in general and a 25% (SD = 13, $p = 0.06$) reduction in death from vascular causes. This trend in decreased cardiac events may be explained by favorable changes in the lipid profile observed after adjuvant tamoxifen therapy for 2 and 5 years (11).

Tamoxifen given to postmenopausal women for 5 years also may preserve bone mineral density in the lumbar region of the spine (12). This effect on bone may eventually translate into a reduction in lumbar spine fractures in women taking tamoxifen for long periods.

Ovarian Ablation

The role of ovarian ablation as an effective form of adjuvant therapy in premenopausal women with breast cancer was a major finding of the 1992 overview (3) and was nicely reviewed by Davidson (13). The 1992 overview found that women younger than 50 years who had an ovarian ablation had a recurrence-free survival rate of 58.5% at 10 years compared with 48.3% in the control group (see Table 6-1).

The overview also examined the effectiveness of chemotherapy plus ovariectomy in women younger than 50 years. By indirect comparison, chemotherapy plus ovariectomy did not seem to yield better results than did ovariectomy alone. Data on the effectiveness of adjuvant ovariectomy with respect to hormone receptor levels were not available in the overview, mainly because these trials were conducted before the era of hormone receptor determination.

Permanent ovarian ablation may be detrimental for younger women. Severe menopausal symptoms such as hot flashes, dysuria, and dyspareunia may develop with the rapid decrease in plasma levels of sex hormones and may be very difficult to alleviate with nonhormonal therapy. Furthermore, suppression of ovarian function for long periods can lead to an increased risk of osteoporosis (14) and ischemic heart disease (15).

Strategies to suppress ovarian function temporarily rather than permanently have been developed recently, with the hope of reducing the incidence and severity of the aforementioned complications. Several ongoing trials are assessing the value of luteinizing hormone–releasing hormone (LHRH) agonists given for 2 to 5 years in premenopausal women with early breast cancer. It is hoped that these trials will help to define the effectiveness of LHRH agonists alone or in combination with chemotherapy. The effectiveness of total estrogen blockade, in which an LHRH agonist is combined with an antiestrogen compound, will also be assessed in some of these trials.

Chemotherapy

According to the 1992 overview (3), polychemotherapy is an effective form of adjuvant therapy for node-positive breast cancer, reducing the annual odds of recurrence and mortality by 30% and 18%, respectively (see Table 6-1). This effect was more pronounced in younger women than in patients older than 50 years and persisted when patients with involvement of four or more axillary nodes were included in the analysis.

The overview clearly indicated that combination chemotherapy is superior to single-agent cytotoxic therapy. Of note, most of the trials of combination chemotherapy included in the overview used cyclophosphamide, methotrex-

ate, and fluorouracil (CMF) (16) or CMF-like regimens.

Role of Anthracyclines

Doxorubicin (17) and its analogue epirubicin (18) are considered the most active cytotoxic drugs against advanced or metastatic breast cancer. When given as single agents at full doses as primary chemotherapy, they prove to be nearly as effective as several standard combinations. In two major trials conducted in patients with metastatic breast cancer, the combination of fluorouracil, doxorubicin, and cyclophosphamide (FAC) was superior to CMF regimens with regard to objective response rate, complete responses, time to progression, and even survival, and fluorouracil, epirubicin, and cyclophosphamide (FEC) produced results comparable to those produced by FAC (19,20).

Anthracyclines were introduced into the adjuvant treatment of node-positive breast cancer more than 20 years ago. However, no firm or definitive conclusions can be drawn today regarding the efficacy of these drugs in the adjuvant setting. This is mainly due to methodologic problems with the design of the published randomized trials, as explained here.

Data from a number of randomized trials comparing anthracycline- with non-anthracycline-containing regimens are presented in Table 6-2 (21–35). Unfortunately, the nonoptimal design of most of these studies has precluded true assessment of the independent value of the anthracyclines as an adjuvant. Since CMF represents the best-studied and most commonly used adjuvant chemotherapy regimen, the utility of anthracyclines would best have been defined by a randomized trial comparing CMF with CAF or CEF; however, no such study has been extensively published so far. Instead, anthracycline-containing regimens have generally been compared with non-anthracycline-containing combinations other than CMF.

The NSABP trials B-11 and B-12 (21) compared a three-drug regimen [melphalan, doxorubicin, and fluorouracil (PAF)] with a two-drug regimen [melphalan and fluorouracil (PF)]. At 6 years of follow-up, PAF was superior to PF in patients younger than 48 years and in patients aged 50 to 59 with negative progesterone receptor status. In women older than 60 years and women aged 50 to 59 with positive progesterone receptor status, PF and PAF

T A B L E **6-2**

Randomized Trials of Anthracycline-Containing Versus Non-Anthracycline-Containing Regimens in Node-Positive Breast Cancer

Design/Group (Reference)	Regimens	No. of Patients	Median Follow-up Time (yr)	Disease-Free Survival Rate (%)			Overall Survival Rate (%)		
				+Aa	−Aa	P	+Aa	−Aa	P
3-Drug vs 2-drug regimen									
National Surgical Adjuvant Breast and Bowel Project (NSABP) B-11 (21)	PAF vs PF	707	5	51	44	0.007	65	59	NS
NSABP B-12 (21)	PAFT vs PFT	1106	5	64	63	NS	77	78	NS
Dissimilar regimens									
Oncofrance (22)	AVCF vs CMF	249	10	54	43	0.04	67	61	0.01
Bordeaux (23)	3 MThVn/3 EVM vs CMF	228	5	78	67	0.05	—	—	NS
NSABP B-15 (24)	4 AC VS 6 CMF	2194	3	62	63	NS	83	82	NS
Sequential vs alternating regimens									
Eastern Cooperative Oncology Group (ECOG) (25)	CMFPT/VAThHT vs CMFPT	533	5	70	63	0.04	77	79	NS
Milan Istituto Nazionale per lo Studio e la Cura dei Tumori (1–3 N+) (26)	8 CMF + 4A vs 12 CMF	486	5	72	74	NS	86	89	NS
Milan Istituto Nazionale per lo Studio e la Cura dei Tumori (≥4 N+) (27,28)	4 A + 8 CMF vs (2 CMF/1A) × 4	403	10	42	28	0.002	58	44	0.002
Similar regimens									
Southeastern Cancer Study Group (SECSG) (29,30)	CAF vs CMF	527	5	—	—	—	74	68	NS
International Cancer Cooperative Group (ICCG) (31,32)	Various FEC vs CMF	760	5	61	58	NS	79	76	NS
National Cancer Institute of Canada (NCI-C) (33)	CEF vs CMF	710	3	73	65	0.03	84	81	NS
Different dose and/or dose intensity									
Cancer and Leukemia	High-dose CAF	513	3.4	74	—	—	92	—	—
Group (CALG)	Moderate-dose CAF	507	—	70	—	—	90	—	—
B-8541 (34)	Lose-dose CAF	509	—	63	—	<0.001	84	—	0.004
NSABP B-22 (35)	Standard-dose AC	746	3	73	—	—	89	—	—
	High-dose AC	737	—	70	—	NS	89	—	NS
	High-dose intensity AC	755	—	74	—	—	87	—	—

+Aa = anthracycline-containing; −Aa = non-anthracycline-containing; A = doxorubicin; C = cyclophosphamide; E = epirubicin; F = fluorouracil; H = fluoxymesterone; M = methotrexate; P = prednisone; T = tamoxifen; Th = thiotepa; V = vincristine; Vn = vindesine; NS = not significant.

plus tamoxifen produced equivalent long-term results. The lack of difference in the latter patient subset could be explained by a negative interaction between tamoxifen and certain anti-neoplastic agents or by reduced effectiveness of anthracycline against well-differentiated steroid receptor–positive tumors.

The Oncofrance trial (22) randomly assigned women to receive either CMF or doxorubicin, vincristine, cyclophosphamide, and fluorouracil (AVCF). With 10-year follow-up, the disease-free and overall survival rates were superior in the subset of premenopausal patients treated with AVCF, but in view of schedule and drug differences and an imbalance in nodal involvement between the two study groups, it is not clear how much of the improvement can be attributed to the use of doxorubicin.

Another French group (23) conducted a trial that randomly assigned women to receive either six courses of CMF intravenously or three courses of mitomycin C, thiotepa, and vindesine followed by three courses of epirubicin, vincristine, and methotrexate. This trial enrolled 228 node-positive, receptor-negative premenopausal patients. Five-year results showed a slightly better relapse-free survival rate in the epirubicin-containing treatment group, but the overall survival rate was similar. The epirubicin-containing regimen was more toxic.

The NSABP trial B-15 (24) examined both the role of doxorubicin in adjuvant therapy and the duration of adjuvant therapy. More than 2000 node-positive breast cancer patients were randomly assigned to receive four courses of doxorubicin and cyclophosphamide (AC) given over 3 months; CMF for 6 months; or four courses of AC given over 3 months followed by reinduction with CMF 6 months later. There were no statistically significant differences in relapse-free or overall survival rates at a median follow-up of 3 years. Given this similar efficacy, short-course AC might be preferable to conventional CMF: AC is better tolerated, so compliance is higher, and AC is also more convenient, as it is given over 3 instead of 6 months. It must be stressed that the shorter duration of AC might have precluded the detection of a difference in treatment outcome in favor of the anthracycline-containing regimen.

The Milan group compared 12 courses of intravenous CMF with eight cycles of CMF followed by four courses of doxorubicin in breast cancer patients with one to three positive nodes

and could not detect any significant difference in outcome after a median follow-up of 5 years (26). The same investigators also tested the Norton-Simon hypothesis of sequential administration of potentially non-cross-resistant chemotherapy regimens in a higher-risk group of patients—those with more than three involved axillary nodes. The investigators observed better relapse-free and overall survival rates with sequential chemotherapy (four courses of doxorubicin followed by eight cycles of CMF) than with alternating chemotherapy (two cycles of CMF followed by one cycle of doxorubicin for a total of 12 courses) (27,28). The promising results with this sequential program warrant confirmatory trials, which are presently under way.

Few randomized trials directly compared the classic CMF regimen with similar cyclophosphamide, doxorubicin, and fluorouracil (CAF) or FEC combinations. At 3 and 5 years of follow-up, the results of the Southeastern Cancer Study Group (29,30), which used "equitoxic" regimens of CMF (cyclophosphamide 600 mg/m^2, methotrexate 60 mg/m^2, and fluorouracil 600 mg/m^2) and CAF (cyclophosphamide 450 mg/m^2, doxorubicin 45 mg/m^2, and fluorouracil 450 mg/m^2), with a lower dose intensity for the CAF regimen, and of the International Cancer Cooperative Group (31,32), which compared various schedules of CMF and FEC, did not clearly show a benefit for anthracycline-containing combinations. However, with a median follow-up of 3 years, the National Cancer Institute of Canada (NCI-C) study of CMF versus CEF, which enrolled premenopausal patients only and used a relatively intensive CEF regimen, demonstrated a significant advantage in relapse-free survival with CEF (33). These results need to be confirmed with a longer follow-up. Meanwhile, the results of another FEC-versus-CMF trial launched by the Danish Breast Cancer Group are eagerly awaited.

The relationship between dose and long-term results remains controversial. With regard to the anthracyclines, only two studies prospectively addressed this question. The results of the Cancer and Leukemia Group B-8541 trial (34) suggested either a dose-response effect or a threshold effect: Inferior results were seen in the low-dose treatment group (cyclophosphamide 300 mg/m^2, doxorubicin 30 mg/m^2, fluorouracil 300 mg/m^2 for four cycles), but similar results were observed so far for the high-dose (cyclophosphamide 600 mg/m^2, doxorubicin $60\,mg/m^2$, fluorouracil $600\,mg/m^2$ for four cycles) and moderate-dose (cyclophosphamide $400\,mg/m^2$, doxorubicin $40\,mg/m^2$, fluorouracil $400\,mg/m^2$ for six cycles) regimens. In fact, the so-called high-dose CAF regimen could be viewed as a standard-dose regimen, whereas the dose and dose intensity of the low-dose treatment group could be viewed as insufficient or inadequate. This potential threshold effect was not detected after a similar follow-up period in the NSABP B-22 protocol (35), which investigated a fixed dose of doxorubicin in combination with more dose-intense or higher-dose cyclophosphamide.

In summary, in spite of 20 years of randomized clinical trials, the role of anthracyclines in adjuvant therapy for node-positive breast cancer remains controversial. Additional randomized trials, longer follow-up of some of the more recent studies, or a meta-analysis of all existing trials will be needed to clarify this important issue. It must be stressed, however, that anthracycline-based regimens have never produced therapeutic results inferior to those produced by CMF regimens. The higher toxicity associated with anthracyclines (discussed later in this chapter) and the remaining uncertainty regarding the long-term survival advantage in the adjuvant setting should raise caution about their widespread use in unselected patients outside the context of randomized clinical trials.

Duration of Adjuvant Chemotherapy

Several prospective, randomized trials addressed the optimal duration of adjuvant chemotherapy (24,36–38). In general, prolonged, relatively low-dose combination regimens for longer than 6 months do not produce better long-term results, and one single perioperative chemotherapy cycle seems to be inadequate (39).

Timing of Adjuvant Chemotherapy

Preclinical models suggest that early initiation of adjuvant chemotherapy may be important to obtain optimal therapeutic results. One study even suggested that perioperative chemotherapy may be a way to prevent accelerated tumor proliferation after surgery (40). Retrospective analyses of the time variable in clinical trials of adjuvant chemotherapy produced conflicting results. In most published studies, adjuvant chemotherapy was required to start within 30 days after surgery. In the prospective trial conducted by the Ludwig Breast Cancer Study Group, the addition of one perioperative course of CMF plus prednisone to six classic CMF-prednisone cycles started 3 to 4 weeks after the surgical procedure did not produce any additional benefit (39).

Primary Chemotherapy

There is clearly renewed interest in primary or "neoadjuvant" chemotherapy following the growing popularity of breast-conserving surgery in the management of breast cancer (41). Numerous trials of primary chemotherapy, most of them nonrandomized, were conducted during the past decade, first in patients with locally advanced but more recently also in patients with operable breast cancer (Table 6-3). Impressive objective response rates and even complete responses were observed in most of these studies, allowing for breast-conserving strategies (42–51). Evaluation of the long-term impact of primary chemotherapy in operable breast cancer, however, must await maturation of ongoing or recently closed randomized clinical trials.

In the meantime, locally advanced breast cancer is the optimal model in which to compare various chemotherapeutic regimens for their potential to induce marked, or even complete, tumor regressions. The European Organization for Research and Treatment of Cancer Breast Cancer Cooperative Group, in collaboration with the NCI-C and the Schweizerische Arbeitsgemeinschaft für Klinische Krebsforschung, has recently closed for accrual a large clinical trial in which patients with locally advanced breast cancer are randomly assigned to receive either a short, "accelerated," and intensive neoadjuvant epirubicin-cyclophosphamide regimen given with granulocyte colony-stimulating factor support or six 1-month cycles of the Canadian "CEF" regimen given without granulocyte colony-stimulating factor. Taxoids are obviously strong candidates for becoming the most widely used drugs in the neoadjuvant chemotherapy setting for these high-risk patients (52).

Sequencing of Chemotherapy and Radiation Therapy

In spite of two decades of clinical trials, the optimal sequence for administering adjuvant

T A B L E   **6-3**

Studies of Primary Chemotherapy in Surgically Resectable Breast Cancer

Group (Reference)	No. of Patients	Type of Elective Locoregional Therapy	Chemotherapeutic Regimen	Response Rate (%)		
				Complete and Partial	Complete	Pathologic Complete
Jacquillat (42)	250	RT	Vinblastine, thiotepa, methotrexate, 5-fluorouracil, ± doxorubicin, ± tamoxifen	75	30	—
Forrest (43)	27	Surgery	Cyclophosphamide, doxorubicin, vincristine, and prednisone	72	NR	NR
Smith (44)	50	Surgery → RT	5-fluorouracil by CI, epirubicin, and cisplatin	98	66	27
Smith (45)	64	RT → Surgery	CMF or MMM	69	17	—
Mauriac (46)	134	RT in patients w/CR	EVM × 3 + MTV × 3	63	33	—
Scholl (47)	153	RT	FAC	82	30	—
Bonadonna (48)	227	Surgery	Doxorubicin or CMF or FAC	78	21	4
Bonadonna (49)	210	Surgery	Doxorubicin	74	12	1.5
Fisher (50)	549	Surgery	Doxorubicin and cyclophosphamide	80	37	NR
Powles (51)	101	Surgery → RT[*]	Methotrexate, mitoxantrone, and tamoxifen ± mitomycin C	85	19	10

NR = not reported; CR = complete response; RT = radiation therapy; CMF = cyclophosphamide, methotrexate, and 5-fluorouracil; MMM = methotrexate, mitoxantrone, and mitomycin C; EVM = epirubicin, vincristine, and methotrexate; MTV = mitomycin C, thiotepa, and vindesine; FAC = fluorouracil, doxorubicin, and cyclophosphamide; CI = continuous infusion.

Source: Adapted from Bonadonna G, Valagussa P, Zucorli R, Salvadori B. Primary chemotherapy in surgically resectable breast cancer. *CA Cancer J Clin* 1995;45:227–243.

[*]Two patients did not receive radiotherapy.

chemotherapy and radiation therapy has not yet been determined. Possible sequence options are chemotherapy followed by radiation therapy, concomitant treatment, sandwich radiation therapy, and radiation therapy followed by chemotherapy (53).

Retrospective data are conflicting. Delaying radiation therapy may result in increased local recurrence rates, and the safety of postponing radiation therapy until the end of chemotherapy in patients who have had lumpectomy or partial mastectomy has not been formally demonstrated. On the other hand, in node-positive breast cancer patients with a high risk of systemic recurrence, early initiation of adjuvant chemotherapy and full-dose chemotherapy may be important, especially in view of the fact that local radiation therapy is unlikely to have a sig-

nificant impact on long-term survival. Several prospective trials were initiated with the hope of clarifying this important sequencing issue.

Results of the first randomized trial assessing the sequence of chemotherapy and radiation therapy after conservative surgery for early breast cancer are now available (54). Two hundred forty-four patients with stage I or II breast cancer, considered to be at substantial risk for systemic metastases, were randomized to receive a 12-week course of chemotherapy either before or after radiation therapy. The 5-year actuarial rates of cancer recurrence at any site and of distant metastases in the radiotherapy-first group and the chemotherapy-first group were 38% and 31% ($p = 0.17$) and 36% and 25% ($p = 0.05$), respectively. The overall survival rates were 73% and 81%

(p = 0.11), respectively. Of interest, a lower chemotherapy dose intensity was delivered to the radiotherapy-first group.

As the authors concluded, the results of this study suggest that it is preferable to give a 12-week course of chemotherapy followed by radiation therapy rather than the opposite sequence. Whether these results can be extrapolated to longer chemotherapy regimens is unknown.

Adjuvant Chemoendocrine Therapy

Several prospective, randomized trials compared the simultaneous administration of adjuvant chemotherapy and hormonal therapy with adjuvant chemotherapy alone or adjuvant hormonal therapy alone. Unfortunately, many of these trials were initiated before determination of tumor hormone receptor status became routine.

In premenopausal women, even when the benefits of ovarian ablation seem to be similar in magnitude to those of chemotherapy, this does not mean that chemotherapy and ovarian ablation are equivalent (3). In the Scottish Cancer Trials Breast Group trial (55), which slowly accrued 332 premenopausal women with node-positive breast cancer and compared ovarian ablation with CMF given for six to eight cycles, there was no statistically significant difference in relapse-free or overall survival rates

T A B L E **6-4**

Randomized Trials of Chemoendocrine Therapy in Postmenopausal Women with Node-Positive Breast Cancer

Group/Trial (Reference)	Regimen	No. of Patients	Median Follow-up Time (yr)	Relapse-free Survival Rate (%)	p	Overall Survival Rate (%)	p
HT vs CHT							
IBCSG (56)	Control	156	7	24	—	47	—
	PT	153	—	36	0.003	51	NS
	CMFP + T	154	—	51	—	57	—
DBCG 82-C (57)	T	458	4	49	—	68	—
	CMF + T	432	—	56	—	66	—
	T + RT	457	—	60	0.03	71	NS
Case Western (58)	T	48	4.6	53	—	78	—
	CMFVP + T	46	—	78	0.04	79	NS
NSABP B-16 (59)	T	376	3	67	—	85	—
	AC + T	377	—	84	0.0004	93	0.04
	T	298	3	66	—	84	—
	MelAF + T	—	—	83	0.0002	84	NS
NCI-C (60)	T	705	7.5	—	—	—	—
	CMF + T	—	—	—	NS	—	NS
CT vs CHT							
NSABP B-09 (61)	MelF	941	5	47	—	67	—
	MelF + T	950	—	52	0.002	67	NS
Crowe (62)	CMF	99	10	36	—	42	—
	CMF + T (+ BCG)	212	—	47	0.02	57	NR
CT vs HT vs CHT							
Southwest Oncology	CMFVP	894	4.3	—	—	78	—
Group (SWOG) (63)	T	—	—	—	NS	77	NS
	CMFVP + T	—	—	—	—	73	—
GROCTA (64,65)	CMF/E	84	3.3	—	—	—	—
	T	89	—	—	0.000	—	0.002
	CMF/E + T	94	—	—	—	—	—

A = doxorubicin; BCG = bacille Calmette-Guérin; C = cyclophosphamide; CHT = combined chemoendocrine therapy; CT = chemotherapy; E = epirubicin; F = fluorouracil; HT = hormonal therapy; Mel = melphalan; M = methotrexate; N/R = not reported; NS = not significant; P = prednisone; RT = radiation therapy; T = tamoxifen; IBCSG = International Breast Cancer Study Group; DBCG = Danish Breast Cancer Group; GROCTA = Breast Cancer Adjuvant Chemo-hormone Therapy Co-operative Group (ITALY).

at 8 years between the two groups. However, ovarian ablation was associated with improved survival in patients with estrogen receptor–rich tumors, and CMF was associated with improved survival in patients with estrogen receptor–poor or –negative tumors.

A number of trials comparing adjuvant chemotherapy and castration (accomplished by surgical ovarian ablation or use of LHRH analogues) either alone or in combination are currently in progress and should help to refine adjuvant therapy for premenopausal patients in the near future. The role of tamoxifen given after chemotherapy is also being explored by the European Organization for Research and Treatment of Cancer Breast Cancer Cooperative Group and by the NCI-C in two parallel ongoing trials.

In postmenopausal women, the addition of chemotherapy to tamoxifen produced conflicting results (Table 6-4). Some of these trials showed that chemoendocrine therapy improves relapse-free survival, but the impact on overall survival is less apparent (56–65). It will be interesting to see whether the next overview of adjuvant therapy trials will confirm the trend in improved relapse-free survival and overall survival for combined chemoendocrine therapy in postmenopausal women that was suggested by the 1992 overview (3). Also, the magnitude of this benefit in relation to hormone receptor status needs to be elucidated.

In any event, many questions related to chemoendocrine therapy remain unanswered: Which patients are most likely to benefit from combined treatment? What is the optimal chemotherapy regimen? Which is more effective—simultaneous or sequential administration of tamoxifen? (Do antagonisms exist between tamoxifen and some cytotoxic drugs?) What is the optimal duration of hormonal therapy?

Until these questions are resolved, a reasonable treatment approach to node-positive breast cancer patients is that recently outlined by an international panel (66).

Adjuvant Therapy for Node-Negative Breast Cancer

About half of all patients newly diagnosed as having breast cancer are node negative, and this proportion is increasing with more aggressive screening (67). Although node-negative patients clearly have a more favorable outlook than

node-positive breast cancer patients, 20% to 30% of node-negative patients will die of their disease.

A well-validated and easily obtainable prognostic factor is the pathologic tumor size. The 5-year survival rate for patients with invasive tumors less than 1 cm in diameter is as high as 98% (68), and such patients have a projected relapse-free survival rate of 88% at 20 years (69). On the other hand, for patients with tumors larger than 2 cm in diameter, the risk of developing distant metastasis is greatly increased (70,71). For tumors between 1 and 2 cm, hormone receptor status, tumor grade, and presence or absence of vascular invasion are currently used to select patients most suitable for adjuvant therapy, but these selection criteria remain unsatisfactory.

There is a crucial need to identify and validate new, powerful prognostic factors and to determine the optimal adjuvant treatment in relation to them. New prognostic factors currently under study are reviewed later in this chapter.

Although the 1992 overview of adjuvant therapy trials (3) showed a statistically significant reduction in relapse-free survival and mortality at 10 years for node-negative patients who received either tamoxifen or polychemotherapy, it should be kept in mind that the majority of patients selected for these trials were those who had tumors larger than 3 cm in diameter or estrogen receptor–negative tumors measuring 1 to 3 cm in diameter.

Future trials for node-negative breast cancer should focus on patients with intermediate-sized tumors (1–2 cm) and the presence of one or more adverse prognostic factors.

Adjuvant Therapy in Older Women with Breast Cancer

The management of breast cancer in older women is becoming a major challenge as the general population ages. Two randomized trials specifically addressed the effectiveness of adjuvant tamoxifen in 170 and 320 women 65 years or older with node-positive breast cancer (72,73). In both trials, patients treated with tamoxifen had a significant improvement in recurrence-free survival but not in overall survival. The lack of significant improvement in overall survival in these two trials is probably due to the small numbers of patients studied.

Indeed, the 1992 overview (3) indicated that the use of tamoxifen improves relapse-free and overall survival rates for postmenopausal women, including those older than 70 years (3). As expected, tamoxifen therapy is of greatest benefit in patients whose primary tumors are estrogen and progesterone receptor positive.

In contrast, adjuvant chemotherapy in older women has been studied only minimally, and therefore the 1992 overview (3) is of little help. In one adjuvant chemotherapy trial in which patients with node-positive breast cancer received a doxorubicin-containing chemotherapy regimen, patients older than 65 years had disease-free and overall survival rates similar to those of their younger counterparts at a median follow-up of 7.3 years (74). Severe leukopenia was the only toxicity found to be more common in older patients (74).

A cost-effectiveness analysis examining total and active life expectancy outcomes in elderly patients receiving chemotherapy for node-negative breast cancer was recently published (75). The authors concluded that a small survival benefit for adjuvant chemotherapy in elderly patients is likely, but the cost associated with this benefit is high.

In summary, there is a clear need to conduct clinical trials of adjuvant chemotherapy for elderly patients, who represent an increasing proportion of breast cancer patients and for whom the benefits and risks of adjuvant therapy have not been properly assessed so far.

Long-Term Side Effects of Adjuvant Therapy

Over the past 5 years, the oncology community has become increasingly aware of possible long-term side effects of adjuvant therapies given to breast cancer patients.

Side Effects of Tamoxifen

Several investigators (8,76,77) reported the occurrence of endometrial cancer in patients taking adjuvant tamoxifen, in the context of several prospective randomized clinical trials (Table 6-5).

A retrospective analysis done on 53 patients with endometrial carcinoma revealed that 15 of these patients had taken tamoxifen for breast carcinoma and that several of these 15 patients presented with high-grade endometrial cancers that had a poor prognosis (78). This aggressive biologic behavior was not observed in patients who developed secondary endometrial cancer within the NSABP B-14 trial (76). A case-control study done in the Netherlands (79) supported the hypothesis that tamoxifen increases the risk of endometrial cancer: A relative risk of 1.3 [95% confidence interval (CI), 0.7–2.4] was found for women using tamoxifen. Furthermore, women who had used tamoxifen for more than 2 years had a relative risk of 2.3 (95% CI, 0.9–5.9) compared with never users. In this study, there was a significant trend for increased endometrial cancer risk with longer tamoxifen use and also with a higher cumulative tamoxifen dose.

Surprisingly, an excess risk of gastrointestinal cancers has also been found in tamoxifen-treated patients (relative risk, 1.9; 95% CI, 1.2–2.9) (77). These data on second cancers obviously need confirmation since they may represent an artifact: Women taking tamoxifen have a prolonged survival and may therefore be at increased risk of developing other neoplasias.

Two other side effects of tamoxifen are worth mentioning: the increased risk of devel-

T A B L E 6-5

Cases of Endometrial Cancer Reported in Randomized Trials of Tamoxifen

Trial (Reference)	No. of Patients	Median Follow-up Time (yr)	Cases of Endometrial Cancer		Relative Risk (95% CI)
			Tamoxifen	Control	
Stockholm Trial (8)[a]	1846	9.5	14	2	6.4 (1.4–28.0)
NSABP B-14 (76)[b]	2843	8	15	0	7.5 (1.7–32.7)
Scandinavian Trials (77)[c]	4914	9	34	8	4.1 (1.9–8.9)

[a] Tamoxifen, 40 mg daily for 2 or 5 yr.

[b] Tamoxifen, 20 mg daily for at least 5 yr.

[c] Tamoxifen, 30 or 40 mg daily for 1 or 2 yr.

oping venous thromboses and tamoxifen-related retinopathy. In the NSABP B-14 trial, 2843 node-negative women were randomly assigned to receive tamoxifen, 20 mg daily, or a placebo (76). Phlebitis was documented in only two patients in the placebo group but in 12 patients receiving tamoxifen, including one patient who died of a pulmonary embolism.

To investigate the incidence and course of ocular toxicity in patients receiving tamoxifen, 20 mg daily, a prospective study (80) was conducted in 63 patients. Retinopathy or keratopathy or both developed in four patients after a median duration of 25 months. In another study, screening of 135 asymptomatic tamoxifen-treated women revealed that two patients had changes consistent with tamoxifen-induced retinopathy (81). The authors of this study concluded that routine ophthalmologic screening was not necessary in tamoxifen-treated patients.

Side Effects of Chemotherapy

In addition to a number of acute side effects such as gastrointestinal distress, hair loss, and myelosuppression, chemotherapy can induce permanent ovarian dysfunction in premenopausal patients, causing menopausal symptoms and resulting in the potential increased risk of developing ischemic heart disease or osteoporosis. Administration of chemotherapy has also been implicated in the development of venous thromboses (82).

Recently, the Milan group reported on the occurrence of second malignancies following their adjuvant treatment program, in which CMF was given to women with resectable breast cancer (83). At 15 years, the cumulative actuarial risk of second malignancies was 6.7% ± 0.8% for the total series. The cumulative risk was 6.4% ± 0.9% in women who had received CMF adjuvant therapy, while it was 8.4% ± 2.9% after local-regional treatment alone, suggesting the lack of an increased risk of second malignancies following CMF chemotherapy. Of note, three cases of acute nonlymphoblastic leukemia developed, all in the chemotherapy group, for a cumulative risk of 0.23% ± 0.15%.

The picture may be somewhat different for patients receiving anthracycline-based chemotherapy. Indeed, several worrisome reports (84–88) of acute myeloid leukemia following anthracycline-based chemotherapy have now been published (Table 6-6). Some of these leukemias showed the typical 11q23 translocation observed with leukemia secondary to topoisomerase II inhibitors. Of note, some cases of acute myeloid leukemia occurring after anthracycline-based therapy for advanced breast cancer have also been reported (89). A synergistic effect in leukemogenesis between anthracyclines and alkylating agents has been proposed but remains hypothetical.

The use of anthracyclines may also be hampered by their potential long-term, drug-related cardiotoxicity—mainly chronic cardiomyopathy,

T A B L E **6-6**

Cases of Acute Myeloid Leukemia (AML) Reported in Breast Cancer Adjuvant Studies

Group (Reference)	Type of Study	Regimen (Dose of Anthracycline in mg/m^2)	No. of Patients Receiving Anthracycline	No. of Cases of AML (Previous RT)	Presence of 11q23	Months Between Study Entry and AML (Median)
Buzdar (84)	Retrospective study	FAC	736	8 (7)	—	68
Riggi (85)	Randomized trials	EC (60 × 2) vs CMF	577	2 (—)	—	22
		FEC (50) vs FEC (75)	621	1 (1)	—	48
Shepherd (86)	Randomized trial	CEF (60 × 2) vs CMF	351	3 (2)[a]	1	18
DeCillis (87)	Randomized trial	AC (60)[b]	2548	6 (2)	3	14
Linassier (88)	Retrospective study	CN (12) F[c]	—	5 (5)[d]	3	16

[a] One case of acute lymphocytic leukemia was also described.

[b] This trial compares different doses of C, i.e., 1200 mg/m^2 × 4 or 2400 mg/m^2 × 2 or 2400 mg/m^2 × 4.

[c] Two patients also received vinblastine.

[d] Four patients received adjuvant chemotherapy, while one received anthracycline for metastatic disease.

RT = radiation therapy; F = fluorouracil; A = doxorubicin; C = cyclophosphamide; E = epirubicin × 2 given on days 1 and 8; M = methotrexate; N = mitoxantrone.

ischemic heart disease, and congestive heart failure. Clear data on anthracycline-induced cardiomyopathy in the adjuvant setting are relatively sparse, and in most of the adjuvant trials performed so far, the incidence of cardiomyopathy was not prospectively or extensively evaluated. With a total cumulative dose of 400 mg/m² or less of doxorubicin or 720 mg/m² or less of epirubicin, the incidence of congestive heart failure was estimated to be about 1%; the incidence was somewhat higher (2%) after both doxorubicin and radiation therapy to the left breast (90). However, additional factors such as the schedule of drug administration (for example, high-dose bolus) and concomitant use of anthracyclines and newer chemotherapy agents, such as the taxoids, could further increase the risk of developing cardiac events. Therefore, monitoring of anthracycline cardiotoxicity will need to be reinforced in the coming years (91).

Future Directions

The latest developments in the field of adjuvant therapy for early breast cancer and some of the highest priorities for future clinical research are discussed.

New Prognostic Factors in Early Breast Cancer

For two decades, clinicians have used information about the number of involved axillary nodes, tumor size, hormone receptor status, and tumor histology as the best but still suboptimal way to predict outcome in patients with early breast cancer. More recently, a rapidly growing number of biologic markers have been proposed as new prognostic factors, but none of them has yet been incorporated into general clinical practice. In addition to problems of quality control in the evaluation of these markers, there are problems in the design of the studies published to date: The new markers were examined individually rather than by multivariate analysis, retrospectively rather than prospectively, and in small trials with a short follow-up period. These important methodologic and statistical problems were extensively discussed by McGuire (92), Gasparini et al (93), and Knoop et al (94).

At present, these new "prognostic factors" should be considered investigational. They include markers related to tumor proliferation (Ki 67, S-phase fraction, thymidine labeling index, and cyclin D1), tumor growth (epidermal growth factor receptor, c-erb B-2 or Neu, insulin-like growth factor, and the H-*ras* oncogene product), growth suppression or metastasis (*p53*, *RB*, and *nm23*), invasion (cathepsin D, urokinase plasminogen activator/plasminogen activator inhibitor 1, and collagenase type IV), adhesion (laminin receptor), and angiogenesis. Table 6-7 summarizes our current knowledge in this developing field.

New Predictive Factors in Early Breast Cancer

A *predictive factor* is defined as a factor allowing the selection of patients most likely to respond to a specific form of therapy. The prototypical predictive factor in breast cancer, known for 20 years, is tumor estrogen receptor content, which correlates with the probability of response to endocrine therapy.

It is only in the past 5 years that other gene products known to play an important role in tumor biology have been investigated as potential predictors of response to hormonal or chemotherapeutic agents. Tumors with pS2 expression were found to be more likely than tumors without pS2 expression to respond to hormonal treatment (95), while tumors expressing c-erb B-2 (96,97), epidermal growth factor receptor (98), or urokinase-type plasminogen activator (99) were poorly responsive to endocrine therapy. P-glycoprotein overexpression was associated with resistance to anthracyclines (100). Of note, all the studies mentioned above were performed in patients with metastatic disease. As far as adjuvant treatment is concerned, Muss et al (101) showed recently that overexpression of c-erb B-2 may identify the subset of patients who are most likely to benefit from higher doses of adjuvant FAC chemotherapy. This elegant study needs additional follow-up and the findings need to be confirmed by other groups (102).

Finally, a number of in vitro studies showed interesting correlations between overexpression of heat shock proteins (103) or mutant-type p53 (104) and decreased sensitivity to chemotherapy.

More studies of this kind in the adjuvant setting are clearly needed: They may spare thousands of patients toxic and costly treatment, and may allow for targeting of specific thera-

T A B L E **6-7**

Examples of Investigational Prognostic Markers in Breast Cancer

Marker	No. of Studies (Median No. of Patients)	Proposed Function	Expression in Breast Tumors, % (Range)	Correlation with Prognosis in Multivariate Analysis (No. of Studies)		Comments
				Yes	No	
erb B-1	13 (212)	Gene product = EGF-R = growth factor receptor	EGF-R: 45 (22–91)	4	4	Conflicting results
erb B-2	38 (380)	Gene product = 185-kd protein p185 = growth factor receptor	erb-B2 gene overexpression: 20–25 p185 positivity: 19 (9–33)	13	13	Conflicting results, poor prognosis in node-positive patients; inverse correlation with ER and PgR; positive correlation with tumor grade, size, and mitotic activity
uPA/PAI1	14 (223)	Local invasiveness marker	High uPA: 42 (29–58)	12	2	High contents of uPA or PAI1 = poor prognosis
p53 (Mutant)	12 (260)	Gene product = 53 kd = suppression of cell proliferation and malignant transformation	p53 positivity: 28 (13–52)	11	0	p53 overexpression = poor prognosis; inverse correlation with ER and PgR; positive correlation with tumor grade
nm23	4 (range; 24–130)	Antimetastatic gene	NR	NR	2	Decreased level of nm23 RNA and nm23 protein = poor prognosis
CD-31 antibody, factor VIII related antigen	14 (73)	Tumor angiogenesis	NR	8	2	Intense neovascularization = poor prognosis

EGF-R = epidermal growth factor receptor; ER = estrogen receptor; NR = not reported; PAI1 = plasminogen activator inhibitor; PgR = progesterone receptor; uPA = urokinase plasminogen activator.

Source: Adapted from Knoop AS, Laenkholm AV, Mirza MR, et al. Prognostic and predictive factors in early breast cancer. ESMO Educational Book, 1994:9–18.

pies to subsets of patients likely to derive the greatest benefit.

New Directions in Adjuvant Endocrine Treatment

In spite of one trial that found that amino-glutethimide as adjuvant endocrine therapy for postmenopausal women was not effective (105), it is likely that the newest aromatase inhibitors, with their increased therapeutic ratio in advanced breast cancer (106), will soon be tested in the adjuvant setting, alone or in combination with tamoxifen.

New antiestrogen products such as toremifene and the pure antiestrogen ICI 182780 may also have a role in the treatment of early breast cancer in view of their well-documented activity in advanced disease (107,108).

Fenretinide, a synthetic retinoid, definitely deserves investigation in the adjuvant setting. Preclinical data demonstrate a decreased incidence of carcinogen-induced mammary tumors with the use of fenretinide and enhanced inhibition of breast carcinogenesis when the drug is combined with ovariectomy (109). Furthermore, fenretinide significantly enhanced the efficacy of tamoxifen against breast cancer growth. A large, placebo-controlled phase III trial, recently closed, will determine the role of fenretinide, if any, in preventing contralateral primary breast cancer (110). The trial enrolled 3000 women with a previous diagnosis of localized breast cancer (110). In the adjuvant setting, trials comparing tamoxifen with tamoxifen plus fenretinide are ready to begin on both sides of the Atlantic Ocean. It is hoped that the combination regimen will increase disease-free and overall survival rates.

New Chemotherapeutic Agents and New Combination Regimens

The past 10 years has witnessed the clinical development of a number of new cytotoxic drugs with innovative mechanisms of action.

Vinorelbine, the taxoids (paclitaxel and docetaxel), thymidylate synthase inhibitors (e.g., tomudex), gemcitabine, and camptothecin analogues (topotecan and irinotecan) have demonstrated interesting activity in advanced breast cancer (52,111,112). One of these compounds, docetaxel, induces unusually high response rates in liver metastases (113). This activity may be of interest in the adjuvant setting: Goldhirsch et al (114) recently showed that adjuvant treatments in current use improve patient outcome mainly by reducing the incidence of first local, regional, or distant soft tissue relapses, while first recurrences in bone or viscera appear to be much less influenced.

Combination regimens that include new, active compounds are now under active investigation against metastatic disease in phase I/II trials. High objective response rates and sometimes high complete remission rates have been reported (115–119). However, these dose-finding studies included very small numbers of patients, and further studies specifically addressing the antitumor activity of these drugs are needed. The role of these new combinations in the management of primary breast cancer should be assessed through properly designed randomized clinical trials.

Renewed Interest in Drug Sequencing

The effects of some chemotherapy regimens are sequence dependent—that is, the effects of the regimens differ depending on the timing of administration of the drugs in the same cycle. When anthracyclines and taxoids are given in combination according to prolonged schedules of drug administration, the observed side effects appear to be dependent on drug sequencing; it is less clear whether the antitumor activity of this combination is sequence dependent. Interestingly, pharmacokinetic studies do not always explain sequence-dependent differences, which suggests that other mechanisms may be operative at the cellular level (120).

Bonadonna et al (28) showed the superiority of sequential versus alternating schedules of doxorubicin and CMF in the adjuvant setting.

Encouraged by this observation, by the feasibility of sequential administration of doxorubicin and high-dose cyclophosphamide, and by the partial non-cross-resistance between paclitaxel and doxorubicin, Memorial Sloan-Kettering Cancer Center launched a study of rapid sequential administration of maximum tolerated doses of doxorubicin, paclitaxel, and cyclophosphamide with granulocyte colony-stimulating factor support in patients with four or more positive nodes (121). This innovative regimen might be a candidate for future prospective randomized clinical trials in the adjuvant setting.

Dose-Intensive Adjuvant Therapy for "High-Risk" Early Breast Cancer

Results of preclinical experiments conducted in mammary tumor models and retrospective analyses of a number of clinical trials in breast cancer patients suggest a possible role for dose-intensive therapies in the treatment of this disease.

While suboptimal doses of adjuvant chemotherapy are associated with inferior results (34,122), the role of high-dose chemotherapy remains controversial (123).

In the past years the results of many small phase I and II trials using high-dose chemotherapy given as single agents or combinations have been published (124,125). The results are promising in comparison with results of historical studies. However, this comparison is seriously hampered by the strict patient selection process for these toxic programs (123,126). Fortunately, randomized clinical trials in patients with stage II disease (five or more positive nodes), stage III disease, and inflammatory breast cancer are currently under way (127). The first results are expected toward the end of this century. Table 6-8 summarizes some important randomized clinical trials in progress.

New Modulating Agents

The former generation of "modulating" agents such as leucovorin, pentoxifylline, toremifene, and cyclosporine has been used in combination with anticancer drugs with the hope of avoiding or overcoming chemotherapy resistance. So far, none of these approaches has been tested in the adjuvant setting, as a clear-cut advantage over conventional treatment could not be shown in advanced disease.

More recently, monoclonal antibodies have been used against the HER-2/neu protein with encouraging preliminary results. Pietras et al (128) showed that a monoclonal antibody to the HER-2/neu receptor can block DNA repair following cisplatin exposure in human breast and ovarian cancer cells. Moreover, this antibody enhanced the cytotoxicity of cisplatin (129), carboplatin (130), and doxorubicin (130) against human breast tumor cells. Paclitaxel was combined with anti–growth factor receptor monoclonal antibodies (anti–epidermal growth factor

TABLE   6-8

Ongoing Randomized Phase III Trials of High-Dose Adjuvant Chemotherapy with Hematopoietic Stem Cell Support

Country (Group)	No. of Involved Axillary Nodes	Induction Regimen	Randomization Arms
USA (CALGB)	>10	CAF × 4	C, B, P* (high dose) vs C, B, P (conventional dose)
USA (ECOG)	>10	CAF × 4	C, T* vs no further therapy
The Netherlands	>10	FEC × 4	C, T, Cb* vs FEC × 1
France (PEGASE 01)	>8	FEC × 4	C, M, Mx* vs no further therapy
Sweden	>5	FEC	C, T, Cb* vs FEC increasing dose + GCSF

*Peripheral stem cell support.

A = doxorubicin; B = carmustine; C = cyclophosphamide; Cb = carboplatin; E = epirubicin; F = fluorouracil; GCSF = granulocyte colony-stimulating factor; M = melphalan; Mx = mitoxantrone; P = cisplatin; T = thiotepa.

TABLE   6-9

Antiangiogenic and Antimetastatic Drugs in Early Clinical Development

Drug	Mechanism of Action	Clinical Experience Mode of Administration	Toxicity
AGM-1470	Inhibition of endothelial cell proliferation	IV	Asymptomatic retinal hemorrhages
r Platelet factor 4	Inhibition of endothelial cell proliferation	Intratumoral or IV	Local pain
Pentosan polysulfate	Inhibition of endothelial cell proliferation	IV or orally	Reversible anticoagulant effects
Razoxane	Antimetastatic	Orally	Neutropenia
BB-2516	Metalloproteinase inhibitor	Orally	Too early to tell

IV = intravenously.

Source: Adapted from Gasparini G, Harris AL. Clinical importance of the determination of tumor angiogenesis in breast carcinoma: much more than a new prognostic tool. *J Clin Oncol* 1995;13:765–782.

receptor ARMA 528, anti–HER 2 ARMA 4 D5) in breast cancer xenografts, with interesting results (131).

A monoclonal antibody against HER-2/neu is presently being investigated in a phase III trial in association with front-line chemotherapy for metastatic breast cancer patients whose tumors overexpress the Neu protein. If this study leads to a prolongation of progression-free survival, it will undoubtedly stimulate the evaluation of this monoclonal antibody in the adjuvant setting.

Differentiating, Antiangiogenic, and Antimetastatic Drugs

Results of several preclinical studies suggest the possible efficacy of novel treatment approaches, including the use of differentiating agents, such as retinoic acid derivatives, and agents interfering with metastasis and angiogenesis (40). Table 6-9 summarizes the early clinical experience with some of the antiangiogenic and antimetastatic drugs (132).

These new agents are not expected to show activity in the presence of bulky disease but may delay tumor progression following response to cytotoxic drugs. The demonstration of such an effect in metastatic disease, if achieved without significant toxicity, would encourage the design of prospective adjuvant clinical trials with these agents.

Conclusions

Systemic adjuvant treatment for early breast cancer is a therapeutic field in constant evolution.

The most important message of this chapter is that "optimal" adjuvant therapy for patients with early-stage breast cancer is adjuvant therapy within the framework of a prospective clinical trial. Too many uncertainties remain about the risk-benefit ratio of the therapies in current use for patients to be treated outside of clinical trials.

The future of adjuvant therapy for breast cancer is promising: A number of innovative treatment approaches based on new cellular targets will soon enter the clinical arena. With improved knowledge of clinical trial methodology, let us hope that these new strategies will benefit from an adequate evaluation early on.

Acknowledgments

The authors want to thank M. Delval and P. Adam for their excellent secretarial work and the Fonds JC Heuson de Recherche en Cancérologie Mammaire and the Fonds National de la Recherche Scientifique (Belgium) for supporting the clinical research fellowships of J. A. Roy, MD, and A. Awada, MD, respectively.

REFERENCES

1. Beatson GT. On the treatment of inoperable cases of carcinoma of the mamma: suggestions for a new method of treatment. *Lancet* 1896;2:104–107, 162–165.

2. Early Breast Cancer Trialists' Collaborative Group. The effects of adjuvant tamoxifen and of cytotoxic therapy on mortality in early breast cancer: an overview of 61 randomised trials among 28,896 women. *N Engl J Med* 1988; 319:1681–1692.

3. Early Breast Cancer Trialists' Collaborative Group. Systemic treatment of early breast cancer by hormonal, cytotoxic or immune therapy. 133 randomized trials involving 31,000 recurrences and 24,000 deaths among 75,000 women. *Lancet* 1992;339:1–15, 71–85.

4. Swedish Breast Cancer Cooperative Group. Randomized trial of 2 versus 5 years of adjuvant tamoxifen in postmenopausal early-stage breast cancer. *Proc Am Soc Clin Oncol* 1996;15:126. Abstract 171.

5. Fisher B, Dignam J, Wieand S, et al. Duration of tamoxifen (TAM) therapy for primary breast cancer: 5 versus 10 years (NSABP B-14). *Proc Am Soc Clin Oncol* 1996;15:113. Abstract 118.

6. Stewart HJ, Forrest AP, Everington D, et al. Randomised comparison of 5 years of adjuvant tamoxifen with continuous therapy for operable breast cancer. *Br J Cancer* 1996;74: 297–299.

7. Fisher B, Costantino J, Redmond C, et al. A randomized clinical trial evaluating tamoxifen in the treatment of patients with node-negative breast cancer who have estrogen-receptor-positive tumors. *N Engl J Med* 1989;320: 479–484.

8. Fornander T, Rutqvist LE, Cedermark B, et al. Adjuvant tamoxifen in early breast cancer: occurrence of new primary cancers. *Lancet* 1989;1:117–120.

9. Rutqvist LE, Matson A, for the Stockholm Breast Cancer Study Group. Cardiac and thromboembolic morbidity among postmenopausal women with early stage breast cancer in a randomized trial of adjuvant tamoxifen. *J Natl Cancer Inst* 1993;85:1398–1406.

10. McDonald CC, Stewart HJ. Fatal myocardial infarction in the Scottish adjuvant tamoxifen trial. The Scottish Breast Cancer Committee. *BMJ* 1991;303:435–437.

11. Love RR, Wiebe DA, Feyzi JM, et al. Effects of tamoxifen on cardiovascular risk factors in postmenopausal women after 5 years of treatment. *J Natl Cancer Inst* 1994;86:1534–1539.

12. Love RR, Barden HS, Mazess RB, et al. Effect of tamoxifen on lumbar spine bone mineral density in postmenopausal women after 5 years. *Arch Intern Med* 1994;154:2585–2588.

13. Davidson NE. Ovarian ablation as treatment for young women with breast cancer. *Monogr Natl Cancer Inst* 1994;16:95–99.

14. Cauley JA, Seeley DG, Ensrud K, et al, for the Study of Osteoporotic Fractures Research Group. Estrogen replacement therapy and fractures in older women. *Ann Intern Med* 1995; 122:9–16.

15. Barrett-Connor E, Bush TL. Estrogen and coronary heart disease in women. *JAMA* 1991;265: 1861–1867.

16. Bonadonna G, Valagussa P, Moliterni A, et al. Adjuvant cyclophosphamide, methotrexate and fluorouracil in node-positive breast cancer. The results of 20 years of follow-up. *N Engl J Med* 1995;332:901–906.

17. Bonadonna G, Valagussa P, Brambilla C, et al. Adjuvant and neoadjuvant treatment of breast cancer with chemotherapy and/or endocrine therapy. *Semin Oncol* 1991;18:515–524.

18. Bonadonna G, Gianni L, Santoro A, et al. Drugs ten years later: epirubicin. *Ann Oncol* 1993; 4:359–369.

19. French Epirubicin Study Group. A prospective randomized phase III trial comparing combination chemotherapy with cyclophosphamide, fluorouracil, and either doxorubicin or epirubicin. *J Clin Oncol* 1988;6:679–688.

20. French Epirubicin Study Group. A prospective randomized trial comparing epirubicin monochemotherapy to two fluorouracil, cyclophosphamide, and epirubicin regimens differing in epirubicin dose in advanced breast cancer patients. *J Clin Oncol* 1991;9:305–312.

21. Fisher B, Redmond C, Wickerham DL, et al. Doxorubicin-containing regimens for the treatment of stage II breast cancer: the National Surgical Adjuvant Breast and Bowel Project Experience. *J Clin Oncol* 1989;7:572–582.

22. Misset JL, Gil-Delgado M, Chollet P, et al. Ten years results of the French trial comparing Adriamycin, vincristine, 5-fluorouracil and cyclophosphamide to standard CMF as adjuvant therapy for node-positive breast cancer. *Proc Am Soc Clin Oncol* 1992;11:54. Abstract 41.

23. Mauriac L, Durand M, Chauvergne J, et al. Randomized trial of adjuvant chemotherapy for operable breast cancer comparing i.v. CMF to an epirubicin-containing regimen. *Ann Oncol* 1992;3:439–443.

24. Fisher B, Brown AM, Dimitrov NV, et al. Two months of doxorubicin-cyclophosphamide with and without interval reinduction therapy compared with 6 months of CMF in positive-node breast cancer patients with tamoxifen-nonresponsive tumors: results from the National Surgical Adjuvant Breast and Bowel Project B-15. *J Clin Oncol* 1990;8:1483–1496.

25. Tormey DC, Gray R, Abeloff MD, et al. Adjuvant therapy with a doxorubicin regimen and long term tamoxifen in premenopausal breast cancer patients: an Eastern Cooperative Oncology Group trial. *J Clin Oncol* 1992;10: 1848–1856.

26. Moliterni A, Bonadonna G, Valagussa P, et al. CMF with or without doxorubicin in the adjuvant treatment of resectable breast cancer with one to three positive axillary nodes. *J Clin Oncol* 1991;9:1124–1130.

27. Buzzoni R, Bonadonna G, Valagussa P, Zambetti M. Adjuvant chemotherapy with doxorubicin plus cyclophosphamide, methotrexate and fluorouracil in the treatment of resectable breast cancer with more than three positive axillary nodes. *J Clin Oncol* 1991;9:2134–2140.

28. Bonnadonna G, Zambetti M, Valagussa P. Sequential or alternating doxorubicin and CMF regimens in breast cancer with more than three positive nodes: ten-year results. *JAMA* 1995; 273:542–547.

29. Carpenter JT, Velez-Garcia E, Aron BS, et al. Prospective randomized comparison of cyclophosphamide, Adriamycin, and fluorouracil (CAF) vs CMF for breast cancer with positive axillary nodes: a Southeastern Cancer Group study. *Proc Am Soc Clin Oncol* 1991;10:45. Abstract 54.

30. Carpenter JT, Velez-Garcia E, Aron BS, et al. Five-year results of a randomized comparison of CAF versus CMF for node positive breast cancer. *Proc Am Soc Clin Oncol* 1994;13:66. Abstract 68.

31. Coombes RC, Bliss JM, Marty M, et al. A randomized trial comparing adjuvant FEC with CMF in premenopausal patients with node positive resectable breast cancer. *Proc Am Soc Clin Oncol* 1991;10:41. Abstract 37.

32. Marty M, Bliss JM, Coombes RC, et al. CMF versus FEC chemotherapy in premenopausal women with node positive breast cancer: results of a randomized trial. *Proc Am Soc Clin Oncol* 1994;13:62. Abstract 50.

33. Levine M, Bramwell V, Bowman D, et al. A clinical trial of intensive CEF versus CMF in premenopausal women with node positive breast cancer. *Proc Am Soc Clin Oncol* 1995;14:103. Abstract 112.

34. Wood WC, Budman DR, Korzun AH, et al. Dose and dose intensity of adjuvant chemotherapy for stage II, node-positive breast carcinoma. *N Engl J Med* 1994;330:1253–1259.

35. Dimitrov N, Anderson S, Fisher B, et al. Dose intensification and increased total dose of adjuvant chemotherapy for breast cancer: findings from NSABP B-22. *Proc Am Soc Clin Oncol* 1994;13:64. Abstract 58.

36. Bonadonna G. Conceptual and practical advances in the management of breast cancer. Karnofsky Memorial Lecture. *J Clin Oncol* 1989;7:1380–1397.

37. Levine MN, Gent M, Hryniuk WM, et al. A randomized trial comparing 12 weeks versus 36 weeks of adjuvant chemotherapy in stage II breast cancer. *J Clin Oncol* 1990;8:1217–1225.

38. Rivkin SE, Green S, Metch B, et al. One versus 2 years of CMVFP adjuvant chemotherapy in axillary node-positive and estrogen receptor-negative patients: a Southwest Oncology Group study. *J Clin Oncol* 1993;11:1710–1716.

39. Ludwig Breast Cancer Study Group. Combination adjuvant chemotherapy for node-positive breast cancer. Inadequacy of a single perioperative cycle. *N Engl J Med* 1988;319:677–683.

40. Folkman J. Angiogenesis in cancer, vascular, rheumatoid and other disease. *Nat Med* 1995;1:27–31.

41. Bonadonna G, Valagussa P, Zucorli R, Salvadori B. Primary chemotherapy in surgically resectable breast cancer. *CA Cancer J Clin* 1995;45:227–243.

42. Jacquillat C, Weil M, Baillet F, et al. Results of neoadjuvant chemotherapy and radiation therapy in the breast conserving treatment of 250 patients with all stages of infiltrative breast cancer. *Cancer* 1990;66:119–129.

43. Forrest AP, Chatty U, Miller WR, et al. A human tumor model. *Lancet* 1986;2:840–842.

44. Smith IE, Jones AL, O'Brien ME, et al. Primary medical (neoadjuvant) chemotherapy for operable breast cancer. *Eur J Cancer* 1993;29A:1796–1799.

45. Smith IE, Walsh G, Jones A, et al. High complete remission rates with primary neoadjuvant infusional chemotherapy for large early breast cancer. *J Clin Oncol* 1995;13:424–429.

46. Mauriac L, Durand M, Avril A, Dilhuydy JM. Effects of primary chemotherapy in conservative treatment of breast cancer patients with operable tumors larger than 3 cm: results of a randomized trial in a single centre. *Ann Oncol* 1991;2:347–354.

47. Scholl SM, Fourquet A, Asselain B, et al. Neoadjuvant versus adjuvant chemotherapy in premenopausal patients with tumors considered too large for breast conserving surgery. Preliminary results of a randomized trial: S6. *Eur J Cancer* 1994;30A:645–652.

48. Bonadonna G. Evolving concepts in the systemic adjuvant treatment of breast cancer. *Cancer Res* 1992;52:2127–2137.

49. Bonadonna G, Valagussa P, Brambilla C, et al. Response to primary chemotherapy increases rates of breast preservation and correlates with prognosis. *Proc Am Soc Clin Oncol* 1994;13:107. Abstract 230.

50. Fisher B, Rockette H, Robidoux A, et al. Effect of preoperative therapy for breast cancer on local-regional disease: first report of NSABP B-18. *Proc Am Soc Clin Oncol* 1994;13:64. Abstract 57.

51. Powles TJ, Hickish TF, Makris A, et al. Randomized trial of chemoendocrine therapy started before or after surgery for treatment of primary breast cancer. *J Clin Oncol* 1995;13:547–552.

52. Piccart MJ. Taxoid compounds in breast cancer: current status and future prospects. In: Muggia FM, ed. *Concepts, mechanisms and new targets for chemotherapy.* Boston: Kluwer Academic, 1995:185–208.

53. Recht A. The integration of radiation and chemotherapy for patients treated with breast

cancer conserving surgery. In: ASCO Educational Book. Philadelphia: American Society of Clinical Oncology, Spring 1994:11–14.

54. Recht A, Come SE, Henderson IG, et al. The sequencing of chemotherapy and radiation therapy after conservative surgery for early-stage breast cancer. *N Engl J Med* 1996;334:1356–1361.

55. Scottish Cancer Trials Breast Group and ICRF Breast Unit, Guy's Hospital, London. Adjuvant ovarian ablation versus CMF chemotherapy in premenopausal women with pathological stage II breast carcinoma: the Scottish trial. *Lancet* 1993;341:1293–1298.

56. Goldhirsch A, Gelber RD. Adjuvant chemoendocrine therapy alone for postmenopausal patients: Ludwig studies III and IV. *Recent Results Cancer Res* 1989;115:153–162.

57. Mouridsen HT, Rose C, Overgaard M, et al. Adjuvant treatment of postmenopausal patients with high risk primary breast cancer. Results from the Danish adjuvant trials DBCG 77C and DBCG 82C. *Acta Oncol* 1988;27:699–705.

58. Pearson OH, Hubay CA, Gordon NH, et al. Endocrine versus endocrine plus five-drug chemotherapy in postmenopausal women with stage II estrogen receptor-positive breast cancer. *Cancer* 1989;64:1819–1823.

59. Fisher B, Redmond C, Legault-Poisson S, et al. Postoperative chemotherapy and tamoxifen compared with tamoxifen alone in the treatment of positive-node breast cancer patients aged 50 years and older with tumors responsive to tamoxifen: results from the National Surgical Adjuvant Breast and Bowel Project B-16. *J Clin Oncol* 1990;8:1005–1018.

60. Pritchard K, Zee B, Paul N, et al. CMF added to tamoxifen as adjuvant therapy in postmenopausal women with node-positive estrogen and/or progesterone receptor positive breast cancer: negative results from a randomized clinical trial. *Proc Am Soc Clin Oncol* 1994;13:65. Abstract 61.

61. Fisher B, Redmond C, Brown A, et al. Adjuvant chemotherapy with and without tamoxifen in the treatment of primary breast cancer: 5-year results from the National Surgical Adjuvant Breast and Bowel Project Trial. *J Clin Oncol* 1986;4:459–471.

62. Crowe JP, Gordon NH, Shenk RR, et al. Short-term tamoxifen plus chemotherapy: superior results in node-positive breast cancer. *Surgery* 1990;108:619–628.

63. Rivkin SE, Green S, Metch B, et al. Adjuvant CMFVP versus tamoxifen versus concurrent CMFVP and tamoxifen for postmenopausal, node-positive, and estrogen receptor-positive breast cancer patients: a Southwest Oncology Group Study. *J Clin Oncol* 1994;12:2078–2085.

64. Boccardo F, Rubagotti A, Bruzzi P, et al. Chemotherapy versus tamoxifen versus chemotherapy plus tamoxifen in node-positive, estrogen receptor-positive breast cancer patients: results of a multicentric Italian study. *J Clin Oncol* 1990;8:1310–1320.

65. Boccardo F, Rubagotti A, Amoroso D, et al. (GROCTA) Chemotherapy versus tamoxifen versus chemotherapy plus tamoxifen in node-positive estrogen-receptor positive breast cancer patients. *Eur J Cancer* 1992;28:673–680.

66. Goldhirsch A, Wood WC, Senn HJ, et al. Meeting highlights: international consensus panel on the treatment of primary breast cancer. *J Natl Cancer Inst* 1995;87:1441–1445.

67. Devesa SS, Blot WJ, Stone BJ, et al. Recent cancer trends in the United States. *J Natl Cancer Inst* 1995;87:175–182.

68. Carter CL, Allen C, Henson DE. Relation of tumor size, lymph node status, and survival in 24,740 breast cancer cases. *Cancer* 1989; 63:181–187.

69. Rosen PP, Groshen S, Saigo PE, et al. Pathological prognostic factors in stage I (T1N0M0) and stage II (T1N1M0) breast carcinoma: a study of 644 patients with a median follow-up of 18 years. *J Clin Oncol* 1989;7:1239–1251.

70. Silvestrini R, Daidone MG, Luisi A, et al. Biologic and clinicopathologic factors as indicators of specific relapse types in node-negative breast cancer. *J Clin Oncol* 1995;13:697–704.

71. Quiet CA, Ferguson DJ, Weichelbaum RR, Hellman S. Natural history of node-negative breast cancer: a study of 826 patients with long-term follow-up. *J Clin Oncol* 1995;13:1144–1151.

72. Cummings FJ, Gray R, Davis T, et al. Adjuvant tamoxifen treatment of elderly women with stage II breast cancer. *Ann Intern Med* 1985;103:324–329.

73. Castiglione M, Gelber RD, Goldhirsch A. Adjuvant systemic therapy for breast cancer in the elderly: competing causes of mortality. *J Clin Oncol* 1990;8:519–526.

74. Muss H, Cooper MR, Hoen H, et al. Adjuvant chemotherapy in older women with node posi-

tive breast cancer: the Piedmont Oncology Association experience. *Proc Am Soc Clin Oncol* 1992;11:147. Abstract 408.

75. Desch CE, Hillner BE, Smith TJ, Retchin SM. Should the elderly receive chemotherapy for node-negative breast cancer? A cost-effectiveness analysis examining total and active life-expectancy outcomes. *J Clin Oncol* 1993;11:777–782.

76. Fisher B, Costantino JP, Redmond CK, et al. Endometrial cancer in tamoxifen-treated breast cancer patients: findings from the National Surgical Adjuvant Breast and Bowel Project (NSABP) B-14. *J Natl Cancer Inst* 1994; 86:527–537.

77. Rutqvist LE, Johansson H, Signomklao T, et al. Adjuvant tamoxifen therapy for early stage breast cancer and second primary malignancies. *J Natl Cancer Inst* 1995;87:645–651.

78. Magriples U, Naftolin F, Schwartz PE, Carcangiu ML. High-grade endometrial carcinoma in tamoxifen-treated breast cancer patients. *J Clin Oncol* 1993;11:485–490.

79. Van Leeuwen FE, Benraadt J, Coebergh JW, et al. Risk of endometrial cancer after tamoxifen treatment of breast cancer. *Lancet* 1994; 343:448–452.

80. Pavlidis NA, Petris C, Briassoulis E, et al. Clear evidence that long-term, low-dose tamoxifen treatment can induce ocular toxicity. A prospective study of 63 patients. *Cancer* 1992; 69:2961–2964.

81. Heier JS, Dragoo RA, Enzenauer RW. Screening for ocular toxicity in asymptomatic patients treated with tamoxifen. *Am J Ophthalmol* 1994;117:772–775.

82. Levine MN, Gent M, Hirsh J, et al. The thrombogenic effect of anti-cancer drug therapy in women with stage II breast cancer. *N Engl J Med* 1988;318:404–407.

83. Valagussa P, Moliterni A, Terenziani M, et al. Second malignancies following CMF-based adjuvant chemotherapy in resectable breast cancer. *Ann Oncol* 1994;5:803–808.

84. Buzdar A, Iwaniec J, Kau S, et al. Secondary leukemia following adjuvant doxorubicin-containing chemotherapy for (stage II or III) breast cancer. *Proc Am Soc Clin Oncol* 1991;10:59. Abstract 112.

85. Riggi M, Riva A. Therapy-related leukemia: what is the role of 4-epi-doxorubicin? *J Clin Oncol* 1993;11:1430–1431.

86. Shepherd L, Ottaway J, Myles J, Levine M. Therapy-related leukemia associated with high dose 4-epi-doxorubicin and cyclophosphamide used as adjuvant chemotherapy for breast cancer. *J Clin Oncol* 1994;12:2514–2515.

87. DeCillis A, Anderson S, Wickerham DL, et al. Acute myeloid leukemia in NSABP B-25. *Proc Am Soc Clin Oncol* 1995;14:98. Abstract 92.

88. Linassier C, Barin C, Brémond JL, et al. Leucémies aiguïs myéloblastiques induites par mitoxantrone dans le cadre d'un traitement pour cancer du sein. *Bull Cancer (Paris)* 1995;82:240. Abstract.

89. Pedersen-Bjergaard J, Sigsgaard TC, Nielsen D, et al. Acute monocytic or myelomonocytic leukemia with balanced chromosome translocations to band 11q23 after therapy with 4-epidoxorubicin and cisplatin or cyclophosphamide for breast cancer. *J Clin Oncol* 1992; 10:1444–1451.

90. Valagussa P, Zambetti H, Biasi S, et al. Cardiac effects following adjuvant chemotherapy and breast irradiation in operable breast cancer. *Ann Oncol* 1994;5:209–216.

91. Shapiro CL, Henderson IC. Late cardiac effects of adjuvant therapy: too soon to tell? *Ann Oncol* 1994;5:196–198. Editorial.

92. McGuire WL. Breast cancer prognostic factors: evaluation guidelines. *J Natl Cancer Inst* 1991; 83:154–155.

93. Gasparini G, Pozza F, Harris AL. Evaluating the potential usefulness of new prognostic and predictive indicators in node-negative breast cancer patients. *J Natl Cancer Inst* 1993; 85:1206–1219.

94. Knoop AS, Laenkholm AV, Mirza MR, et al. Prognostic and predictive factors in early breast cancer. ESMO European Society for Medical Oncology, Lugano (Switzerland) 1994: 9–18.

95. Schwartz LH, Koerner FC, Edgerton SM, et al. pS2 expression and response to hormonal therapy in patients with advanced breast cancer. *Cancer Res* 1991;51:624–628.

96. Leitzel K, Teramoto Y, Konrad K, et al. Elevated serum c-erbB-2 antigen levels and decreased response to hormone therapy of breast cancer. *J Clin Oncol* 1995;13:1129–1135.

97. Gusterson BA, Gelber RD, Goldhirsch A, et al. Prognostic importance of c-erbB-2 expression in breast cancer. *J Clin Oncol* 1992;10:1049–1056.

98. Nicholson S, Sainsburg JRC, Halcrow P, et al. Expression of epidermal growth factor receptors associated with lack of response to endocrine therapy in recurrent breast cancer. *Lancet* 1989;1:182–185.

99. Foekens JA, Look MP, Peters HA, et al. Urokinase-type plasminogen activator and its inhibitor PAI-1: predictors of poor response to tamoxifen therapy in recurrent breast cancer. *J Natl Cancer Inst* 1995;87:751–756.

100. Gasparini G, Bevilacqua P, Pozza F, et al. P-Glycoprotein expression predicts response to chemotherapy in previously untreated advanced breast cancer. *Breast* 1993;2:27–32.

101. Muss HB, Thor AD, Berry DA, et al. c-ErbB-2 expression and response to adjuvant therapy in women with node-positive early breast cancer. *N Engl J Med* 1994;330:1260–1266.

102. Goldhirsch A, Gelber R. Understanding adjuvant chemotherapy for breast cancer. *N Engl J Med* 1994;330:1308–1309.

103. Giocca DR, Fuqua SAW, Lock-Lim S, et al. Response of human breast cancer cells to heat shock and chemotherapeutic drugs. *Cancer Res* 1992;52:3648–3654.

104. Lowe SW, Ruley HE, Jacks T, Housman DE. p53-dependent apoptosis modulates the cytotoxicity of anticancer agents. *Cell* 1993;74:957–967.

105. Jones AL, Powles TJ, Law M, et al. Adjuvant aminoglutethimide for postmenopausal patients with primary breast cancer: analysis at 8 years. *J Clin Oncol* 1992;10:1547–1552.

106. Goss PE, Gwyn KMEH. Current perspectives on aromatase inhibitors in breast cancer. *J Clin Oncol* 1994;12:2460–2470.

107. Vogel CL, Shemano I, Schoenfelder J, et al. Multicenter phase II efficacy trial of toremifene in tamoxifen-refractory patients with advanced breast cancer. *J Clin Oncol* 1993;11:345–350.

108. Howell A, DeFriend D, Robertson J, et al. Response to a specific antiestrogen (ICI 182780) in tamoxifen-resistant breast cancer. *Lancet* 1995;345:29–30.

109. McCormick DL, Mehta RG, Thompson CA, et al. Enhanced inhibition of mammary carcinogenesis by combined treatment with N-(4-hydroxyphenyl) retinamide and ovariectomy. *Cancer Res* 1982;42:508–512.

110. Costa A, Formelli F, Chiesa F, et al. Prospects of chemoprevention of human cancers with the synthetic retinoid fenretinide. *Cancer Res* 1994;54(suppl 7):2032s–2037s.

111. Hortobagyi GN. Future directions for vinorelbine (Navelbine). *Semin Oncol* 1995;22(suppl 5):80–87.

112. Piccart M. Docetaxel. A new defence in the management of breast cancer. *Anticancer Drugs* 1995;6(suppl 4):7–11.

113. Awada A, Cvitovic E, Piccart MJ. Cancer du sein et métastases hépatiques: nouveaux espoirs? *Bull Cancer (Paris)* 1995;82:478. Abstract.

114. Goldhirsch A, Gelber RD, Price KN, et al. Effect of systemic adjuvant treatment on first sites of breast cancer relapse. *Lancet* 1994;343:377–381.

115. Gianni L. Use of paclitaxel with other anticancer agents. *Proc EORTC Early Drug Development Meeting* 1995:54-55.

116. Tolcher AW, Gelmon KA. Interim results of a phase I/II study of biweekly paclitaxel and cisplatin in patients with metastatic breast cancer. *Semin Oncol* 1995;22(suppl 8):28–32.

117. Dieras V, Gruia G, Pouillart P, et al. Phase I study of the combination of docetaxel (D) and doxorubicin (DX) in 1st line CT treatment of metastatic breast cancer (MBC). *Eur J Cancer* 1995;31A(suppl 5):s194. Abstract 935.

118. Fumoleau P, Delecroix V, Gentin M, et al. Docetaxel in combination with vinorelbine as 1st line chemotherapy in patients with MBC: phase I dose finding study. *Eur J Cancer* 1995;31A(suppl 5):s195. Abstract 938.

119. Friedman MA. New directions for breast cancer therapeutic research. *Hematol Oncol Clin North Am* 1994;8:113–119.

120. Roy JA, Awada A, Kusenda Z, Piccart MJ. Sequence dependent effect (SDE) of chemotherapy (CT agents): a review. Presented at the 19th International Congress of Chemotherapy, Montreal, July 1995.

121. Seidman AD, Hudis CA, Norton L. Memorial Sloan-Kettering Cancer Center experience with paclitaxel in the treatment of breast cancer: from advanced disease to adjuvant therapy. *Semin Oncol* 1995;22(suppl 8):3–8.

122. Henderson IC, Hayes DF, Gelman R. Dose response with treatment of breast cancer: a critical review. *J Clin Oncol* 1988;6:1501–1515.

123. Hortobagyi GN. High-dose chemotherapy is not an established treatment for breast cancer. ASCO Educational Book, Springer 1995:341–346.

124. Antman KH, Souhami RL. High-dose chemotherapy in solid tumours. *Ann Oncol* 1993;4(suppl 1):529–544.

125. Antman KH. Dose intensive adjuvant therapy in breast cancer. ASCO Educational Book, 1994: 80–83.

126. Crump M, Pruice M, Goss PE. Outcome of extensive evaluation of women with ≥10 positive axillary lymph nodes prior to adjuvant therapy for breast cancer. *Proc Am Soc Clin Oncol* 1995;13:102. Abstract 107.

127. Smigel K. Phase III ABMT studies under way. *J Natl Cancer Inst* 1995;87:952–955.

128. Pietras RJ, Fendly BM, Chazin VR, et al. Antibody to HER-2/neu receptor blocks DNA repair after cisplatin in human breast and ovarian cancer cells. *Oncogene* 1994;9:1829–1838.

129. Hancock MC, Langton BC, Chan T, et al. A monoclonal antibody against the c-erbB-2 protein enhances the cytotoxicity of cis-diamminedichloroplatinum against human breast and ovarian tumor cell lines. *Cancer Res* 1991;51: 4575–4580.

130. Pegram MD, Pietras RJ, Slamon DJ. Monoclonal antibody to HER-2/neu gene product potentiates cytotoxicity of carboplatin and doxorubicin in human breast tumor cells. *Proc Am Assoc Cancer Res* 1992;23:442. Abstract 2639.

131. Baselga J, Norton L, Coplan K, et al. Antitumor activity of paclitaxel in combination with anti-growth factor receptor monoclonal antibodies in breast cancer xenografts. *Proc Am Assoc Cancer Res* 1994;35:380. Abstract 2262.

132. Gasparini G, Harris AL. Clinical importance of the determination of tumor angiogenesis in breast carcinoma: much more than a new prognostic tool. *J Clin Oncol* 1995;13:765–782.

Radiotherapy for Breast Cancer

SEYMOUR H. LEVITT

*R*adiotherapy has been an integral part of the management of breast cancer since the discovery of the therapeutic benefits of radiation in the late 1800s. The evolution of the use of radiotherapy for breast cancer treatment since that time has been well described (1). The early use of radiotherapy, either alone or in conjunction with radical mastectomy, was based on the premise that breast cancer spreads in an orderly fashion from the primary tumor through the lymph nodes. This halstedian paradigm, named after the surgeon who initially described this view of the disease, suggested that some early disease is curable if adequate local treatment is given. Based on this view, several modifications to mastectomy have been tried, including extended radical mastectomy and the incorporation of postmastectomy radiotherapy, to better ensure local disease control. Several randomized clinical trials clearly proved, and long-term results confirmed, that the addition of radiotherapy after mastectomy significantly improves local control (2–5). However, whether the addition of radiotherapy produces a survival benefit is less clear, and this fact continues to generate questions about the importance of controlling local disease.

In the 1970s, several developments in breast cancer research had a strong impact on the role of radiotherapy in the treatment of breast cancer. Studies by Stjernsward and Cuzick (6–8) suggested that postmastectomy radiotherapy may actually decrease survival, studies on the use of chemotherapy showed survival benefits (9,10), and a new paradigm was introduced that viewed breast cancer as a systemic disease (11). All of these changes converged to call into question the importance of controlling local disease in curing disease and to call into question the role of radiotherapy.

Throughout these years, retrospective studies (12) and critical assessments of the Stjernsward and Cuzick studies (13) argued for a positive effect of local control on survival. Recent long-term follow-up of some of these trials (2,14), along with emerging biologic data on breast tumors (15), gave rise to the most recent paradigm, which maintains that some early disease is curable if adequate local treatment is given. This paradigm, newly named the *sequential view* of the disease (16), resurrects the importance of local disease control and therefore the importance of adequate radiotherapy in curing some disease.

Regardless of the continual debate over the impact of local control on survival, reducing the risk of or delaying local recurrence is generally supported as an essential goal of patient care because of the psychological trauma of disease recurrence.

Because the successful treatment of breast cancer depends on the integration of different treatment modalities, improved dialogue between surgeons, radiation oncologists, and medical oncologists is needed, beginning at the time of diagnosis. This seems common sense, yet all too often radiation oncologists are not included in the diagnostic evaluation of a patient and see a patient only after surgery and after systemic therapies have been initiated. One implicit purpose of this chapter is to show that the essential role of radiotherapy in the treatment of breast cancer mandates the inclusion of radiation oncologists in the initial treatment planning for breast cancer patients.

Treatment by Stage of Disease

Ductal Carcinoma In Situ

Increased diagnosis of ductal carcinoma in situ (DCIS) in recent years has led to increased focus on the best treatment for this type of breast carcinoma. Although mastectomy is the traditional treatment, excision alone or with radiotherapy has become more widely used because of the good results obtained with conservative surgery for early invasive disease. Results of retrospective and randomized studies suggest that the addition of radiotherapy improves local disease control. The average local failure rate is about 20% in studies of excision alone versus 10% in studies of excision with irradiation (17). The National Surgical Adjuvant Breast and Bowel Project (NSABP) trial B-17, a large randomized trial comparing these two treatments (18), as well as a meta-analysis of 12 trials comparing wide excision alone versus wide excision with radiotherapy versus mastectomy (19), found similar results. Recently published long-term findings of a collaborative international study from nine institutions of 259 patients with DCIS treated with conservative surgery and irradiation revealed an actuarial rate of local failure of 19% and an actuarial cause-specific survival rate of 96% at 15 years (20) (Table 7-1). Studies currently under way will help better determine the role of radiotherapy in the treatment of DCIS (17).

Although conservative surgery and irradiation is becoming more widely accepted and is used for the majority of women with DCIS, certain features may indicate the need for mastectomy. These features include diffuse or high-grade lesions and young patient age (17). For women in whom conservative surgery is indicated, several pathologic and histologic features of the tumor are used to determine whether radiotherapy is needed. Of the histologic subtypes—micropapillary, papillary, solid, cribriform, and comedo—the comedo type suggests the most aggressive disease and a higher probability of recurrence and malignant changes. Margin status and lesion size are important pathologic indicators of the risk of recurrence (17). The role of radiotherapy as determined by these prognostic factors is shown in Figure 7-1, which outlines a fairly standard current approach to treating DCIS. Although a standard prognostic classification system for DCIS has yet to be identified, attempts have been made to classify patients according to whether they are candidates for mastectomy, excision with radiation, or excision alone (21).

Early Disease: Stages I and II

Conservative surgery (lumpectomy) followed by radiotherapy is now considered standard treatment for many women with early breast cancer. Long-term results of randomized studies showing comparable survival between patients treated with mastectomy and patients treated with conservative surgery plus irradiation (Table 7-2) (22–28) led in 1990 to the following statement by the National Cancer Institute: "Breast conservation treatment is an appropriate

T A B L E   **7-1**

Actuarial Outcome Data at 5, 10, and 15 Years for Patients with Ductal Carcinoma In Situ Treated with Conservative Surgery and Radiotherapy

Outcome	At 5 Years		At 10 Years		At 15 Years	
	%	**95% CI**	**%**	**95% CI**	**%**	**95% CI**
Overall survival	98	97–100	94	91–97	87	81–93
Cause-specific survival	99	98–100	97	95–99	96	93–99
Freedom from distant metastases	99	98–100	97	95–99	96	94–99
Local failure	7	4–10	16	11–21	19	13–25
Contralateral breast cancer	2	0–4	6	3–9	9	4–13

CI = confidence interval.

Source: Reproduced by permission from Solin LJ, Kurz J, Fourquet A, et al. Fifteen year results of breast conserving surgery and definitive breast irradiation for the treatment of ductal carcinoma in situ (intraductal carcinoma) of the breast. *J Clin Oncol* 1996;14:757.

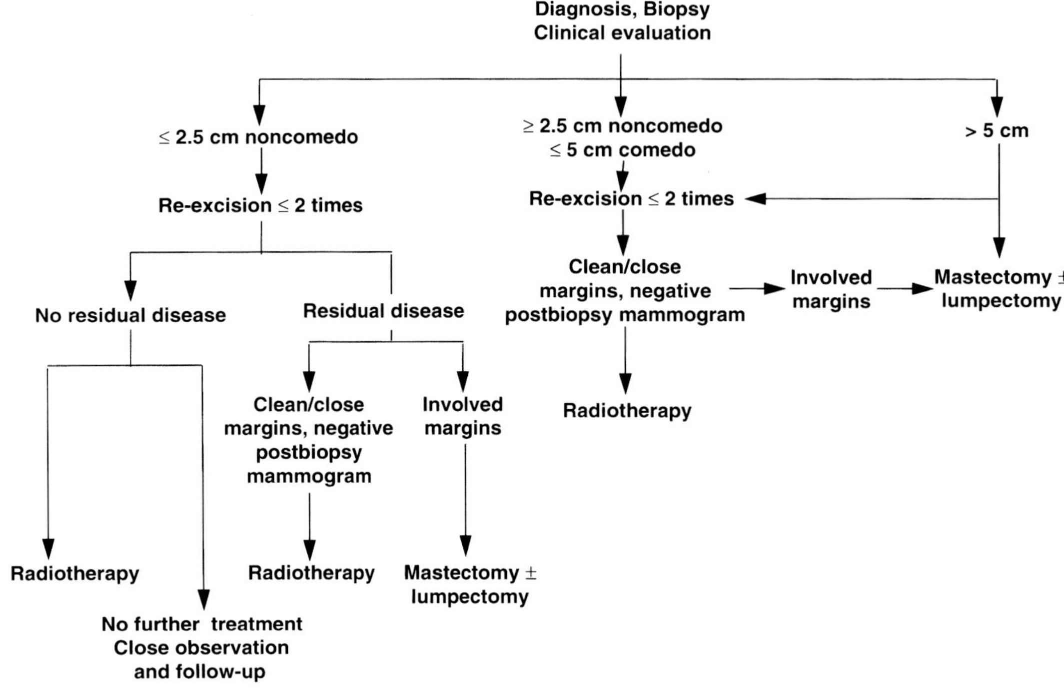

F I G U R E   **7-1**

Management of ductal carcinoma in situ.

method of primary therapy for the majority of women with stage I-II breast cancer and is preferable because it provides survival rates equivalent to those of total mastectomy and axillary dissection while preserving the breast" (29).

Although the majority of stage I and II breast cancer patients are eligible for breast-conserving surgery, the potential increased risk of local failure for some patients requires careful patient selection. A report on standards of care for breast-conserving therapy issued in 1992 by a joint committee of the American College of Surgeons, the American College of Radiology, the College of American Pathologists, and the Society of Surgical Oncology outlines both absolute and relative contraindications for breast-conserving therapy (30). Absolute contraindications include two or more gross tumors in separate quadrants of the breast, diffuse indeterminate or malignant-appearing microcalcifications, and previous irradiation of the region. Breast-conserving therapy is also contraindicated in women in the first or second trimester of pregnancy. Relative contraindications include a large tumor-to-breast ratio, large breast size, tumor located beneath the nipple, and a history

of connective tissue disease. Several of these relative contraindications—for example, large breasts and nipple involvement—are predictors of poorer cosmetic results. The variation between women in expectations and wishes regarding cosmetic outcome makes these contraindications truly relative (31).

Other controversial contraindications potentially associated with increased risk of recurrence are young age, family history of breast cancer, and certain pathologic features of the tumor (32). Two important pathologic features are margin status and the presence of extensive intraductal component (EIC). Figure 7-2 shows a fairly standard approach to the treatment of patients with early disease. Patients with clear margins and those with close margins without EIC are candidates for radiotherapy. Patients with involved margins are generally treated with mastectomy with or without reconstruction, with additional postmastectomy chest wall irradiation given to patients at high risk for recurrence (33). Whether involved margins and the presence of EIC are associated with increased local failure rates remains open to debate, however. A clear and uniform classification

T A B L E   **7-2**

Randomized Trials of Mastectomy Versus Conservative Surgery and Radiotherapy

Trial (Years) (No. of Patients)	Local Recurrence Rate		Survival Rate		Length of Follow-up (Survival)
	M	CS + RT	M	CS + RT	
Gustave-Roussy (22) (1972–1979) (n = 179)	14%*	9%*	65%	73%	15 y
NCI Milan (23,24) (1973–1980) (n = 701)	2%	4%	69%	71%	13 y
NSABP B-06 (25) (1976–1984) (n = 1843)	8%	10%	71%	76%	8 y
NCI (26) (1979–1987) (n = 237)	6%	20%	85%	89%	5 y
EORTC (27) (1980–1986) (n = 903)	9%	13%	75%	75%	7 y
Danish Breast Cancer Group (1983–1987) (n = 905)	4%	3%	82%	79%	6 y

*First cause of failure.

CS = conservative surgery; EORTC = European Organization for Research and Treatment of Cancer; M = mastectomy; NCI = National Cancer Institute; NSABP = National Surgical Adjuvant Breast and Bowel Project; RT = radiotherapy.

Source: Reproduced by permission from Harris JR, Morrow M. Treatment of early-stage breast cancer. In: Harris JR, Morrow M, Hellman S, eds. *Diseases of the breast.* Philadelphia: Lippincott-Raven, 1996:492–493.

system for margin status is still lacking among treatment centers (32), and while the results of several studies indicate that EIC is associated with increased local failure rates (34,35), other findings do not (36).

Regardless of the extent of excision (mastectomy or lumpectomy), the addition of radiotherapy significantly improves local disease control and results in a demonstrated survival benefit. This is confirmed by long-term results from the Stockholm trial of postmastectomy irradiation (4) (Table 7-3) and by the more recent studies on conservative surgery (24,37–39). In addition, the extent to which radiotherapy is needed to achieve local control is reflected in data from the NSABP B-06 trial, which showed a significantly higher rate of mastectomies among node-negative patients initially treated with lumpectomy alone than among patients treated with lumpectomy and irradiation (84% versus 66%, $p = 0.006$) (40). Maintenance of

local control is clearly important because it spares patients the physical and psychological hardships associated with a recurrence. The effect of local control on survival, although highly controversial, appears to grow over time, and recent findings strongly suggest a small but clinically important survival benefit with radiation (41,42) (Tables 7-3 and 7-4).

Of current interest is the definition of subgroups of patients with early breast cancer in whom radiotherapy may not be needed. Since systemic adjuvant therapies are now a standard part of treatment for patients with breast disease of all stages, even node-negative disease, it is important to be able to identify patients in whom further adjuvant treatment is unnecessary to avoid the unnecessary psychological, economic, and physical costs of extra treatment. To date, subgroups of patients in whom radiotherapy can safely be withheld have not been identified (43).

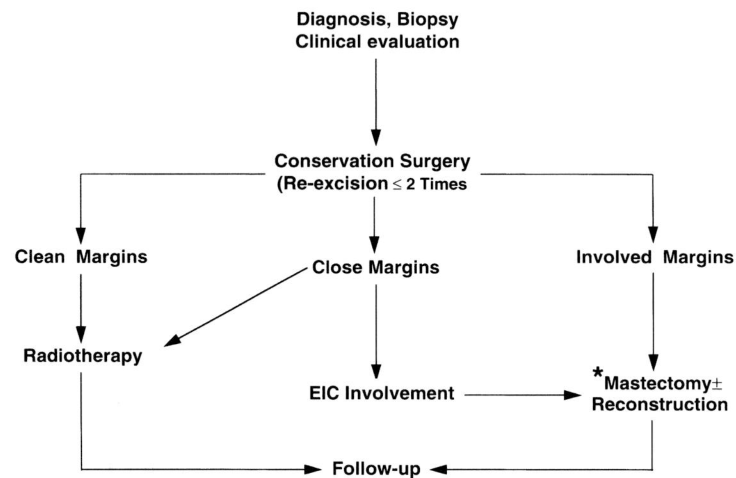

F I G U R E   **7-2**

Management of early breast cancer. *Postmastectomy radiation for selected patients

T A B L E   **7-3**

Stockholm Trial of Postoperative Radiotherapy

Event	Postoperative Radiotherapy		Surgery Alone		Rate Ratio (95% Confidence Interval)	*p* Value (Log-Rank)
	Patients	Events (%)	Patients	Events (%)		
Pathologically negative nodes	204		197			
Treatment failure*		74 (36%)		99 (50%)	0.65 (0.48–0.88)	<0.01
Local-regional recurrence		10 (5%)		45 (23%)	0.25 (0.15–0.42)	<0.001
Distant metastases		52 (26%)		49 (25%)	1.02 (0.69–1.50)	0.94
Death		66 (33%)		74 (38%)	0.87 (0.63–1.21)	0.40
Breast cancer death		47 (23%)		43 (22%)	1.05 (0.70–1.59)	0.80
Pathologically positive nodes	118		120			
Treatment failure*		76 (64%)		94 (78%)	0.64 (0.47–0.87)	<0.01
Local-regional recurrence		18 (15%)		58 (48%)	0.29 (0.18–0.45)	<0.001
Distant metastases		61 (52%)		83 (69%)	0.66 (0.48–0.92)	0.02
Death		72 (61%)		84 (70%)	0.82 (0.60–1.12)	0.21
Breast cancer death		59 (50%)		81 (68%)	0.70 (0.50–0.98)	0.04

*Treatment failure defined as local-regional recurrence, distant metastases, or death without recurrence.

Source: Reproduced by permission from Harris JR, Morrow M. Treatment of early-stage breast cancer. In: Harris JR, Morrow M, Hellman S, eds. *Diseases of the breast*. Philadelphia: Lippincott-Raven Publishers, 1996:514. Data from Ruqvist L, Pettersson D, Johansson M. Adjuvant radiation therapy versus surgery alone in operable breast cancer: long-term follow-up in a randomized clinical trial. *Radiat Oncol* 1993;26:104.

Locally Advanced Disease

The current standard treatment for locally advanced disease favors a multimodal approach that combines primary chemotherapy, adjuvant radiotherapy, and either mastectomy or lumpectomy. Several studies indicate the increased benefit to locoregional control and survival with multimodality therapy. A study by Klefstrom et al of 120 stage III breast cancer patients randomized into three different treatment schemes, surgery plus chemotherapy, surgery plus radiotherapy, and surgery plus radiotherapy plus chemotherapy, reported a 5-year disease-free survival of 30%, 22%, and 67%, respectively (44). Another study by Perez et al, which examined three different treatment schemes of combined mastectomy and radiotherapy with or

TABLE 7-4

Five-Year Survival Benefit with the Addition of Radiotherapy to Lumpectomy in Node-Negative Breast Cancer Patients: Combined Results of Uppsala-Orebro, Canadian, and NSABP B-06 Trials*

Treatment	Overall Survival	Difference in Survival	Probability of a Positive Treatment Effect	Annual Mortality Rate	Relative Reduction in Annual Mortality Rate (SE)
Lumpectomy	87.5%	—	—	2.7%	—
Lumpectomy + RT	88.7%	1.27%	79%	2.4%	9.6% (±13.7%)

RT = radiotherapy; SE = standard error.

*Based on bayesian analysis.

Source: Reproduced by permission from Levitt SL, Aeppli DM, Nierengarten ME. The impact of radiation on early breast carcinoma survival: a bayesian analysis. *Cancer* 1996;78:1038.

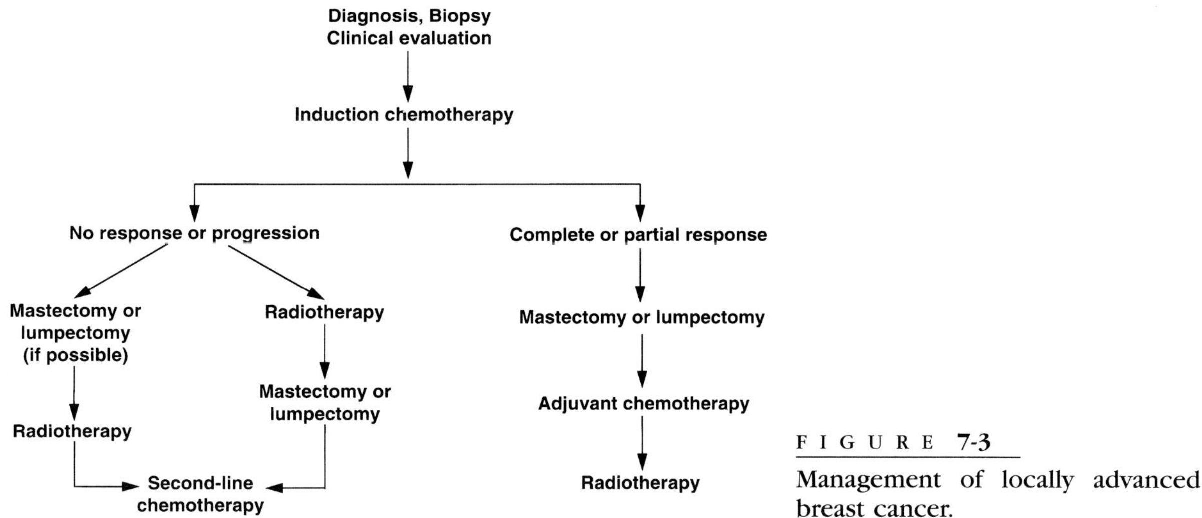

FIGURE 7-3

Management of locally advanced breast cancer.

without chemotherapy in locally advanced non-inflammatory breast cancer patients, reported locoregional tumor control at 5 years of 91% for combined chemotherapy, radiotherapy, and mastectomy, 80% for irradiation and mastectomy, 54% for irradiation and chemotherapy, and 31% for irradiation alone. Corresponding actuarial 10-year disease-free survival rates were 36%, 19%, 10%, and 11% (45). The benefit of treating patients with adjuvant irradiation in combination with systemic therapy and surgery is further highlighted in a recent study by Fisher et al that examined the significance of extracapsular nodal extension (ECE) on locoregional failure and survival in 82 stage II or III breast cancer patients treated by systemic chemotherapy or hormonal therapy without locoregional radiation (46). Based on the patterns of failure of these patients, the authors recommended breast/chest wall and supraclavicular radiation for all patients with pathological evidence of ECE who have had a level I and II axillary dis-section regardless of the number of positive axillary nodes.

The use of induction chemotherapy followed by surgery and radiation is another approach to treating locally advanced patients. The use of primary chemotherapy developed after trials of radiation alone failed to provide optimal treatment because of increased complications stemming from the need for higher radiation dose to control gross disease (47–49). Good tumor shrinkage with the use of induction chemotherapy resulted in trials that examined whether adjuvant radiotherapy or mastectomy offered better local control. Two randomized trials failed to show any significant difference in relapse rates or survival between the two treatments when they were combined with chemotherapy (50,51).

The sequencing of mastectomy and radiation after primary chemotherapy for advanced disease is uncertain. Many centers perform surgery first after chemotherapy and reserve

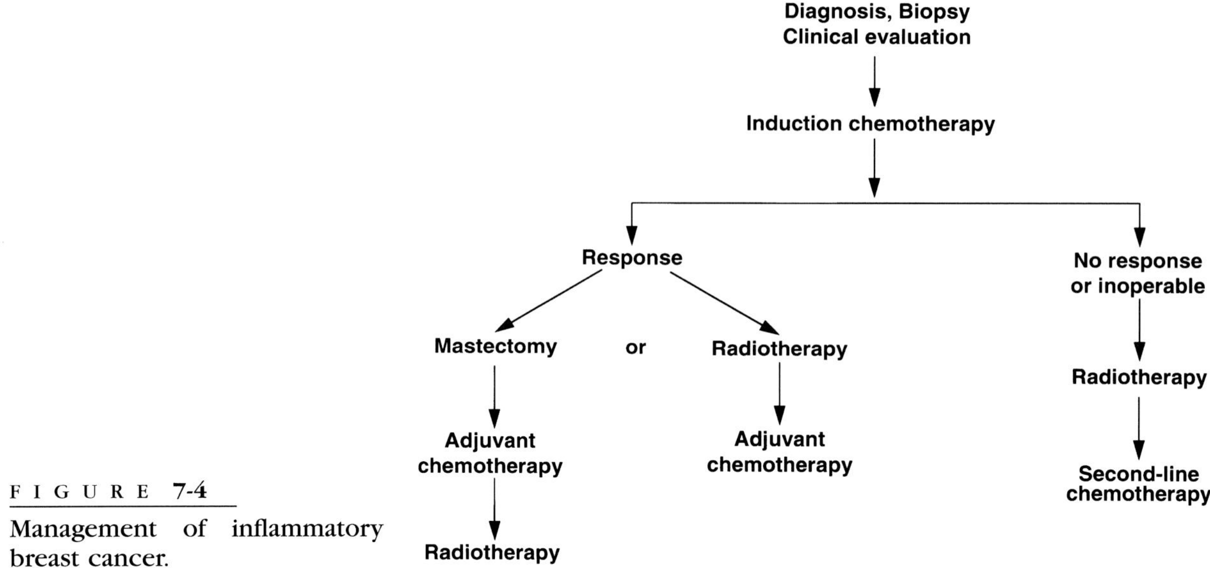

F I G U R E **7-4**

Management of inflammatory breast cancer.

radiotherapy to the chest wall and nodal areas until the completion of chemotherapy (52). Results from the National Cancer Institute of Italy and the University of Texas M. D. Anderson Cancer Center suggest the inclusion of maintenance chemotherapy after this regimen to improve outcomes (53,54). A fairly standard approach to treating locally advanced disease is shown in Figure 7-3. A similar combined-modality approach is used for patients with inflammatory disease and is shown in Figure 7-4.

Other approaches under investigation for the treatment of advanced disease also suggest an important role for radiotherapy. Breast-conserving therapy followed by radiation is one approach that has produced favorable results in carefully selected patients. Studies from the M. D. Anderson Cancer Center demonstrated local recurrence rates of less than 10% in carefully selected patients who respond well to systemic chemotherapy (55–58). In these studies, patient selection for breast-conserving therapy after neoadjuvant chemotherapy was based on tumor size (solitary primary tumor of 4 cm or less or two primary tumors within a sphere of 4 cm); the absence of skin involvement or tumor fixation to the chest wall; a tumor-to-breast ratio favorable for cosmetic outcomes; the absence of palpable or small, low, mobile axillary lymph nodes; the absence of collagen vascular disease; and the absence of extensive lymphatic involvement in the breast (58). Total excision of the gross tumor in these patients allowed for a reduced radiation dose to avoid cosmetic complications. Other studies also indicate breast-conserving therapy for some patients with locally advanced disease (59), although recommendations for standard care in these patients must await long-term results.

The combined use of radiotherapy and autologous bone marrow transplantation after conventional or high-dose chemotherapy is another treatment under investigation for advanced disease. Early results from a pilot study by the Cancer and Leukemia Group B of stage II and III patients with 10 or more positive nodes treated with mastectomy followed by conventional-dose plus high-dose chemotherapy with autologous bone marrow transplantation and radiotherapy indicate that the addition of radiotherapy helps to lower the frequency of chest wall and regional lymph node recurrence (60,61). The pilot study concluded that radiotherapy is an important component of this treatment regimen. Later analysis demonstrated that the high frequency of hematologic toxicity found with the addition of radiotherapy in this study was primarily due to the lower blood cell counts of patients prior to radiotherapy (62).

Specific Issues in Radiotherapy for Breast Cancer

Node-Negative Patients

Studies are examining whether breast-conserving surgery without radiotherapy is indicated in certain subsets of node-negative patients. Results so far do not indicate a group of patients in whom adjuvant radiotherapy can be omitted without compromise of optimal local disease control (43).

Pregnant Patients

Radiotherapy is contraindicated in pregnant patients because it is not possible to shield the fetus from internal radiation scatter. Lumpectomy and axillary dissection during the third trimester followed by radiotherapy after delivery is possible (52).

Older Women

Different treatment for older women based on age has not yet been indicated. For early-stage disease, conservative surgery with radiotherapy is a viable option, as it is in younger patients. Because disease is often more indolent in women older than 65, studies are under way to determine whether less aggressive treatment is adequate for these women. The Cancer and Leukemia Group B is conducting a study to assess whether radiotherapy can be omitted in some of these women with early-stage T1-2 disease (63).

Radiotherapy after Local Recurrence

For most women treated initially with mastectomy, the treatment of a local recurrence with radiotherapy results in complete disease regression. However, a large number of women still have a further locoregional recurrence, which may be due to delayed radiotherapy or inadequate technique (4,64,65). One good argument for the use of prophylactic irradiation after mastectomy is the difficulty of controlling locoregional disease once it recurs. The 16-year follow-up of the Stockholm study of adjuvant radiotherapy versus surgery alone found that the overall proportion of patients with locoregional disease at death or last follow-up was significantly higher among patients treated with surgery alone than it was among patients treated with adjuvant radiotherapy (16% versus 6%, $p < 0.01$) (4).

The importance of adequate technique is highlighted by a series of patients treated with radiotherapy for recurrence at the Mallinckrodt Institute of Radiology. The 5-year failure rate was 25% when adequate chest wall irradiation was given but 64% when only small fields were treated. An adequate radiation technique significantly reduced the risk of further recurrence in the supraclavicular nodes from 16% in untreated patients to 6% in irradiated patients (64). This study showed that achievement of long-term local control is highly dependent on the volume of disease remaining at the time of irradiation (Table 7-5). For gross disease that precludes excision, a proper radiation dose is necessary to achieve local control. A detailed discussion of the appropriate radiation technique for achieving long-term control after recurrence can be found elsewhere (66).

Studies on the use of radiotherapy to treat recurrences in patients treated initially with mastectomy and irradiation are few and small, although the results do indicate some palliative benefit from limited doses of radiation. Similarly, there is little information on the use of

T A B L E **7-5**

Chances of In-field Tumor Recurrence According to Radiation Dose and Extent of Surgery*

Dose (Gy)	Complete Excision	Residual Tumor ≤ 3 cm	Tumor > 3 cm or Diffuse or Multiple Tumors
≤49.99	1/9 (11%)	2/7 (29%)	7/8 (88%)
50–54.99	1/26 (4%)	1/5 (20%)	7/15 (47%)
55–59.99	1/21 (5%)	2/9 (22%)	2/11 (18%)
60–64.99	4/22 (18%)	0/9 (0%)	10/20 (50%)
≥65	0/2 (0%)	0/6 (0%)	7/15 (47%)

*Patients treated to small fields excluded.

Source: Reproduced by permission from Recht A, Hayes DF, Eberkin TJ, Sadowsky NL. Local-regional recurrence after mastectomy or breast conserving therapy. In: Harris JR, Lippman ME, Morrow M, Hellman S, eds. *Diseases of the breast*. Philadelphia: Lippincott-Raven, 1996:653. Data from Halvorson KJ, Perez CA, Kuske RR, et al. Isolated local-regional recurrence of breast cancer following mastectomy: radiotherapeutic management. *Int J Radiat Oncol Biol Phys* 1990;19:851.

radiotherapy to treat recurrences after breast-conserving surgery either alone or with irradiation, with several small studies reporting inconclusive results (66). Five recent randomized trials of the combined use of radiotherapy and hyperthermia to treat recurrent breast cancer revealed promising results for control of local disease (67).

Complications

Many of the acute complications of modern radiotherapy, such as erythema, edema, and mild tiredness, are short-term conditions that become neither chronic nor life-threatening. Chronic, more serious conditions such as arm edema, decreased arm mobility, soft tissue necrosis, rib fractures, radiation pneumonitis, and brachial plexopathy are possible but occur very infrequently when an appropriate radiation technique is used (31). Improved radiation techniques have also minimized radiation-induced cardiac morbidity and carcinogenesis, which were major complications prior to modern radiotherapy. Cause-specific mortality data from the updated Cuzick meta-analysis show that cardiac deaths accounted for increased mortality in the older trials that used orthovoltage techniques (2). The updated Cuzick meta-analysis and a combined analysis of the Stockholm and Oslo trials (14) showed that increased cardiac morbidity and mortality were not evident with the use of modern megavoltage techniques. A further study from Stockholm showed that patients who received the highest volume of irradiation had the most increased risk of cardiac mortality (68).

The risk of radiation-induced cancers, including sarcomas, leukemia, and lung cancer, has substantially decreased with the current technique of treating only the tangential breast fields. Among breast cancer patients currently treated with radiotherapy, the excess risk of death due to radiation-induced cardiac mortality or secondary cancers is estimated to be less than 1%. Patients younger than 45 at the time of diagnosis and treatment have a higher risk of radiation-related contralateral breast cancer, whereas patients older than 45 have little if any risk (69,70).

A fairly new concern is the development of breast cancer after chest irradiation for Hodgkin's disease. A recent study indicated a high risk for women treated with radiotherapy for childhood Hodgkin's disease (71). Women who were 16 years or younger at the time of treatment had the highest risk of developing breast cancer.

Radiotherapy and Systemic Therapies

For both early and advanced breast cancer, study results indicate improved local control and survival with the combined use of adjuvant radiotherapy and chemotherapy after breast-conserving surgery or mastectomy. This is especially true for patients with four or more positive nodes. Studies reported a locoregional recurrence rate of 10% in patients with one to three positive nodes treated with chemotherapy alone compared with 20% to 30% in patients with four or more positive nodes or primary tumors 5 cm or larger (72–75). For these women at high risk, the combination of chemotherapy and radiotherapy produces better locoregional control and disease-free survival rates than either adjuvant modality alone does (76,77).

The proper sequencing of radiotherapy and chemotherapy after surgery remains an important and controversial aspect of treatment. A recently published trial by the Joint Center for Radiation Therapy examined this question in a subgroup of patients considered at increased risk for systemic metastases (i.e., nearly all the patients had positive nodes). In that trial, 244 stage I and II patients treated with breast-conserving surgery were randomly assigned to receive a 12-week course of chemotherapy either before or after radiotherapy (78). At a median follow-up in surviving patients of 58 months, the authors found an increased risk of local recurrence in the group who received chemotherapy first (14% versus 5%) and an increased risk of distant recurrence in the group who received radiotherapy first (32% versus 20%). These results suggest that a 12-week course of chemotherapy before radiotherapy may result in a better outcome for patients at increased risk for systemic metastases. Although the possible detrimental effects of delaying radiotherapy were not addressed in this study, an earlier study by the same authors found that delaying radiotherapy for more than 16 weeks after surgery resulted in a 5-year actuarial local control rate of 28% versus 5% in patients treated within 16 weeks (79). Similarly, another study reported a significant increase in the relapse rate at 5 years for women in whom radiotherapy was not delivered until at least 120 days after surgery (80). Other studies, however, found no difference in local control rates based on the timing of radiation delivery (81,82).

Quality of Life

Survival remains the primary goal of breast cancer treatment, but it is not the only goal. This fact is emphasized by the shift from radical mastectomy to breast-conserving therapy for many women with early breast cancer. Many women who opt for breast-conserving therapy rather than mastectomy have a better body image and sexual functioning without an increased fear of recurrence (83). However, in some women the fear of recurrence associated with breast-conserving surgery outweighs the possible benefit of improved cosmesis (84). Addressing the different expectations and desires of each woman in her treatment choice is integral to incorporating quality-of-life considerations into the decision-making process. In addition, good communication between physician and patient is important to help manage the anxiety and depression that frequently accompany the diagnosis and treatment of this disease and that diminish the quality of life. A pilot study that assessed the main treatment factors affecting quality of life in breast cancer patients found that patient-centered care (tailoring treatment choice to fit the particular needs and wishes of each patient), good communication between physician and patient, psychological support from the physician, the availability of additional services to help provide emotional support, and continuity of care affected quality of life during treatment (85). A compendium of different tests to measure quality of life in breast cancer patients was recently published (86).

Conclusions

Radiotherapy is an integral part of breast cancer management. Radiotherapy after mastectomy or conservative surgery significantly improves local control rates and has a demonstrated ability to improve survival. Appropriate radiotherapy technique is critical for optimal disease control and improved survival, as reflected in the better outcomes of trials that employed modern radiotherapy techniques. Essential to a good radiation oncology center is a state-of-the-art team of radiation oncologists, medical physicists, and technicians, as well as state-of-the-art equipment, including linear accelerators, simulators, and treatment-planning computers. With improved treatment planning and delivery, radiotherapy is becoming increasingly effective in delivering optimal doses to the tumor while minimizing doses to normal tissue. In breast cancer management, the incidence of complications following chest wall irradiation has been drastically reduced, as has the incidence of radiation-induced malignancies.

Acknolwedgments

I wish to thank Mary Beth Nierengarten for editorial assistance.

REFERENCES

1. Mansfield CM. *Early breast cancer: its history and results of treatment. Experimental biology and medicine: monographs on interdisciplinary topics*, vol. 5. Basel: S. Karger, 1976.

2. Cuzick J, Stewart H, Rutqvist L, et al. Cause-specific mortality in long-term survivors of breast cancer who participated in trials of radiotherapy. *J Clin Oncol* 1994;12:447–453.

3. Host H, Brennhovd IO. The effect of post-operative radiation therapy in breast cancer. *Int J Radiat Oncol Biol Phys* 1977;2:1061–1067.

4. Rutqvist LE, Pettersson D, Johansson H. Adjuvant radiation therapy versus surgery alone in operable breast cancer: long-term follow-up of a randomized clinical trial. *Radiother Oncol* 1993;26:104–110.

5. Uematsu M, Boarnstein BA, Recht A, et al. Long-term results of post-operative radiation therapy following mastectomy with or without chemotherapy in stage I-III breast cancer. *Int J Radiat Oncol Biol Phys* 1993;25:765–779.

6. Cuzick J, Stewart H, Peto R, et al. Overview of randomized trials comparing radical mastectomy without radiotherapy against simple mastectomy with radiotherapy in breast cancer. *Cancer Treat Rep* 1987;71:7–14.

7. Cuzick J, Stewart H, Peto R, et al. Overview of randomized trials of postoperative adjuvant radiotherapy in breast cancer. *Cancer Treat Rep* 1987;71:15–25.

8. Stjernsward J. Can survival be decreased by postoperative irradiation? *Int J Radiat Oncol Biol Phys* 1977;2:1171–1175.

9. Bonadonna G, Brusamolino E, Valagussa P, et al. Combination chemotherapy as an adjuvant treatment in operable breast cancer. *N Engl J Med* 1976;294:405–410.

10. Fisher B, Redmond C, Elias EG, et al. Adjuvant chemotherapy for breast cancer: an overview of NSABP findings. *Int Adv Surg Oncol* 1982;5:65–90.

11. Fisher B. Laboratory and clinical research in breast cancer—a personal adventure: the David A. Karnofsky Memorial Lecture. *Cancer Res* 1980;40:3863–3874.

12. Fletcher GH, McNeese MD, Owald MJ. Long-range results for breast cancer patients treated by radical mastectomy and postoperative radiation without adjuvant chemotherapy: an update. *Int J Radiat Oncol Biol Phys* 1989;17:11–14.

13. Levitt SH. Is there a role for post-operative adjuvant radiation in breast cancer? Beautiful hypothesis versus ugly facts. 1987 Gilbert H. Fletcher Lecture. *Int J Radiat Oncol Biol Phys* 1988;14:787–796.

14. Auquier A, Rutqvist LE, Host H, et al. Postmastectomy megavoltage radiotherapy: the Oslo and Stockholm trials. *Eur J Cancer* 1992;28:433–437.

15. Tubiana M. Postoperative radiotherapy and the pattern of distant spread in breast cancer. In: Fletcher GH, Levitt SH, eds. *Non-disseminated breast cancer: controversial issues in management.* Berlin: Springer, 1993:11–26.

16. Hellman S. Karnofsky Memorial Lecture. Natural history of small breast cancers. *J Clin Oncol* 1994;12:2229–2234.

17. Wood WC. Management of lobular carcinoma in situ and ductal carcinoma in situ of the breast. *Semin Oncol* 1996;23:446–452.

18. Fisher ER, Constantino J, Fisher B, et al. Pathologic findings from the National Surgical Adjuvant Breast Project (NSABP) protocol B-17. *Cancer* 1995;75:1310–1319.

19. Bradley SJ, Weaver DW, Bouwman DL. Alternatives in the surgical management of in situ breast cancer. A meta-analysis of outcome. *Am Surg* 1990;56:428–432.

20. Solin LJ, Kurz J, Fourquet A, et al. Fifteen year results of breast conserving surgery and definitive breast irradiation for the treatment of ductal carcinoma in situ (intraductal carcinoma of the breast). *J Clin Oncol* 1996;14:754–763.

21. Silverstein MJ, Poller DN, Waisman JR, et al. Prognostic classification of breast ductal carcinoma-in-situ. *Lancet* 1995;345:1154–1157.

22. Arriagada R, Le MG, Rochard F, Contesso G. Conservative treatment versus mastectomy in early breast cancer: patterns of failure with 15 years of follow-up results. *J Clin Oncol* 1996;14:1558–1564.

23. Veronesi U, Banfi A, Salvadori B, et al. Breast conservation is the treatment of choice in small breast cancer: long-term results of a randomized clinical trial. *Eur J Cancer* 1990;26:668–670.

24. Veronesi U, Luini A, Galimberti V, Zurrida S. Conservation approaches for the management of stage I/II carcinoma of the breast: Milan Cancer Institute trials. *World J Surg* 1994;18:70–75.

25. Fisher B, Redmond C, Poisson R, et al. Eight-year results of a randomized clinical trial comparing total mastectomy and lumpectomy with or without irradiation in the treatment of breast cancer. *N Engl J Med* 1989;320:822–828.

26. Lichter A, Lippman M, Danforth D, et al. Mastectomy versus breast conserving therapy in the treatment of stage I and II carcinoma of the breast: a randomized trial at the National Cancer Institute. *J Clin Oncol* 1992;10:976–983.

27. van Dongen JA, Bartelink H, Fentiman IS, et al. Randomized clinical trial to assess the value of breast-conserving therapy in stage I and II breast cancer: EORTC 10801 trial. *Monogr Natl Cancer Inst* 1992;11:15–18.

28. Blichert-Toft M, Rose C, Andersen J, et al. Danish randomized trial comparing breast conservation therapy with mastectomy: six years of life-table analysis. *Monogr Natl Cancer Inst* 1992;11:19–25.

29. NIH Consensus Conference. Treatment of early-stage breast cancer. *JAMA* 1991;265:391–395.

30. Winchester D, Cox J. Standards for breast conservation treatment. *CA Cancer J Clin* 1992;42:134–162.

31. Harris JR, Morrow M. Local management of invasive breast cancer. In: Harris JR, Lippman ME, Morrow M, Hellman S, eds. *Diseases of the breast.* Philadelphia: Lippincott-Raven, 1996:487–547.

32. Recht A. Selection of patients with early stage invasive breast cancer for treatment with conservative surgery and radiation therapy. *Semin Oncol* 1996;23:19–30.

33. Love S, Parker B, Ames M, et al. Practice guidelines for breast cancer. *Cancer J Sci Am* 1996;2(suppl 3A):S7–S21.

34. Paterson DA, Anderson TJ, Jack WJL, et al. Pathological features predictive of local recur-

rence after management by conservation of invasive breast cancer: importance of noninvasive carcinoma. *Radiother Oncol* 1992;25:176–180.

35. Vicini FA, Recht A, Abner A, et al. Recurrence in the breast following conservative surgery and radiation therapy for early-stage breast cancer. *Monogr Natl Cancer Inst* 1992;11:33–39.

36. Solin LJ, Fowble BL, Schultz DJ, Goodman RL. The significance of the pathology margins of the tumor excision on the outcome of patients treated with definitive irradiation for early stage breast cancer. *Int J Radiat Oncol Biol Phys* 1991;21:279–287.

37. Fisher B, Anderson S, Redmond CK, et al. Reanalysis and results after 12 years of follow-up in a randomized clinical trial comparing total mastectomy with lumpectomy with or without irradiation in the treatment of breast cancer. *N Engl J Med* 1995;333:1456–1461.

38. Liljegren G, Holmberg L, Adami HO, et al. Sector resection with or without postoperative radiotherapy for stage I breast cancer: five-year results of a randomized trial. Uppsala-Orebro Breast Cancer Study Group. *J Natl Cancer Inst* 1994;86:717–722.

39. Whelan T, Clark R, Roberts R, et al. Ipsilateral breast tumor recurrence postlumpectomy is predictive of subsequent mortality: results from a randomized trial. Investigators of the Ontario Clinical Oncology Group. *Int J Radiat Oncol Biol Phys* 1994;30:11–16.

40. Kemperman H, Borger J, Hart A, et al. Prognostic factors for survival after breast conserving therapy for stage I and II breast cancer. The role of local recurrence. *Eur J Cancer* 1995;31A: 690–698.

41. Levitt SH, Aeppli DM, Nierengarten ME. The impact of radiation on early breast carcinoma survival: a bayesian analysis. *Cancer* 1996;78: 1035–1042.

42. National Cancer Institute. Reanalysis of the NSABP protocol B06, Emmes Corporation. CancerNet, National Cancer Institute, April 11, 1994.

43. Morrow M, Harris JR, Schnitt SJ. Local control following breast-conserving surgery for invasive cancer: results of clinical trials. *J Natl Cancer Inst* 1995;87:125–129.

44. Klefstrom P, Grohn P, Heinonen E, et al. Adjuvant postoperative radiotherapy, chemotherapy, and immunotherapy in stage III breast cancer. II. 5-year results and influence of levamisole. *Cancer* 1987;60:936–942.

45. Perez CA, Graham ML, Taylor ME, et al. Management of locally advanced carcinoma of the breast. I. Non-inflammatory. *Cancer* 1994;74: 453–465.

46. Fisher BJ, Perera FE, Cooke AL, et al. Extracapsular axillary extension in patients receiving adjuvant systemic therapy: an indication for radiotherapy. *Int J Radiat Oncol Biol Phys* 1982; 8:31–36.

47. Bedwinek J, Rao D, Perez C. Stage III and localized stage IV breast cancer: irradiation alone vs. irradiation plus surgery. *Int J Radiat Oncol Biol Phys* 1982;8:31–36.

48. Sheldon T, Hayes DF, Cady B, et al. Primary radiation for locally advanced breast cancer. *Cancer* 1987;60:1219–1225.

49. Spanos W, Montague E, Fletcher G. Late complications of radiation only for advanced breast cancer. *Int J Radiat Oncol Biol Phys* 1980;6: 1473–1476.

50. DeLena M, Varini M, Zucali R. Multimodal treatment for locally advanced breast cancer. *Cancer Clin Trials* 1981;4:229–236.

51. Perloff M, Lesnick G, Korzun A. Combination chemotherapy with mastectomy or radiotherapy for stage III breast carcinoma: a Cancer and Leukemia Group B study. *J Clin Oncol* 1988; 6:261–269.

52. Harris JR, Morrow M, Bonadonna G. Cancer of the breast. In: De Vita VT, Hellman S, Rosenberg SA, eds. *Cancer: principles and practices of oncology.* 4th ed. Philadelphia: JB Lippincott, 1993:1264–1332.

53. Hortobagyi GN. Comprehensive management of locally advanced breast cancer. *Cancer* 1990; 66:1367–1391.

54. Valagussa P, Zambetti M, Bonadonna G. Prognostic factors in locally advanced noninflammatory breast cancer. Long-term results following primary chemotherapy. *Breast Cancer Res Treat* 1990;15:137–147.

55. Feldman LD, Hortobagyi GN, Buzdar AU, et al. Pathological assessment of response to induction chemotherapy in breast cancer. *Cancer Res* 1986;46:2578–2581.

56. Hortobagyi GN, Blumenschein GR, Spanos W, et al. Multimodal treatment of locoregionally advanced breast cancer. *Cancer* 1983;51: 763–768.

57. Segel MC, Paulus DD, Hortobagyi GH. Advanced primary breast cancer: assessment at

mammography of response to induction chemotherapy. *Radiology* 1988;169:49–54.

58. Singletary SE, McNeese MD, Hortobagyi GN. Feasibility of breast-conservation surgery after induction chemotherapy for locally advanced breast carcinoma. *Cancer* 1992;69:2849–2852.

59. Kuske RR, Farr GH, Harris K, et al. Is breast preservation possible in women with large, locally advanced breast cancers? *J La State Med Soc* 1993;145:165–167.

60. Marks LB, Halperin EC, Prosnitz LR, et al. Post-mastectomy radiotherapy following adjuvant chemotherapy and autologous bone marrow transplantation for breast cancer patients with ≤10 positive axillary lymph nodes. *Int J Radiat Oncol Biol Phys* 1992;23:1021–1026.

61. Peters WP, Ross M, Vredenburgh JJ, et al. High-dose chemotherapy and autologous bone marrow support as consolidation after standard-dose adjuvant therapy for high-risk primary breast cancer. *J Clin Oncol* 1993;11:1132–1143.

62. Marks LB, Rosner GL, Prosnitz LR, et al. The impact of conventional plus high dose chemotherapy with autologous bone marrow transplantation on hematologic toxicity during subsequent local-regional radiotherapy for breast cancer. *Cancer* 1994;74:2964–2971.

63. Shank B. Ageism or acumen—the treatment of older women with breast cancer. *Int J Radiat Oncol Biol Phys* 1996;34:753–754.

64. Halverson KJ, Perez CA, Kuske RR, et al. Isolated local-regional recurrence of breast cancer following mastectomy: radiotherapeutic management. *Int J Radiat Oncol Biol Phys* 1990;19:851–858.

65. Kenda R, Lozza L, Zucali R. Results of irradiation in the treatment of chest wall recurrent breast cancer. *Radiother Oncol* 1992;24:S41. Abstract.

66. Recht A, Hayes DF, Eberlein TJ, Sadowsky NL. Local-regional recurrence after mastectomy or breast-conserving therapy. In: Harris JR, Lippman ME, Morrow M., Hellman S, eds. *Diseases of the breast*. Philadelphia: Lippincott-Raven, 1996:649–667.

67. Vernon CC, Hand JW, Field SB, et al. Radiotherapy with or without hyperthermia in the treatment of superficial localized breast cancer: results from five randomized controlled trials. *Int J Radiat Oncol Biol Phys* 1996;35:731–744.

68. Rutqvist LE, Lax I, Fornander T, Johansson H. Cardiovascular mortality in a randomized trial of adjuvant radiation versus surgery alone in primary breast cancer. *Int J Radiat Oncol Biol Phys* 1992;22:887–896.

69. Boice JD Jr, Harvey EB, Blettner M, et al. Cancer in the contralateral breast after radiotherapy for breast cancer. *N Engl J Med* 1992;326:781–785.

70. Shapiro CL, Recht A. Late effects of adjuvant therapy for breast cancer. *Monogr Natl Cancer Inst* 1994;16:101–112.

71. Bhatia S, Robison LL, Oberlin O, et al. Breast cancer and other second neoplasms after childhood Hodgkin's disease. *N Engl J Med* 1996;334:745–751.

72. Fowble B. The role of postmastectomy adjuvant radiotherapy for operable breast cancer. In: Fowble B, Goodman RL, Glick JH, Rosato EF, eds. *Breast cancer treatment: a comprehensive guide to management*. St. Louis: Mosby-Year Book, 1991:289–309.

73. Griem KL, Henderson IC, Gelman R, et al. The 5-year results of a randomized trial of adjuvant radiation therapy after chemotherapy in breast cancer patients treated with mastectomy. *J Clin Oncol* 1987;5:1546–1555.

74. Stefanik D, Goldberg R, Byrne P, et al. Local-regional failure in patients treated with adjuvant chemotherapy for breast cancer. *J Clin Oncol* 1985;3:660–665.

75. Sykes HF, Sim DA, Wong CJ, et al. Local-regional recurrence in breast cancer after mastectomy and Adriamycin-based adjuvant chemotherapy: evaluation of the role of postoperative radiotherapy. *Int J Radiat Oncol Biol Phys* 1989;16:641–647.

76. Overgaard M, Christensen JJ, Johansen H, et al. Evaluation of radiotherapy in high-risk breast cancer patients: report from the Danish Breast Cancer Cooperative Group (DBCG 82) trial. *Int J Radiat Oncol Biol Phys* 1990;19:1121–1124.

77. Ragaz J, Jackson SM, Plenderleith IH, et al. Can adjuvant radiotherapy improve the overall survival of breast cancer patients in the presence of adjuvant chemotherapy? 10 year analysis of the British Columbia randomized trial. *Proc Am Soc Clin Oncol* 1993;12:10. Abstract.

78. Recht A, Come SE, Henderson IC, et al. The sequencing of chemotherapy and radiation therapy after conservative surgery for early-stage breast cancer. *N Engl J Med* 1996;334:1356–1361.

79. Recht A, Harris JR, Come SE. Sequencing of irradiation and chemotherapy for early-stage breast cancer. *Oncology* 1994;8:19–28.

80. Hartsell WF, Recine DC, Griem KL, Murthy AK. Delaying the initiation of intact breast irradiation for patients with lymph node positive breast cancer increases the risk of local recurrence. *Cancer* 1995;76:2497–2503.

81. McCormick B, Norton L, Yao TJ, et al. The impact of the sequence of radiation and chemotherapy on local control after breast-conserving surgery. *Cancer J Sci Am* 1996;2:39–45.

82. Wallgren A, Bernier J, Gelber RD, et al. Timing of radiotherapy and chemotherapy following breast-conserving surgery for patients with node-positive breast cancer. *Int J Radiat Oncol Biol Phys* 1996;35:649–659.

83. Hietanen PS. Measurement and practical aspects of quality of life in breast cancer. *Acta Oncol* 1996;35:39–42.

84. Fallowfield LJ, Baum M, Maguire GP. Effects of breast conservation on psychological morbidity associated with diagnosis and treatment of early breast cancer. *BMJ* 1986;293:1331–1334.

85. Hietanen P, ed. Finnish Hospital League. *The quality of life in a breast cancer patient.* Jyvaskyla, Finland: Gummelius Press, 1990.

86. Fallowfield LJ. Assessment of quality of life in breast cancer. *Acta Oncol* 1995;34:689–694.

CHAPTER 8

Advanced Breast Carcinoma, Locoregional Recurrences, and Distant Metastases

S. EVA SINGLETARY
AMAN U. BUZDAR
ELENI DIAMANDIDOU

Although the frequency of locally advanced breast cancer has decreased to less than 5% of breast cancers detected in mammographically screened populations, it represents 30% to 50% of newly diagnosed breast cancer cases in medically underserved areas of the United States and in many other countries (1,2). Because the greatest risk for patients with locally advanced breast cancer is the development of distant metastases and subsequent death, the goals of surgery are maximal locoregional control with minimal disfigurement and accurate staging to determine prognosis and thus the need for postoperative adjuvant therapy. Close cooperation between the medical and surgical oncologists and the reconstructive surgeon is required to determine the feasibility of breast preservation and to assess the advisability of major resections of either persistent advanced primary disease or locoregional recurrences. If life expectancy is very short, as with patients who have bulky visceral disease or metastases nonrespondent to multiple chemotherapy regimens, the true benefit of a complex but technically feasible operation should be evaluated carefully. However, in selected patients, surgery may achieve quality palliation of the local symptoms of pain, hemorrhage, and malodorous ulceration.

Locally Advanced Disease

Evolution of Standard Treatment

In 1943, on the basis of the outcomes of 1135 breast cancer patients treated with radical mastectomy from 1915 to 1942, Haagensen and Stout (3) defined the clinical features of locally advanced breast cancer that predicted a 50% or higher chance of local recurrence and a 0% five-year survival rate: extensive edema involving more than two thirds of the breast, satellite skin nodules, "inflammatory" carcinoma, and edema of the arm. Patients with less extensive skin edema (one third of the breast), skin ulcerations, a tumor fixed to the chest wall, or fixed axillary lymph nodes had a local recurrence rate of 40%, with a long-term survival rate of less than 5%. Because surgery alone for locally advanced breast cancer produced such poor results, high-dose radiotherapy subsequently replaced surgery as the local therapy of choice, producing an overall 5-year survival rate of 21% in combined series (4–6). Unfortunately, high-dose radiotherapy was often associated with severe side effects such as fibrosis and skin ulceration, brachial plexopathy, and lymphedema of the arm. During the 1960s and early 1970s, procedures designed to lower the total dose of radiation—preoperative radiotherapy followed by radical mastectomy or, conversely, a debulking extended simple mastectomy followed within 2 to 3 weeks by irradiation—became the standard treatment for patients with locally advanced breast cancer treated at major institutions in this country (7).

In the early 1970s, the paradigm that survival from breast cancer depends on the eradication of occult micrometastases was introduced. This concept led to the integration of systemic chemotherapy into a combined-modality approach with local therapy. Today, with the increasing use of induction (preoperative) chemotherapy, the extent of surgery, if any, that is necessary after downstaging of the tumor remains unclear.

Role of Surgery Following Induction Chemotherapy

In a Cancer and Leukemia Group B study (8), 87 patients with locally advanced breast cancer were randomly assigned to receive radiotherapy or mastectomy after downstaging with a doxorubicin-based induction chemotherapy regimen. Locoregional relapse rates and duration of disease control were not significantly different between the mastectomy and radiotherapy groups (19% and 29 months versus 27% and 24 months, respectively). Survival was equivalent regardless of the modality of local therapy used. In the Milan study (9) with a follow-up of 10 years, for patients who had a complete remission with preoperative doxorubicin-based combination chemotherapy, the locoregional recurrence rate was 40% in 65 patients treated with surgery alone and 51% in 95 patients treated with radiotherapy alone.

A recent update of the National Cancer Institute's pilot trial (10), in which 43% of patients had inflammatory breast cancer, revealed a 16% local failure rate in 31 patients treated with radiotherapy but no surgery who had complete responses with induction chemotherapy as confirmed by needle biopsies. The actuarial 5-year rate of local recurrence as the first sign of relapse was 23%. Similarly, Jacquillat et al (11) reported a locoregional recurrence rate of 13% [subsequently updated to 18% (12)] for 98 patients with stage III disease treated with doxorubicin-based induction chemotherapy and both external and interstitial radiotherapy but no surgery. Eighty percent of patients were described as having an excellent or good cosmetic result. However, the late complications of radiation alone as treatment for advanced breast cancer may create considerable long-term morbidity in patients who have chemosensitive tumors and survive for a long time (13).

For the past 20 years, patients with primary breast cancers larger than 5 cm in diameter (T3), with skin or chest wall involvement (T4), or with matted or fixed axillary lymph nodes (N2) have been treated at The University of Texas M. D. Anderson Cancer Center with a multimodal approach comprising induction chemotherapy followed by surgery or irradiation or both.

In the first M. D. Anderson clinical trial of this multimodal approach, induction combination chemotherapy was administered to 174 evaluable patients (191 registered) with noninflammatory stage III breast cancer. Seventeen percent of the patients had a complete remission and 71% had a partial remission after three cycles of 5-fluorouracil, doxorubicin, and cyclophosphamide (FAC) therapy (14). Radiation alone was then given to the chest wall and regional lymph nodes of patients with an excellent tumor response and minimal residual disease. A combination of irradiation and complete mastectomy with limited axillary lymph node dissection was used for patients who had residual tumor of substantial volume. After completion of locoregional therapy, FAC was reinitiated and continued until the total dose of 450 mg/m^2 of doxorubicin was reached, at which time treatment with cyclophosphamide, methotrexate, and 5-fluorouracil (CMF) was instituted for a total treatment period of 2 years. The induction chemotherapy was well tolerated, and the surgical procedures were completed without an increased rate of infection or delayed wound healing (15).

A histologically confirmed response in the mastectomy specimen after induction chemotherapy was an excellent prognostic factor for survival (16,17). The number of positive axillary nodes after induction chemotherapy was also an excellent prognostic factor for survival, with actuarial 5-year survival rates of 70% for patients with negative lymph nodes, 62% for patients with 1 to 3 positive lymph nodes, 47% for patients with 4 to 10 positive lymph nodes, and 21% for patients with more than 10 positive lymph nodes (Fig. 8-1) (17). The 5-year disease-free survival rates were 72%, 46%, 35%, and 6%, respectively. When subsets of patients with four or more positive lymph nodes were combined, the overall survival rate at 5 years was 38%, and the disease-free survival rate was only 20%. Of the subset of 22 patients whose tumors showed a minor or no clinical response to induction chemotherapy in this protocol,

F I G U R E **8-1**

Actuarial survival of patients with locally advanced breast cancer by the number of axillary lymph nodes still positive for metastatic disease after induction chemotherapy. (Reproduced by permission from McCready DR, Hortobagyi GN, Kau SW, et al. The prognostic significance of lymph node metastases after preoperative chemotherapy for locally advanced breast cancer. *Arch Surg* 1989; 124:21–25.).

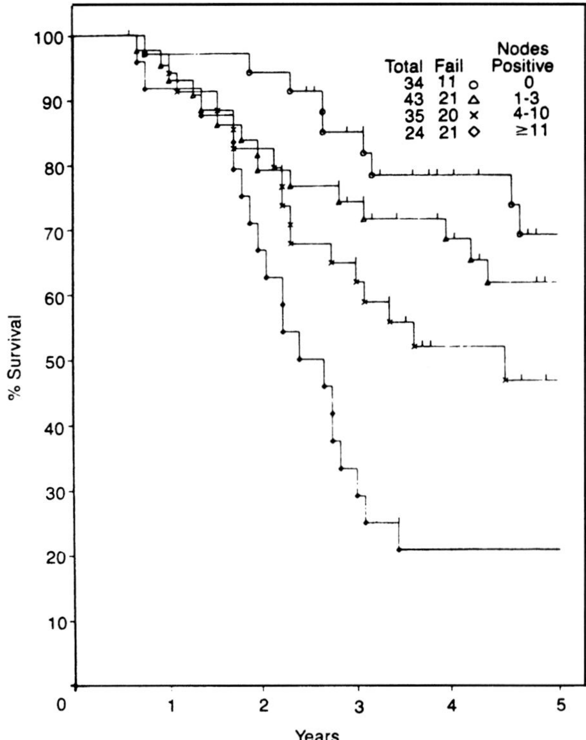

only 7 were alive at 5 years, for a disease-free survival rate of 16% (18). This dismal survival rate associated with macroscopic residual disease after induction chemotherapy parallels M. D. Anderson results obtained with mastectomy and postoperative irradiation but no systemic therapy for locally advanced breast carcinoma (19). An alternative treatment option for patients with four or more positive lymph nodes after induction chemotherapy is enrollment in a randomized trial of standard chemotherapy (e.g., FAC) with or without consolidation therapy with high-dose chemotherapy regimens (e.g., cisplatin, etoposide, and cyclophosphamide) or a crossover chemotherapy regimen of promising new agents such as paclitaxel (20,21).

The next M. D. Anderson clinical trial (1985–1989) was designed to determine whether the extent of residual disease in the mastectomy specimen after induction chemotherapy could be used as a guide to plan postoperative adjuvant treatment. Three cycles of vincristine, doxorubicin, cyclophosphamide, and prednisone (VACP) were administered at 21-day intervals, and then a modified radical mastectomy (complete removal of all breast tissue including the nipple-areolar complex, and axillary lymph node dissection) was performed. Patients with histologically confirmed complete remission and those with less than $1\,cm^3$ of residual tumor received five additional cycles of VACP; those with no response to induction chemotherapy were crossed over to receive five cycles of methotrexate, 5-fluorouracil, and vinblastine (MFVb). Patients with partial responses were randomly assigned to receive five additional cycles of either VACP or MFVb. All patients received radiation to the chest wall and regional lymph nodes. Eight patients whose tumors remained inoperable after initial induction chemotherapy underwent irradiation before mastectomy and MFVb. The irradiation had a minimal effect on wound healing as long as wound tension and thin skin flaps were avoided. If mastectomy resulted in a large defect, flap coverage consisting of healthy autogenous tissue was preferred to the use of skin grafts.

Of 193 evaluable patients in this trial (200 registered), 161 had a partial or greater clinical response to the three cycles of induction chemotherapy. No statistically significant difference ($p = 0.64$) was detected in the 4-year survival rates for the MFVb and VACP groups (75% and 58%, respectively) (22). Of the 32 patients in this study whose tumors showed a minor or no response to induction chemotherapy, only 16 remain alive (8 are disease free) at the time of writing. The lack of impact on survival of the crossover regimen was probably due to the absence of effective second-line therapy in this study. However, the downstaging observed—17 mastectomy specimens had no evidence of residual tumor, and 54 mastectomy specimens had less than $1\,cm^3$ of tumor—led us to consider the possibility of performing breast preservation surgery for locally advanced disease.

Breast Preservation Surgery

To assess the feasibility of breast preservation surgery after tumor downstaging, we performed a retrospective review that correlated the clinical and mammographic responses with the histologic findings in the mastectomy specimen and with subsequent locoregional relapse (23). Of the 161 patients with chemoresponsive tumors, 18 were excluded either because they refused total mastectomy (n = 8) or because their tumor response could not be fully analyzed (n = 10). The tumors of the remaining 143 patients who had either a complete response (16%) or a partial response (84%) were then staged according to the 1988 American Joint Committee on Cancer staging system (24): 17% were stage IIB (T3, N0), 36% were stage IIIA (T1-3, N2), 41% were stage IIIB (T4, N0-3), and 6% were stage IV (positive supraclavicular lymph nodes). According to strict eligibility criteria for breast preservation (Table 8-1), 33 (23%) of the 143 patients who responded to induction chemotherapy could

T A B L E   **8-1**

Criteria for Breast Preservation Surgery after Induction Chemotherapy for Locally Advanced Breast Cancer

Complete resolution of skin edema (peau d'orange)
Residual tumor size <5 cm
Absence of extensive intramammary lymphatic invasion
Absence of extensive suspicious microcalcifications
No known evidence of multicentricity
Patient's desire for breast preservation

have had a segmental mastectomy (wide local excision) and axillary node dissection rather than a modified radical mastectomy. None of the total mastectomy specimens from these 33 patients were found to have tumor in other quadrants of the breast, and at a median follow-up of 34 months, none of the patients had experienced a chest wall recurrence. In contrast, of 110 patients who were not considered to be good candidates for breast preservation surgery, 55 (50%) had tumor in other quadrants: 22 (40%) involving two quadrants, 9 (16%) involving three quadrants, and 24 (44%) involving the entire breast.

The factors most commonly associated with multiple-quadrant involvement were persistent skin edema (65%), residual tumor size larger than 4 cm (56%), extensive intramammary lymphatic invasion (20%), and known mammographic evidence of multicentric disease (16%). Of the 110 patients who were not candidates for breast preservation, 17 (15%) had recurrence in the chest wall after radiotherapy. Of these 17 patients, 13 (76%) had persistent skin edema before mastectomy, 2 (12%) had known extensive intramammary lymphatic invasion, and 2 (12%) had extensive multicentric disease. These findings led to the objective of the third M. D. Anderson clinical trial (1989–1992): to determine prospectively what fraction of patients with locally advanced breast cancer become eligible for breast preservation surgery after tumor downstaging with induction chemotherapy and choose that alternative. Of 203 evaluable patients with stage IIA through stage IV breast cancer who completed four cycles of induction chemotherapy (FAC) from 1989 to 1991, 51 (25%) elected breast preservation and the procedure was performed (Fig. 10-2). The breast preservation rate for patients with ulcerative lesions or dermal lymphatic involvement (stage IIIB) was only 6%. With a median follow-up time of longer than 43 months (range, 29–61 months), only 4 patients had relapses in the breast, and at the time of this report 2 of these patients remained disease free after mastectomy.

Schwartz et al (25) reported that 39% of stage II and III patients who received induction chemotherapy until maximum clinical response was achieved underwent breast preservation surgery. With a median follow-up time of 29 months, only one patient had developed recurrent disease in the breast. Since 1990, these

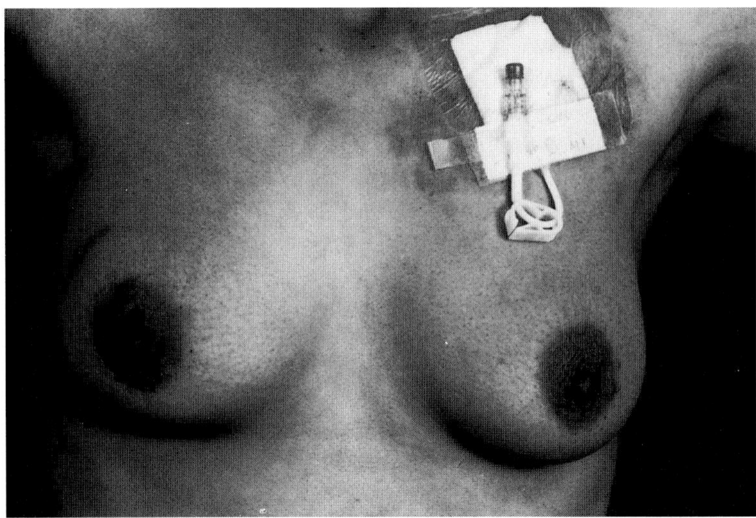

A 39-year-old woman with T2, N2, M0 carcinoma of the right breast who underwent segmental mastectomy and axillary lymph node dissection after four cycles of induction chemotherapy with 5-fluorouracil, doxorubicin, and cyclophosphamide (FAC). No residual tumor was found in the breast or axillary nodes. Postoperatively, she completed five additional cycles of FAC followed by radiation to the breast and peripheral lymphatics. She was free of disease at her 5-year follow-up.

investigators have performed breast preservation in approximately three fourths of their patients who responded to induction chemotherapy.

To determine whether induction chemotherapy yields higher survival and breast preservation rates than does postoperative adjuvant chemotherapy in patients with large primary breast tumors, Scholl et al (26) randomly assigned 390 premenopausal patients with T2-3, N0-1, M0 breast cancer to receive either four cycles of induction chemotherapy with FAC followed by irradiation, surgical excision of any persistent tumor, and an axillary node dissection (n = 200), or irradiation with or without surgery followed by four cycles of adjuvant chemotherapy with FAC (n = 190). Of the 153 patients in the induction chemotherapy arm who were evaluable after four cycles of FAC, 82% experienced tumor regression of greater than 50%. Sixty-one percent of patients with residual disease after four cycles of FAC achieved a complete response with irradiation. Thirty percent of the patients in this treatment arm underwent limited excision, and 18% of these patients underwent mastectomy, for a breast preservation rate of 82%. Of the 143

evaluable patients in the postoperative adjuvant treatment arm, 85% experienced tumor regression of greater than 50% with irradiation. Thirty percent of the patients then underwent limited excision, and 23% underwent mastectomy, for a breast preservation rate of 77%. At a median follow-up time of 54 months, the 5-year survival probability was higher in patients who received induction chemotherapy than in those who received postoperative adjuvant therapy (86% versus 78%, $p = 0.039$). However, no differences in disease-free intervals or local recurrence rates were detected between the induction chemotherapy and adjuvant chemotherapy groups.

Recently, this approach of induction chemotherapy has been used even in patients with smaller primary tumors (2–5 cm). In the pilot study of Bonadonna et al (27) of 227 women with primary tumors at least 3 cm in largest diameter without skin or chest wall involvement, patients whose tumors were downstaged by induction chemotherapy to less than 3 cm at the time of surgery underwent quadrantectomy (minimum margin of 2 cm) and irradiation (5 fractions per week for a total dose of 60 Gy in 6 weeks). One of five different drug regimens was used for three to four cycles preoperatively, with additional postoperative chemotherapy (two to three cycles) given to patients with positive nodes or with negative nodes but estrogen receptor–negative tumors. Clinical response was determined by palpation prior to surgery. Of 200 evaluable patients, 21% had complete responses, 57% had partial responses, 15% had objective improvement, and 3% had progressive disease. Response rates were unrelated to the drug regimen used. Breast preservation was possible in 91% of patients with an initial tumor size of 3 to 5 cm (n = 183) and in 73% of patients with an initial tumor size larger than 5 cm (n = 37). At a median follow-up time from completion of induction chemotherapy of 30 months, the local recurrence rate was 2%, and the overall survival rate was 93%. These encouraging preliminary results suggest that breast preservation may be an appropriate treatment option for selected patients with locally advanced breast cancer.

If breast preservation surgery is performed, radiopaque hemoclips should be placed at the base of the excision defect in the breast to guide the radiotherapist in planning the radiation fields (28).

Currently, regardless of whether the breast is preserved or removed, a level I and II axillary lymph node dissection (removal of lymph nodes lateral and posterior to the pectoralis minor muscle) is included for histologic assessment of tumor response to the induction chemotherapy and for identification of patients who may qualify for dose-intensive chemotherapy programs (i.e., patients with four or more positive nodes after induction chemotherapy). The necessity of axillary lymph node dissection and its future role in treatment are being addressed in clinical trials. For example, in the current clinical trial at M. D. Anderson, patients with T2-3, N0-1 breast cancer are initially randomized to receive either paclitaxel or standard FAC preoperatively. After the completion of induction chemotherapy, patients who have become candidates for breast preservation and who have clinically negative axilla are further randomly assigned to undergo either observation of the axilla or a standard level I and II axillary lymph node dissection (Fig. 8-3). This is then followed by completion of systemic therapy and breast irradiation that includes the lower axilla and the supraclavicular fossa in patients with a nondissected axilla.

Treatment Options for Unresectable Tumors

Patients whose tumors remain unresectable after doxorubicin-based induction combination chemotherapy and preoperative irradiation should be offered systemic therapy. The optimal regimen is determined by patient and tumor characteristics. Patients with strongly positive estrogen or progesterone receptor status and especially those with a long tumor history or well-differentiated tumor histology should be given a course of hormonal therapy. In this

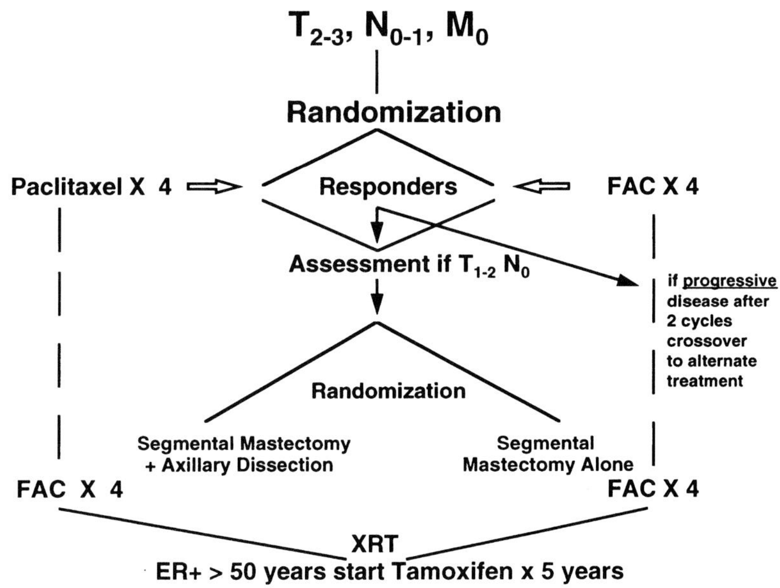

FIGURE 8-3

Treatment schema for T2-3, N0-1 breast carcinoma comparing 5-fluorouracil, doxorubicin, and cyclophosphamide (FAC) with paclitaxel. Patients who become candidates for breast preservation surgery after induction chemotherapy are randomly assigned to segmental mastectomy either with or without axillary node dissection. ER+ = estrogen receptor positive; XRT = radiation therapy.

setting, tamoxifen (29,30) would be the initial choice for both postmenopausal and premenopausal patients, although surgical oophorectomy (31) or administration of a luteinizing hormone–releasing hormone analogue (32) might be an acceptable substitute in the latter patients. All other patients should be offered second-line cytotoxic therapy or participation in clinical trials of investigational agents (33–35). Paclitaxel has become the de facto second-line regimen in the United States as there is no cross-resistance of this agent with doxorubicin. The probability of response with paclitaxel is 20% to 30% in patients previously treated with doxorubicin (19,20,36,37). Other agents with potential usefulness in this situation include the vinca alkaloids [vinblastine and vinorelbine (Navelbine)] used as single agents or in combination with other drugs, such as methotrexate, mitomycin, and 5-fluorouracil with folinic acid (33,35). When used as second-line therapy for metastatic breast cancer, these regimens result in response rates of 30% to 40%, but their activity in patients with anthracycline-resistant and radioresistant tumors remains to be defined. Another option to be considered is the use of intra-arterial chemotherapy. Investigators (38,39) reported a high response rate and very rapid responses after intra-arterial administration of chemotherapy, even in patients with recurrent breast cancer or tumors refractory to standard chemotherapy. Mitoxantrone, fluoropyrimidines, and mitomycin are agents frequently used for intra-arterial therapy. However, intra-arterial therapy requires a team with extensive experience in this type of treatment because of the toxicities and complications related to this procedure.

Several novel therapies are being explored for the treatment of breast cancer. Among new cytotoxic agents, docetaxel (Taxotere), vinorelbine, the anthrapyrazoles (losoxantrone and others), and new folate antagonists (edatrexate) have demonstrated activity against breast cancer, while many others are in phase I/II trials (33,34). Monoclonal antibodies, radioimmunoconjugates, immunotoxins, and several forms of gene therapy are proceeding through early clinical development (40–42). Patients with unresectable tumors after induction chemotherapy and radiotherapy are encouraged to participate in these clinical trials when possible.

If the tumor becomes operable after second-line systemic therapy, completion of locoregional therapy with surgical resection is advisable for optimal local and systemic control.

High-dose chemotherapy is being investigated in patients with high-risk primary breast cancer, including those with locally advanced breast cancer (43). However, one of the lessons learned from the high-dose chemotherapy protocols for metastatic breast cancer was that patients with previously demonstrated resistance to chemotherapy do not benefit from this procedure (44). Therefore, patients with no response or progression of disease after induction chemotherapy are not advised at this time to participate in high-dose chemotherapy programs outside of clinical trials.

Reconstructive Surgery

In some patients with locally advanced breast cancer who need or elect to have standard mastectomy, breast reconstructive surgery for cosmesis is often delayed until completion of both adjuvant chemotherapy and irradiation. As most locoregional recurrences are in the skin or subcutaneous tissue of the chest wall (45,46), a flat postmastectomy chest wall often makes irradiation technically easier than does a reconstructed breast mound.

Because of loss of skin elasticity and fibrosis of underlying tissues after irradiation, tissue expansion for implant reconstruction in an irradiated field has had disappointing results, with a high complication rate as well as patient discomfort and dissatisfaction (47,48). In contrast, the use of a myocutaneous flap for breast reconstruction, either before or after irradiation, has not interfered with the resumption of chemotherapy or the ability to detect locoregional recurrence (49–51). Irradiation of the reconstructed breast mound flap has not impaired the flap's blood supply or significantly affected the cosmetic result (52). Thus, in selected patients with an excellent response to chemotherapy or when palliative debulking surgical procedures are needed, the preference is to use an autogenous flap to create a breast mound or to provide skin coverage of the operative defect without the use of skin grafts. The two most frequently used tissue flaps are the myocutaneous flaps based on the latissimus dorsi and rectus abdominis muscles and their blood supplies.

The latissimus dorsi myocutaneous flap consists of an elliptical island of skin carried on the latissimus dorsi muscle (28). This muscle has a single dominant vascular pedicle from the thoracodorsal artery at its insertion and, at its origin, multiple segmental pedicles originating from some of the lumbar and lower six intercostal arteries. The advantages of the latissimus dorsi flap include its reliable blood supply and the relative rarity of donor-site morbidity. It also is a relatively thin flap, so it matches the thickness of the native chest wall skin fairly closely and is therefore excellent for providing coverage of a soft tissue defect (Fig. 8-4). The chief disadvantage of the latissimus dorsi flap is its limited size; an implant is usually required if the patient desires a reconstructed breast mound. The amount of available surplus skin varies from patient to patient, but in general, the latissimus dorsi flap is never more than 10 cm wide or 20 cm long.

The rectus abdominis myocutaneous flap (53,54) is an abdominal skin island flap based on the rectus abdominis muscle, whose blood supply is normally provided by the superior epigastric vessels at the junction of the costal margin and the xiphoid process. However, if a free flap is used, the inferior epigastric vessels are usually anastomosed to the thoracodorsal vascular bundle in the axilla. Rectus abdominis flaps can be quite large and are therefore most useful for defects too large to repair with a latissimus dorsi flap. Their chief disadvantage is that they tend to be bulky, so they do not match the thickness of the native chest wall skin well. This thickness, however, can occasionally become an advantage if the defect is located directly over a missing breast (Fig. 8-5). In such a case, the surgeon can simultaneously cover the wound and use the excess flap bulk to reconstruct a breast.

There are two main types of rectus abdominis flaps: the transverse rectus abdominis myocutaneous (TRAM) flap and the vertical rectus abdominis myocutaneous (VRAM) flap. The TRAM flap has a greater arc of rotation and a more symmetric and easily concealed donor site. The VRAM flap leaves a more noticeable donor scar but is technically easier to construct and has a more reliable blood supply. In general, the TRAM flap is used most often when cosmetic considerations are important or when

A 42-year-old patient presented with an 8 × 10-cm carcinoma of the left breast that involved the overlying skin (*A, B*). The patient refused induction chemotherapy or radiation therapy. To provide coverage of the skin defect after a modified radical mastectomy (*C*), an island of skin carried on the latissimus dorsi muscle was used as a myocutaneous flap (*D*). The patient had excellent range of motion 10 days after surgery (*E*). (Reproduced by permission from Singletary SE. Breast surgery. In: Roh MS, Ames FC, eds. *Atlas of advanced oncologic surgery*. New York: Gower Medical, 1993:14.1–14.9.).

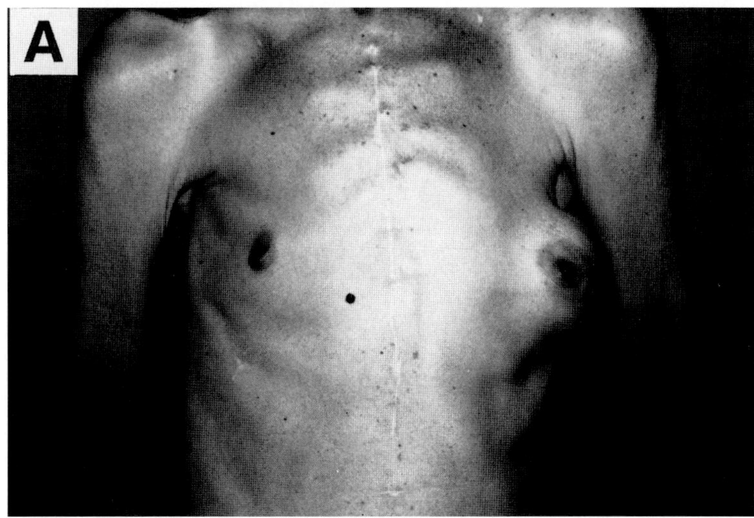

F I G U R E **8-4**

Continued

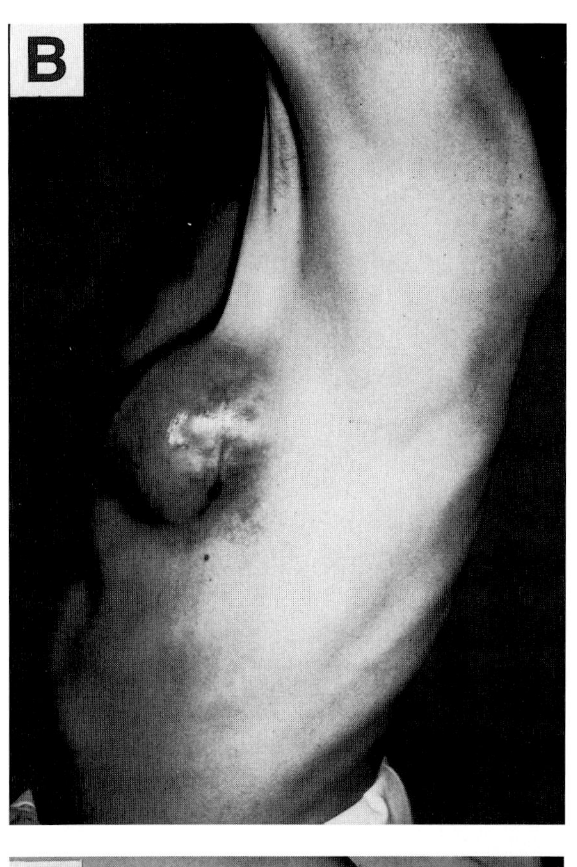

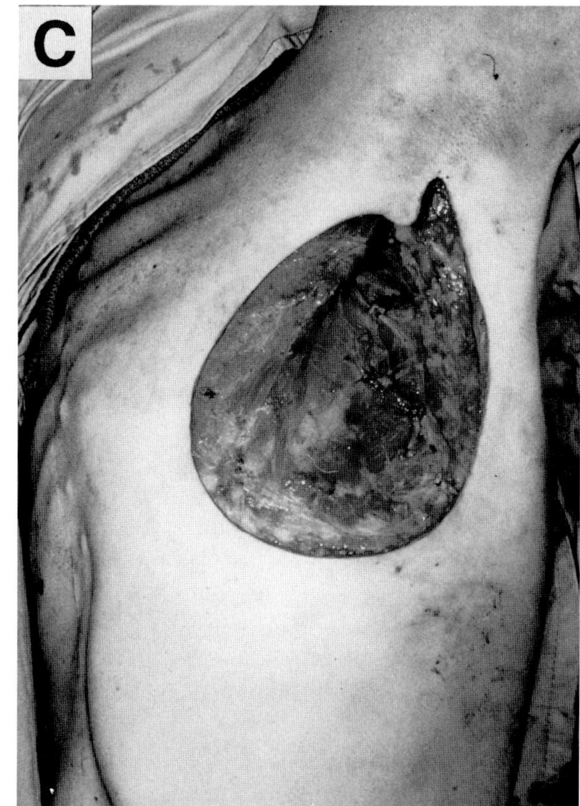

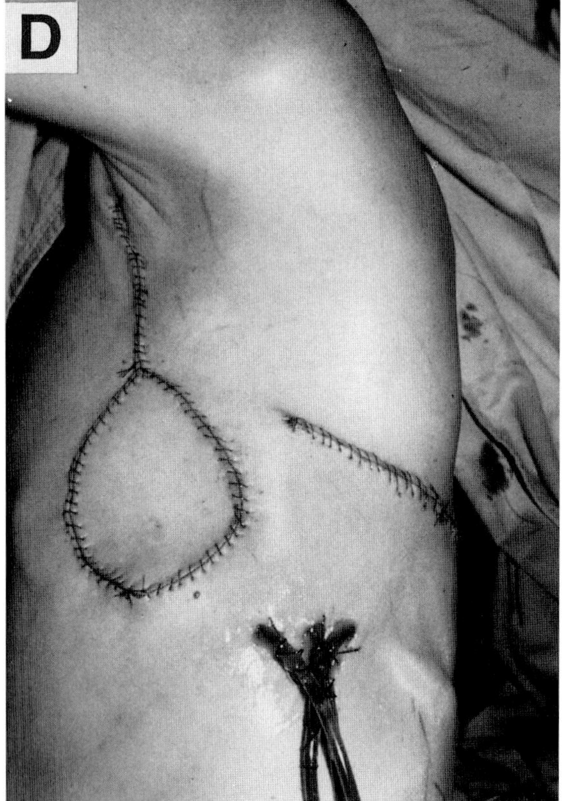

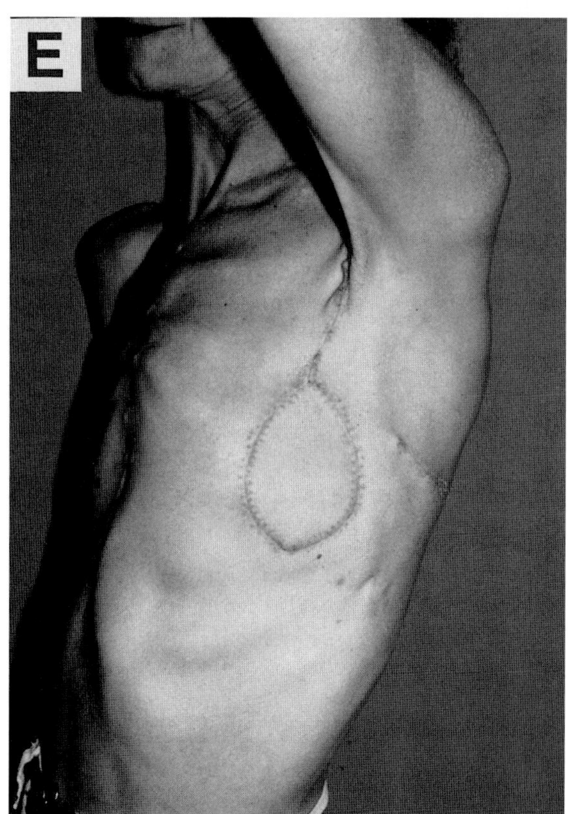

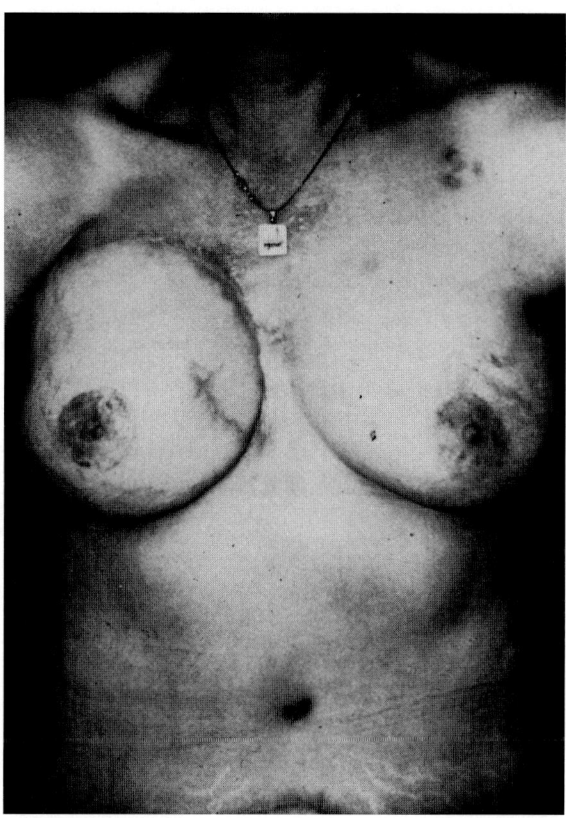

Soft tissue and skin coverage provided by a transverse rectus abdominis myocutaneous flap after a debulking mastectomy for locally advanced carcinoma of the right breast. Nipple reconstruction was performed 6 weeks later by tattooing.

the surgeon is trying to reconstruct a breast. Use of the VRAM flap is more common when cosmesis is unimportant and wound coverage is the only goal.

When patients have a history of heavy smoking, lower abdominal scarring, or diabetes or require a larger lateral flap, the skin island flap should be placed more cephalad on the abdominal wall to improve the flap's blood supply; alternatively, a double-pedicled or microsurgically augmented flap should be considered.

Chest Wall Resections

The availability of tissue flaps carrying their own blood supply has improved surgeon's ability to perform complex chest wall resections for persistent advanced primary disease or locoregional recurrences. The indications for full-thickness chest wall resection are control of

local symptoms, removal of a site of sepsis, and osteoradionecrosis (55). The defect must be covered with a well-vascularized flap of nonirradiated tissue, but the blood supply to the flap itself may have been irradiated before flap transfer (52). In the M. D. Anderson series (56) of 61 patients with locally recurrent breast cancer or radionecrosis infection of the chest wall, prior irradiation of the internal mammary artery, the nutrient vessel to the rectus abdominis flap, or the thoracodorsal artery, which provides blood to the latissimus dorsi flap, did not compromise the viability of any of the flaps used for wound coverage. It is best to cover the wound with the largest flap that can be raised without creating excessive tension when the donor site is closed. In patients with radionecrosis, the surgical defect to be covered is often 50% to 75% larger than the actual size of the resected area, owing to retraction of the edges of the surgical wound as the irradiation-induced contracture or scarring is released. Moreover, it is often advisable to resect additional damaged but viable tissue at the margin of the radionecrosis provided that the size of the flap is sufficient to cover the resulting wound. This reduces the incidence of wound complications and prevents further progression of the radionecrosis.

The rectus abdominis flap is capable of covering a wide area from the clavicle to the costal margin and from the sternum to the midaxillary line. The bulkiness of this flap provides enough chest wall stability that up to five ribs or the entire sternum can be resected without the need for prosthetic mesh. When there is a defect of three or more ribs, however, it may be advisable to stabilize the defect with mesh anyway. Although the mesh is not necessary for survival, its use improves chest wall mechanics and reduces the duration of ventilator dependence and hospital stay. Provided that the mesh is covered by well-vascularized tissue, the risk of infection and extrusion is relatively small (57). Marlex, a nonabsorbable durable mesh, can be used for flat surfaces of the chest wall. For larger defects, a "sandwich" of Marlex mesh and methyl methacrylate can be formed to create a more anatomically normal contour (58).

Other alternatives to the latissimus dorsi and rectus abdominis flaps include the pectoralis major myocutaneous flap (59) and the omental flap (60). These flaps are rarely used today because they require split-thickness skin grafts, they give a less satisfactory cosmetic result, and they lack inherent strength.

Locoregional Recurrences

Local recurrence after mastectomy is defined as the recurrence of breast cancer on the chest wall at the site of a previous mastectomy, either in the skin flaps or along the surgical scar. *Regional recurrence* after primary treatment is defined as recurrence of breast cancer in the regional lymphatics in the axilla or in the internal mammary nodal chain. Tumor involvement of the supraclavicular nodal basin is now categorized as distant disease (M1) by the American Joint Committee on Cancer (24).

Risk factors for locoregional recurrence are four or more positive axillary nodes, primary tumor size larger than 5 cm, macroscopic extranodal disease in the axilla, and extensive dermal lymphatic invasion (61–63). The type of mastectomy (radical, modified radical, or extended simple) has not been shown to affect the locoregional recurrence rate (45). Although systemic chemotherapy may lower the incidence of locoregional recurrence as compared with surgery alone, adding radiotherapy to chemotherapy after mastectomy for patients with operable stage III disease lowered the locoregional recurrence rate from 18% to only 8% (45). Similarly, radiation decreased the rate of locoregional relapse following mastectomy and FAC adjuvant therapy from 14% to 5% in patients with 4 to 10 positive nodes and from 21% to 8% in patients with more than 10 positive nodes (45).

Of 367 evaluable patients registered (n = 391) in M. D. Anderson protocols (21) for locally advanced breast cancer (1974–1989) in which a doxorubicin-based induction combination chemotherapy regimen plus local surgery or irradiation, or both, was used, only 57 (16%) patients developed a locoregional recurrence as a first site of relapse (chest wall, 72%; regional nodal basins including the supraclavicular area, 21%; or both, 7%). The initial tumor stage was T2 in 2% of patients, T3 in 17%, and T4 in 81%. Matted axillary nodes (N2) had been present in 37%. Eleven of the 57 patients had shown resistance to prior induction chemotherapy. Surgery (usually a total mastectomy with level I and/or II axillary node dissection) had been performed in 51 patients, and consolidation therapy with irradiation had been performed in 29 patients.

Five patients had received irradiation only without mastectomy.

Unfortunately, 17 of these patients with locoregional recurrences also had synchronous distant metastasis; their median survival time from the first recurrence (regional or distant) was 5 months. The median survival time from recurrence for the 40 patients whose first relapse was locoregional only was 16 months (range, 1–109 months); only 1 patient was still alive without disease at the time of this writing (21).

Although locoregional recurrence has historically been considered a harbinger of distant metastases and subsequent death, selected patients experience a long disease-free interval and occasionally long-term survival (64–66). A multifactorial analysis (67) of prognostic variables for survival following locoregional recurrence of operable breast cancer demonstrated 5-year actuarial overall survival rates of 44% to 49% for patients with isolated chest wall or nodal disease as compared with 21% to 24% for patients with multiple or concomitant locoregional recurrences. In a subset of patients whose chest wall recurrences were excised or were less than 3 cm and who had a disease-free interval of at least 2 years from primary treatment, the 5-year disease-free and overall survival rates were 54% and 67%, respectively. Other investigators also observed that solitary recurrences of tumor of limited volume with a long interval between primary treatment and relapse may identify a subset of patients with a favorable prognosis (68–70).

Thus, for selected patients, surgical attempts to render the patient free of disease may influence the course of the disease. For the majority of patients with locoregional recurrences, however, improvement in survival will require the development of more effective systemic approaches.

Systemic treatment for patients with locoregional recurrence depends on several factors. Patients who develop recurrent disease while receiving induction or postoperative adjuvant chemotherapy or within 6 months of the last chemotherapy treatment are considered to have a tumor that is resistant to front-line therapy. Consequently, their best option would be second-line chemotherapy or, in patients with estrogen receptor–positive tumors, hormonal therapy.

Patients who have relapses more than 6 months after the last dose of front-line chemotherapy may still benefit from the same regimen used for reinduction chemotherapy. In fact, the longer the interval between the last dose of adjuvant chemotherapy and relapse, the higher the probability of response to reinduction with the same regimen. Maintenance of optimal dose intensity appears to be important during adjuvant chemotherapy and probably during induction and reinduction therapy too. Hematopoietic growth factors (granulocyte colony-stimulating factor and granulocyte-macrophage colony-stimulating factor) are excellent aids in the maintenance of dose intensity, even in patients with prior exposure to chemotherapy and radiotherapy (71).

For patients who respond well to reinduction therapy, consolidation therapy with high-dose chemotherapy [with autologous bone marrow (ABM) or peripheral blood stem cell (PBSC) support] represents an exciting investigational option (72). However, to date, no definite survival benefit has been demonstrated for this procedure. The observation that high tumor grade and c-*erb* B-2 overexpression may help predict which patients are more likely to respond to high-dose chemotherapy still needs to be confirmed (73,74).

No conclusive data are available to show that radiotherapy alters survival duration; instead, radiotherapy may only reduce the frequency of local failure as the first site of relapse. However, many studies showed that irradiation can effectively control local recurrences in only 50% to 60% of patients not treated by primary radiation (75,76). To avoid symptomatic local recurrence and its emotional sequelae, irradiation should be considered for patients at high risk for recurrent disease.

Systemic Therapy for Metastatic Disease

The incidence of breast cancer has risen steadily over the past decades. Approximately 100,000 women die each year in Western Europe and North America as a result of breast cancer; in the United States alone, 46,000 women died of breast cancer in 1995 (77).

While early disease is frequently curable with combined-modality therapy, the prognosis of patients with recurrent disease is not as favorable. With currently available therapy, a high fraction of patients with recurrent disease have objective tumor shrinkage but only a small frac-

tion of patients who have complete remission remain in remission (78–80).

In patients with metastatic breast cancer, the optimal selection of therapy for individual patients is guided by several factors: the extent of disease, the pattern and aggressiveness of the recurrence, estrogen and progesterone receptor status, and the patient's menstrual status. For patients with rapidly progressive disease, chemotherapy can often produce objective responses more quickly than other treatment modalities can. For less aggressive disease and for patients with no vital organ involvement and positive estrogen and progesterone receptor status, endocrine therapies should be considered.

Combinations of hormonal agents with chemotherapy (81), rotation of chemotherapeutic regimens (82), and more recently, high-dose chemotherapy with or without the support of ABM transplantation or PBSC transplantation (43,44,83–85) may result in higher objective response rates, but it is still unclear whether these treatments result in improved long-term survival rates.

Patients who have a relapse after a disease-free interval of longer than 2 years with the dominant site of the metastasis in bones or soft tissue and whose tumor is estrogen or progesterone receptor positive have much longer median survival times (83 months) than do patients with the same characteristics but with the site of relapse in a visceral organ (56 months). The median survival of patients who either have a relapse in less than 2 years or have a tumor that is estrogen or progesterone receptor negative is much worse (15–29 months), particularly if the site of the metastases is visceral (86).

Prior adjuvant chemotherapy and response to anthracycline-based regimens play an important role in subsequent responses to secondary chemotherapies and overall survival. Most first-line chemotherapy regimens for metastatic disease include CMF or FAC combinations (87,88). These regimens produce response rates in untreated patients in the range of 50% to 80%, with a median survival time of 2 years (89,90).

Anthracycline-containing combinations are considered the most active agents presently available for advanced breast cancer, with response rates ranging from 20% to 75% (the higher response rates are observed in patients who have not received prior anthracycline chemotherapy or have chemoresponsive tumors) (91–93). Evidence for a dose-response relationship for anthracyclines has also been described (94–96). Patients previously treated with anthracycline-based chemotherapy whose tumors did not respond or recurred soon after completion of chemotherapy usually have lower response rates (20%–27%) to second-line chemotherapy (97). Patients with anthracycline-resistant tumors represent a particularly difficult clinical situation with limited therapeutic options and poor prognosis (98,99).

Vinorelbine (Navelbine), a new vinca alkaloid, is one of the chemotherapeutic drugs shown to produce acceptable response rates (16%–40%) when used as a second-line regimen even in anthracycline-resistant tumors (100–104).

Several other drugs have been used alone or in combination in the setting of salvage therapy, including mitomycin C, vinblastine, 5-fluorouracil (weekly, continuous infusion, or bolus every 3 weeks), methotrexate, and mitoxantrone (105–112). Response rates with these agents have ranged from 7% to 40% (105–112).

Taxanes

Taxanes (paclitaxel and docetaxel) recently became available for the treatment of patients resistant to first-line therapy, and both drugs have significant antitumor activity in this patient population. These drugs have a novel and unique mechanism of action.

For patients with metastatic disease who have received prior adjuvant treatment, paclitaxel is often used as a first-line treatment. Multiple schedules of administration were tested in phase I trials, but in most of the current regimens, the drug is administered over 3, 24, or 96 hours. Response rates in patients who have not previously received anthracycline-based chemotherapy but whose tumors responded to prior therapy range from 32% to 62%. The drug doses evaluated have ranged from 135 to 250 mg/m^2 given over 3 to 24 hours (21,113,114). In patients with anthracycline-resistant tumors, response rates have ranged from 15% to 48% (17,115–117).

Docetaxel, a semisynthetic taxoid, promotes the polymerization of tubulin into stable microtubules. Docetaxel given by 1-hour infusion in patients with metastatic breast cancer and with three or fewer previous chemotherapy regimens produced response rates between 31% and 70% (118,119).

Combinations of paclitaxel or docetaxel with anthracyclines, cyclophosphamide, cisplatin, vinorelbine, 5-fluorouracil, and other agents are under investigation, and some triple-drug regimens have also been studied. Recently, the results of a study using combinations of paclitaxel and doxorubicin were published (120). Reported response rates were as high as 90%, but there was associated higher cardiotoxicity (120).

Other New Cytotoxic Drugs

Several new chemotherapeutic drugs have been developed over the past 5 to 10 years and are presently being evaluated for the treatment of metastatic breast cancer.

Camptothecin, a plant alkaloid with broad-spectrum activity, was isolated from *Camptotheca acuminata* more than two decades ago. More recently, several novel semisynthetic and synthetic analogues designed to be less toxic and to overcome the problems associated with pharmaceutical formulations of natural products have appeared. These analogues inhibit both DNA and RNA synthesis by topoisomerase I–mediated effects (121). Topotecan and irinotecan (CPT-11) were given to patients with metastatic breast cancer who had received minimal or no prior chemotherapy and produced response rates (mainly partial remissions) of 23% to 36% (122,123). There are no sufficient data for duration of response.

Gemcitabine is a pyrimidine antimetabolite. It inhibits DNA synthesis and has a long accumulation phase. Gemcitabine was given to patients with minimally treated metastatic breast cancer and produced response rates of 29% (all partial remissions) (124).

High-Dose Chemotherapy

Breast cancer is now the most common disease for which high-dose chemotherapy with ABM or PBSC support is performed in the United States.

In 1984, Hryniuk and Bush (125) introduced the concept of dose intensity (drug dose administered expressed as mg/m^2/wk) to quantify dose-response effects using breast cancer as a model. They hypothesized that dose intensity correlates with response, which in turns correlates with survival. However, for some drugs, there may be little or no advantage to dose escalation. For example, for vinblastine, the dose-response curve for antitumor activity plateaus after a small dose escalation, but its sensitivity and toxicity to normal tissues continue to increase with further dose escalations (126). On the other hand, for alkylating agents at a dose level within the intrinsic tumor resistance range, dose escalations will not be effective. However, once the resistance level is exceeded, dose escalation may prove to be much more effective in killing tumor cells. This concept led to the initiation of high-dose chemotherapy regimens for patients with breast cancer.

Even prior to initiation of high-dose chemotherapy with ABM or PBSC support, Bonadonna and Valagussa (127) showed that patients who received adjuvant chemotherapy at higher doses had significantly better disease-free and overall survival rates. Later, studies using high-dose combination alkylating agents with ABM/PBSC support demonstrated a high frequency of objective responses, especially complete responses, even in very heavily pretreated patients with refractory metastatic disease (128). The encouraging early results prompted Peters et al (129) to conduct a trial of high-dose combination alkylating agents with ABM support as consolidation for patients with metastatic breast cancer who experienced a complete remission after intensive doxorubicin-based induction therapy. Patients had documented metastatic disease and estrogen and progesterone receptor–negative tumors. Approximately half of these patients were premenopausal, and half of them had not received prior adjuvant chemotherapy. The performance status of all patients was excellent (Zubrod scale score of 0–1). The results of this study were updated at the 1996 American Society of Clinical Oncology meeting (130). The reported overall survival rate for all randomized patients with complete tumor responses was 25% at 5 years. Patients randomly assigned to undergo observation followed by transplantation at the time of relapse had a superior overall survival time compared with patients who received transplants immediately (3.2 years versus 1.9 years, $p = 0.04$).

The drawback for the ABM/PBSC trials is the lack of an appropriate control group of patients who received standard chemotherapy for metastatic breast cancer. One of the most controversial points is the selection criteria for patients entering the ABM/PBSC studies. In the high-dose trials, most patients were chemosensitive during induction therapy. This is not always the case in patients treated with standard chemotherapy. In addition, patients in the high-dose trials usually had more limited disease, good performance status, and minimal comorbidity, all of which are features predicting superior survival.

Interestingly, the results of a 10-year follow-up study of premenopausal women with metastatic breast cancer treated with standard doxorubicin-based chemotherapy showed an overall median survival time of 35 months (131). Subgroup analysis showed that estrogen receptor–negative patients had a shorter overall median survival time than did estrogen receptor–positive patients (30 months compared to 42 months). These results indicate that premenopausal women with metastatic breast cancer treated with standard chemotherapy have a survival time comparable to that in most recently reported ABM/PBSC-treated groups (130). In addition, patients treated with standard chemotherapy have significantly fewer side effects from chemotherapy, better quality of life, and owing to the lower cumulative cyclophosphamide dose, a lower risk of treatment-related leukemias (132).

Endocrine Therapy

Endocrine therapy is an option for the treatment of estrogen or progesterone receptor–positive advanced disease. Hormonal therapy has been shown to be effective in 25% to 30% of unselected patients; in patients with receptor-positive status, the response rate is approximately 50%.

The goal of endocrine therapy for breast cancer is to decrease or stop the growth of estrogen-dependent tumors by reducing estrogen levels or blocking the interaction of estrogen with its receptor (133). Prediction of response to endocrine therapy is based on the presence of hormone receptors in the tumor. For patients with both estrogen and progesterone receptor positivity, response rates can be as high as 70%, compared with 30% in patients whose tumor is positive for either receptor and 11% in patients whose tumor is negative for both receptors (134). Previous response to endocrine therapy is a useful indication that the tumor is hormone dependent and that the likelihood of response to a second-line hormonal therapy is therefore high. Hormonal receptors are also more likely to be present in tumors of postmenopausal women (approximately 63%) than in tumors of premenopausal women (approximately 45%).

Currently, the most commonly applied endocrine manipulations include surgical oophorectomy or radiation castration (in premenopausal women), antiestrogens, progestins, luteinizing hormone–releasing hormone agonists (in premenopausal women), and aromatase inhibitors.

Tamoxifen

Tamoxifen is now the most prescribed hormonal treatment for patients with primary and metastatic breast cancer. Tamoxifen has been the standard first-line therapy for metastatic breast cancer in postmenopausal women since the late 1970s.

Tamoxifen has also been used in premenopausal women with receptor-positive metastatic disease. Tamoxifen was compared to oophorectomy in two trials (135,136). The difference in median survival between patients treated with tamoxifen and those treated with oophorectomy did not reach statistical significance. However, in both studies, hormone receptor status was not available for all of the patients.

Progestins

Progestins have been used for the treatment of metastatic breast cancer for more than three decades (137,138). The response rates appear to be similar to those seen with other endocrine therapies. An overall response rate of 25% was reported for megestrol acetate as second-line therapy in advanced disease (139).

Luteinizing Hormone–Releasing Hormone Agonists

Luteinizing hormone–releasing hormone agonists have most commonly been used in premenopausal women with metastatic breast cancer. In large studies, the reported response rates ranged from 33% (hormone receptor–negative patients) to 49% (hormone receptor–positive patients) (140,141).

Aromatase Inhibitors

Selective aromatase inhibitors, including anastrozole, letrozole, formestane, and trilostane,

have been developed over the years in an attempt to reduce associated side effects, eliminate the need for concomitant steroid supplementation, and increase the specificity while retaining clinical efficacy.

Anastrozole is a competitive and highly selective nonsteroidal inhibitor of aromatase. It has no activity against desmolase or other enzymes involved in steroid biosynthesis. The recommended dose of 1 mg/day is based on the results of two large randomized trials (142,143). The doses tested were 1 mg/day (which completely suppresses estradiol but not estrone) and 10 mg/day (which suppresses both estradiol and estrone). These two doses were compared with 40 mg of megestrol acetate four times a day. There was no statistically significant difference in median time to objective progression among the three treatment groups or between the two dose levels. Given the similar efficacy and favorable safety profile, oral nonsteroidal aromatase inhibitors such as anastrozole should be considered in patients who are candidates for further hormonal therapy after tamoxifen treatment.

REFERENCES

1. Seidman H, Gell SK, Silverberg E, et al. Survival experience in the Breast Cancer Detection Demonstration Project. *CA Cancer J Clin* 1987; 37:258–290.

2. Zeichner GI, Mohar BA, Ramirez UMT. Epidemiologia del cancer de mama en el Instituto Nacional de Cancerologia (1989–1990). *Cancerologia* 1993;39:1825–1830.

3. Haagensen CD, Stout AP. Carcinoma of the breast. II. Criteria of operability. *Ann Surg* 1943; 118:859–870, 1032–1051.

4. Baclesse F. Roentgen therapy alone as the method of treatment of cancer of the breast. *AJR Am J Roentgenol* 1949;62:311–319.

5. Fletcher GH, Montague ED. Radical irradiation of advanced breast cancer. *AJR Am J Roentgenol* 1965;93:573–584.

6. Harris JR, Sawicka J, Gelman R, Hellman S. Management of locally advanced carcinoma of the breast by primary radiation therapy. *Int J Radiat Oncol Biol Phys* 1983;9:345–349.

7. Rodger A, Montague ED, Fletcher G. Preoperative or postoperative irradiation as adjunctive treatment with radical mastectomy in breast cancer. *Cancer* 1983;51:388–392.

8. Perloff M, Lesnick GJ, Korzun A, et al. Combination chemotherapy with mastectomy or radiotherapy for stage III breast carcinoma: a Cancer and Leukemia Group B study. *J Clin Oncol* 1988;6:261–269.

9. Valagussa P, Zambetti M, Bonadonna G, et al. Prognostic factors in locally advanced noninflammatory breast cancer: long-term results following primary chemotherapy. *Breast Cancer Res Treat* 1990;15:137–147.

10. Pierce LJ, Lippman M, Ben-Baruch N, et al. The effect of systemic therapy on local-regional control in locally advanced breast cancer. *Int J Radiat Oncol Biol Phys* 1992;23:949–960.

11. Jacquillat CL, Baillet F, Weil M, et al. Results of a conservative treatment combining induction (neoadjuvant) and consolidation chemotherapy, hormonotherapy, and external and interstitial irradiation in 98 patients with locally advanced breast cancer (IIIA–IIIB). *Cancer* 1988;61: 1977–1982.

12. Baillet F, Housset M, Weil M, et al. Study of 58 local-regional failures after conservative treatment involving neoadjuvant chemotherapy and exclusive radiotherapy in 304 breast cancer patients. In: *Fourth International Congress on Anti-Cancer Chemotherapy. Paris, France* 1993; 23:63.

13. Spanos WJ Jr, Montague ED, Fletcher GH. Late complications of radiation only for advanced breast cancer. *Int J Radiat Oncol Biol Phys* 1980;6:1473–1476.

14. Hortobagyi GN, Ames FC, Buzdar AU, et al. Management of stage III primary breast cancer with primary chemotherapy, surgery, and radiation therapy. *Cancer* 1988;62:2507–2516.

15. Broadwater JR, Edwards MJ, Kuglen C, et al. Mastectomy following preoperative chemotherapy. *Ann Surg* 1991;213:126–129.

16. Feldman LD, Hortobagyi GN, Buzdar AU, et al. Pathological assessment of response to induction chemotherapy in breast cancer. *Cancer Res* 1986;46:2578–2581.

17. McCready DR, Hortobagyi GN, Kau SW, et al. The prognostic significance of lymph node metastases after preoperative chemotherapy for locally advanced breast cancer. *Arch Surg* 1989;124:21–25.

18. Singletary SE, Hortobagyi GN, Kroll SS. Surgical and medical management of local-regional treatment failures in advanced primary breast cancer. *Surg Oncol Clin N Am* 1995;4:671–684.

19. Strom EA, McNeese MD, Fletcher GH, et al. Results of mastectomy and postoperative irradiation in the management of locoregionally advanced carcinoma of the breast. *Int J Radiat Oncol Biol Phys* 1991;21:319–323.

20. Rowinsky EK, Casenave LA, Donehower RC. Taxol: a novel investigational antimicrotubule agent. *J Natl Cancer Inst* 1990;82:1247–1259.

21. Holmes FA, Walters RS, Theriault RL, et al. Phase II trial of taxol, an active drug in the treatment of metastatic breast cancer. *J Natl Cancer Inst* 1991;83:1797–1805.

22. Hortobagyi GN, Singletary SE, Buzdar AU, et al. Primary chemotherapy for breast cancer: M. D. Anderson experience. In: Banzet P, ed. *Proceedings of the 3rd international congress on neo-adjuvant chemotherapy.* New York: Springer, 1991:145–148.

23. Singletary SE, McNeese MD, Hortobagyi GN. Feasibility of breast conservation surgery after induction chemotherapy for locally advanced carcinoma. *Cancer* 1992;69:2849–2852.

24. American Joint Committee on Cancer. *Manual for staging of cancer.* 3rd ed. Philadelphia: JB Lippincott, 1988:145–150.

25. Schwartz GF, Birchansky CA, Komarnicky LT, et al. Induction chemotherapy followed by breast conservation for locally advanced carcinoma of the breast. *Cancer* 1994;73:362–369.

26. Scholl SM, Fourquet A, Asselain B, et al. Neoadjuvant versus adjuvant chemotherapy in premenopausal patients with tumours considered too large for breast conserving surgery: preliminary results of randomised trial: S6. *Eur J Cancer* 1994;30A:645–652.

27. Bonadonna G, Veronesi U, Brambilla C, et al. Primary chemotherapy for resectable breast cancer. *Recent Results Cancer Res* 1993;127: 113–117.

28. Singletary SE. Breast surgery. In: Roh MS, Ames FC, eds. *Atlas of advanced oncologic surgery.* New York: Gower Medical, 1993:14.1–14.9.

29. Kiang DT, Kennedy BJ. Tamoxifen (antiestrogen) therapy in advanced breast cancer. *Ann Intern Med* 1977;87:687–690.

30. Jaiyesimi IA, Buzdar AU, Decker DA, Hortobagyi GN. Use of tamoxifen for breast cancer: twenty-eight years later. *J Clin Oncol* 1995; 13:513–529.

31. Kennedy BJ, Fortuny IE. Therapeutic castration in the treatment of advanced breast cancer. *Cancer* 1964;17:1197–1202.

32. Manni A, Santen R, Harvey H, et al. Treatment of breast cancer with gonadotrophin-releasing hormone. *Endocr Rev* 1986;7:89–94.

33. Hortobagyi GN. Overview of new treatments for breast cancer. *Breast Cancer Res Treat* 1992;21:3–13.

34. Chevallier B, Fumoleau P, Kerbrat P, et al. Docetaxel is a major cytotoxic drug for the treatment of advanced breast cancer: a phase II trial of the clinical screening cooperative group of the European Organization for Research and Treatment of Cancer. *J Clin Oncol* 1995;13:314–322.

35. Toussaint C, Izzo J, Spielmann S, et al. Phase I/II trial of continuous infusion vinorelbine for advanced breast cancer. *J Clin Oncol* 1994;12:2102–2112.

36. Pazdur R, Kudelka AP, Kavanagh JJ, et al. The taxoids: paclitaxel (Taxol) and docetaxel (Taxotere). *Cancer Treat Rev* 1993;19:351–386.

37. Seidman AD, Reichman BS, Crown JPA, et al. Paclitaxel as second and subsequent therapy for metastatic breast cancer: activity independent of prior anthracycline response. *J Clin Oncol* 1995;13:1152–1159.

38. Smith IE, Walsh G, Jones A, et al. High complete remission rates with primary neoadjuvant infusional chemotherapy for large early breast cancer. *J Clin Oncol* 1995;13:424–429.

39. Schneebaum S, Walker MJ, Young D, et al. The regional treatment of liver metastases from breast cancer. *J Surg Oncol* 1994;55:26–32.

40. Goodman GE, Hellstrom I, Brodzinsky L, et al. Phase I trial of murine monoclonal antibody L6 in breast, colon, ovarian and lung cancer. *J Clin Oncol* 1990;8:1083–1092.

41. Baselga J, Norton L, Masui H, et al. Antitumor effects of doxorubicin in combination with anti-epidermal growth factor receptor monoclonal antibodies. *J Natl Cancer Inst* 1993;85:1327–1333.

42. Trail PA, Willner SJ, Lasch AJ, et al. Cure of xenografted human carcinomas by BR96-doxorubicin immunoconjugates. *Science* 1993;261:212–215.

43. Peters WP, Ross M, Vredenburgh JJ, et al. High-dose chemotherapy and autologous bone marrow support as consolidation after standard-dose adjuvant therapy for high-risk primary breast cancer. *J Clin Oncol* 1993;11:1132–1143.

44. Dunphy FR, Spitzer G, Buzdar AU, et al. Treatment of estrogen receptor negative or hormonally refractory breast cancer with double high-dose chemotherapy intensification and bone marrow support. *J Clin Oncol* 1990;8:1207–1216.

45. Buzdar AU, McNeese MD, Hortobagyi GN, et al. Is chemotherapy effective in reducing the local failure rate in patients with operable breast cancer? *Cancer* 1990;65:394–399.

46. Ung O, Langlands AO, Barraclough B, Boyages J. Combined chemotherapy and radiotherapy for patients with breast cancer and extensive nodal involvement. *J Clin Oncol* 1995;13:435–443.

47. Halpern J, McNeese MD, Kroll SS, Ellerbrock N. Irradiation of prosthetically augmented breasts: a retrospective study on toxicity and cosmetic results. *Int J Radiat Oncol Biol Phys* 1990;18:189–191.

48. Rosato RM, Dowden RV. Radiation therapy as a cause of capsular contracture. *Ann Plast Surg* 1994;32:342–345.

49. Kroll SS, Ames FC, Singletary SE, Schusterman MA. The oncologic risks of skin preservation at mastectomy when combined with immediate reconstruction of the breast. *Surg Gynecol Obstet* 1991;172:17–20.

50. Schusterman MA, Kroll SS, Miller MJ, et al. The free transverse rectus abdominis musculocutaneous flap for breast reconstruction: one center's experience with 211 consecutive cases. *Ann Plast Surg* 1994;32:234–242.

51. Slavin SH, Love SM, Goldwyn RM. Recurrent breast cancer following immediate reconstruction with myocutaneous flaps. *Plast Reconstr Surg* 1994;93:1191–1204.

52. Kroll SS, Schusterman MA, Reece GP, et al. Breast reconstruction with myocutaneous flaps in previously irradiated patients. *Plast Reconstr Surg* 1994;93:460–469.

53. Hartrampf CR, Scheflan M, Black PW. Breast reconstruction with a transverse abdominal island flap. *Plast Reconstr Surg* 1982;69:216–224.

54. Ishii CH, Bostwick J, Raine TJ, et al. Double-pedicled transverse abdominis myocutaneous flap for unilateral breast and chest wall reconstruction. *Plast Reconstr Surg* 1985;76:901–907.

55. McKenna RJ, McMurtrey MJ, Larson DL, Mountain CF. A perspective on chest wall resection in patients with breast cancer. *Ann Thorac Surg* 1984;38:482–486.

56. McKenna RJ, Mountain CF, McMurtrey MJ, et al. Current techniques for chest wall reconstruction: expanded possibilities for treatment. *Ann Thorac Surg* 1988;46:508–512.

57. Kroll SS, Walsh G, Ryan B, King RC. Risks and benefits of using Marlex mesh in chest wall reconstruction. *Ann Plast Surg* 1993;31:303–306.

58. McCormack PM, Bains MS, Burt ME, et al. Local recurrent mammary carcinoma failing multimodality therapy. *Arch Surg* 1989;124:158–161.

59. Starzynski TE, Snyderman RK, Beattie EJ Jr. Problems of major chest wall reconstruction. *Plast Reconstr Surg* 1969;44:525–535.

60. Jurkiewicz MJ, Arnold PG. The omentum: an account of its use in the reconstruction of the chest wall. *Ann Surg* 1977;185:548–554.

61. Fowble B, Gray R, Gilchrist K, et al. Identification of a subgroup of patients with breast cancer and histologically positive axillary nodes receiving adjuvant chemotherapy who may benefit from postoperative radiotherapy. *J Clin Oncol* 1988;6:1107–1117.

62. Valagussa P, Bonadonna G, Veronesi U. Patterns of relapse and survival following radical mastectomy. *Cancer* 1978;41:1170–1178.

63. Aberizk WJ, Silver B, Henderson IC, et al. The use of radiotherapy for treatment of isolated regional recurrence of breast cancer after mastectomy. *Cancer* 1986;58:1214–1218.

64. Bedwinek JM, Lee J, Fineberg B, Ocwieza M. Prognostic indicators in patients with isolated local-regional recurrence of breast cancer. *Cancer* 1981;47:2232–2235.

65. Griem KL, Henderson IC, Gelman R, et al. The 5-year results of a randomized trial of adjuvant radiation therapy after chemotherapy in breast cancer patients treated with mastectomy. *J Clin Oncol* 1987;5:1546–1555.

66. Holmes FA, Buzdar AU, Kau S-W, et al. Combined-modality approach for patients with isolated recurrences of breast cancer (IV-NED). The M. D. Anderson experience. *Breast Dis* 1994; 7:7–20.

67. Halverson KJ, Perez CA, Kuske RR, et al. Survival following locoregional recurrence of breast cancer: univariate and multivariate analysis. *Int J Radiat Oncol Biol Phys* 1992;23:285–291.

68. Crowe JP Jr, Gordon NH, Antunez AR, et al. Local-regional breast cancer recurrence following mastectomy. *Arch Surg* 1991;126:429–432.

69. Janjan NA, McNeese MD, Buzdar AU, et al. Management of locoregional recurrent breast cancer. *Cancer* 1986;58:1552–1556.

70. Probstfeld MR, O'Connell TX. Treatment of locally recurrent breast carcinoma. *Arch Surg* 1989;124:1127–1130.

71. Neidhart JA. Dose-intensive treatment of breast cancer supported by granulocyte-macrophage colony-stimulating factor. *Breast Cancer Res Treat* 1991;20(suppl):S15–S23.

72. Neidhart JA, Morris DM, Herman TS. Dose-intensification chemotherapy for patients with advanced breast cancer. *Semin Radiat Oncol* 1994;4:236–241.

73. Muss HB, Thor AD, Berry DA, et al. c-erb B-2 expression and response to adjuvant therapy in women with node-positive early breast cancer. *N Engl J Med* 1994;330:1260–1266.

74. Resnick JM, Sneige N, Kemp BL, et al. p53 and c-erb B-2 expression and response to preoperative chemotherapy in locally advanced breast cancer. *Breast Dis* 1995;8:149–158.

75. Pierce LJ, Lichter AS, Archer P. Indications, integration, and technical aspects of local-regional irradiation in the management of advanced breast cancer. *Semin Radiat Oncol* 1994;4: 242–253.

76. Singletary SE. Surgical management of locally advanced breast cancer. *Semin Radiat Oncol* 1994;4:254–259.

77. Wingo PA, Tong T, Bolden S. Cancer statistics. *CA Cancer J Clin* 1995;45:8–30.

78. Garber JE, Henderson IC. The use of chemotherapy in metastatic breast cancer. *Hematol Oncol Clin North Am* 1989;3:807–821.

79. Greengerg PAC, Hortobagyi GNH, Smith T, et al. Long-term follow-up of patients with complete remission following combination chemotherapy for metastatic breast cancer. *J Clin Oncol* 1996;14:2197–2205.

80. Sledge GW Jr, Antman KH. Progress in chemotherapy for metastatic breast cancer. *Semin Oncol* 1992;19:317–332.

81. Paridaens R, Heuson JC, Julien JC, et al. Assessment of estrogenic recruitment before chemotherapy in advanced breast cancer: preliminary results of a double-blind randomized study of the EORTC Breast Cancer Cooperative Group. *J Steroid Biochem Mol Biol* 1990;6:1109–1113.

82. Paridaens R, Van Zijl J, Van der Merwe J, et al. Comparison between the alternating and the sequential administration of three different chemotherapy regimens in advanced breast cancer. A randomized study of the EORTC Breast Cancer Cooperative Group. Communication at the 5th EORTC Breast Cancer Working Conference, Leuven, Belgium, September 3–6, 1991.

83. Jones RB, Shpall EJ, Shogan J, et al. The Duke AFM program. Intensive induction chemotherapy for metastatic breast cancer. *Cancer* 1990; 66:431–436.

84. Antman K, Gale RP. Advanced breast cancer, high-dose chemotherapy and bone marrow autotransplants. *Ann Intern Med* 1988;108: 570–574.

85. Wallerstein R Jr, Spitzer G, Dunphy F, et al. A phase II study of mitoxantrone, etoposide, and thiotepa with autologous bone marrow support for patients with relapsed breast cancer. *J Clin Oncol* 1990;8:1782–1788.

86. Vogel CL, Azevedo S, Hilsenbeck S, et al. Survival after first recurrence of breast cancer: the Miami experience. *Cancer* 1992;70:129–135.

87. Hayes DF, Henderson IC, Shapiro CL. Treatment of metastatic breast cancer: present and future prospects. *Semin Oncol* 1995;22:5–21.

88. Henderson IC, Harris JR, Kinne DW, et al. Cancer of the breast. In: De Vita VT Jr, Hellman S, Rosenberg SA, eds. *Cancer: principles and practice of oncology.* 3rd ed. Philadelphia: JB Lippincott, 1989:1197–1258.

89. Henderson IC. Chemotherapy for metastatic disease. In: Harris JR, Hellman S, Henderson IC, Kinne DW, eds. *Breast diseases.* 2nd ed. Philadelphia: JB Lippincott, 1991:604–665.

90. Mouridsen HT. Systemic therapy of advanced breast cancer. *Drugs* 1992;44:17–28.

91. Neidhart JA, Gochnour D, Roach R, et al. A comparison of mitoxantrone and doxorubicin in breast cancer. *J Clin Oncol* 1986;4:672–677.

92. Henderson IC, Allegra JC, Woodcock T, et al. Randomized clinical trial comparing mitoxantrone with doxorubicin in previously treated patients with metastatic breast cancer. *J Clin Oncol* 1989;17:560–571.

93. Jain KK, Casper ES, Geller NL, et al. A prospective randomized comparison of epirubicin and doxorubicin in patients with advanced breast cancer. *J Clin Oncol* 1985;3:818–826.

94. Hortobagyi GN, Bodey GP, Buzdar AU, et al. Evaluation of high-dose versus standard FAC chemotherapy for advanced breast cancer in protected environment units, a prospective randomized study. *J Clin Oncol* 1987;5:254–364.

95. Habeshaw T, Paul J, Jones R, et al. Epirubicin at two dose levels with prednisolone as treatment for advanced breast cancer, the results of a randomized trial. *J Clin Oncol* 1991;9:295–304.

96. Piccart M, van der Schueren E, Bruningx P, et al. High-dose-intensity (DI) chemotherapy (CT) with epiadriamycin (E), cyclophosphamide (C) and r-metHuG-CSF (AMGEN) in breast cancer (BC) patients. *Eur J Cancer* 1991;27:S56.

97. Porkka K, Blomquvist C, Rissanen P, et al. Salvage therapies in women who fail to respond to first-line treatment with fluorouracil, epirubicin, and cyclophosphamide for advanced breast cancer. *J Clin Oncol* 1994;12:1639–1647.

98. Buzdar AU. Chemotherapeutic approaches to advanced breast cancer. *Semin Oncol* 1988; 15:65–70.

99. Buzdar AU, Legha SS, Hortobagyi GN, et al. Management of breast cancer patients failing adjuvant chemotherapy with Adriamycin-containing regimens. *Cancer* 1981;47:1798–2802.

100. Weber B, Vogel C, Jones S, et al. A U.S. multicenter phase II trial of Navelbine in advanced breast cancer. *Proc Am Soc Clin Oncol* 1993; 12:61. Abstract.

101. Agostara B, Gebbia V, Testa A, et al. Mitomycin-C and vinorelbine as second line chemotherapy for metastatic breast carcinoma. *Tumori* 1994; 80:33–36.

102. Jones S, Winer E, Vogel C. A randomized comparison of vinorelbine and melphalan in anthracycline-refractory advanced breast cancer. *J Clin Oncol* 1995;13:2567–2574.

103. Degardin M, Bonneterre J, Hecquet B, et al. Vinorelbine (Navelbine) as a salvage treatment for advanced breast cancer. *Ann Oncol* 1994; 15:423–426.

104. Gasparini G, Caffo O, Barni S, et al. Vinorelbine is an active antiproliferative agent in pretreated advanced breast cancer patients: a phase II study. *J Clin Oncol* 1994;12:2094–2101.

105. Stoger H, Schmid M, Bauernhofer T, et al. A phase II trial of weekly high-dose folinic acid and 5-fluorouracil in combination with epirubicin as salvage chemotherapy in advanced breast cancer. *Oncology* 1994;51:518–522.

106. Ingle JN, Mailliard JA, Schaid DJ, et al. Randomized trial of doxorubicin alone or combined with vincristine and mitomycin-C in women with metastatic breast cancer. *Am J Clin Oncol* 1989;12:474–480.

107. Sedlacek SM. First-line and salvage therapy of metastatic breast cancer with mitomycin/vinblastine. *Oncology* 1993;50:16–23.

108. Francini G, Petrioli R, Aquino A, et al. Advanced breast cancer treatment with folinic

acid, 5-fluorouracil, and mitomycin C. *Cancer Chemother Pharmacol* 1993;32:359–364.

109. Konits PH, Aisner J, Van Echo DA, et al. Mitomycin C and vinblastine chemotherapy for advanced breast cancer. *Cancer* 1981;48:1295–1298.

110. Garewal HS, Brooks RJ, Jones SE, et al. Treatment of advanced breast cancer with mitomycin C combined with vinblastine or vindesine. *J Clin Oncol* 1983;1:772–775.

111. Radford JA, Knight RK, Rubens RD. Mitomycin C and vinblastine in the treatment of advanced breast cancer. *Eur J Cancer Clin Oncol* 1985;21:1475–1477.

112. Cameron DA, Gabra H, Leonard RC. Continuous 5-fluorouracil in the treatment of breast cancer. *Br J Cancer* 1994;70:120–124.

113. Reichman BS, Seidman AD, Crown JPA, et al. Paclitaxel and recombinant human granulocyte colony-stimulating factor as initial chemotherapy for metastatic breast cancer. *J Clin Oncol* 1993;11:1943–1951.

114. Mamounas E, Brown A, Fisher DL, et al. Three-hour high-dose taxol infusion in advanced breast cancer: an NSABP phase II study. *Proc Am Soc Clin Oncol* 1995;14:127. Abstract.

115. Seidman AD, Tiersten C, Hudis M, et al. Phase II trial of paclitaxel by 3-hour infusion as initial and salvage chemotherapy for metastatic breast cancer. *J Clin Oncol* 1995;13:2575–2581.

116. Wilson WH, Berg SL, Bryant G, et al. Paclitaxel in doxorubicin-refractory breast cancer: a phase I/II trial of 96-hour infusion. *J Clin Oncol* 1994;12:1621–1629.

117. Abrams JS, Vena DA, Baltz J, et al. Paclitaxel activity in heavily pretreated breast cancer: a National Cancer Institute treatment referral center trial. *J Clin Oncol* 1995;13:2056–2065.

118. Ten Bokkel Huinink WW, Prove AM, Piccart M, et al. A phase II trial with docetaxel (Taxotere) in second line treatment with chemotherapy for advanced breast cancer. *Ann Oncol* 1994;5:527–532.

119. Valero V, Holmes FA, Walters RS, et al. Phase II trial of docetaxel: a new highly effective antineoplastic agent in the management of patients with anthracycline resistant metastatic breast cancer. *J Clin Oncol* 1995;13:2886–2894.

120. Gianni L, Munzone E, Capri G, et al. Paclitaxel by 3-hour infusion in combination with bolus doxorubicin in women with untreated metastatic breast cancer: high antitumor efficacy and cardiac effects in a dose-finding and sequence-finding study. *J Clin Oncol* 1995;13:2688–2699.

121. Slichenmeyer WJ, Rowinsky EK, Donehower RC, et al. The current status of camptothecin analogues as antitumor agents. *J Natl Cancer Inst* 1993;85:271–291.

122. Chang AY, Garrow G, Boros L, et al. Clinical and laboratory studies of topotecan in breast cancer. *Proc Am Soc Clin Oncol* 1995;14:105. Abstract.

123. Bonneterre J, Pion JM, Adenis A, et al. A phase II study of a new camptothecin analogue CPT-11 in previously treated advanced breast cancer patients. *Proc Am Soc Clin Oncol* 1993;12:94. Abstract.

124. Carmichael J, Possinger K, Philip P, et al. Difluorodeoxycytidine (gemcitabine): a phase II study in patients with advanced breast cancer. *Proc Am Soc Clin Oncol* 1993;12:64. Abstract.

125. Hryniuk WM, Bush H. The importance of dose intensity in chemotherapy of metastatic breast cancer. *J Clin Oncol* 1984;2:1281–1287.

126. Bruce WR, Meeker BE, Valeriote FA. Comparison of the sensitivity of normal hematopoietic and transplanted lymphoma colony-forming cells to chemotherapeutic agents administered in vivo. *J Natl Cancer Inst* 1966;37:233–245.

127. Bonadonna G, Valagussa P. Dose-response effect of adjuvant chemotherapy in breast cancer. *N Engl J Med* 1981;304:10–15.

128. Lazarus HM, Herzig RH, Graham-Pole J, et al. Intensive melphalan chemotherapy and cryopreserved autologous bone marrow transplantation for the treatment of refractory cancer. *J Clin Oncol* 1983;2:359–367.

129. Peters WP, Ross M, Vredenburgh JJ, et al. High-dose chemotherapy and autologous bone marrow support as consolidation after standard-dose adjuvant therapy for high-risk primary breast cancer. *J Clin Oncol* 1993;11:1132–1143.

130. Peters WP, Jones RB, Vredenburgh J, et al. A large, prospective, randomized trial of high-dose combination alkylating agents (CPB) with autologous cellular support (ABMS) as consolidation for patients with metastatic breast cancer achieving complete remission after intensive doxorubicin-based induction therapy (AFM). *Proc Am Soc Clin Oncol* 1996;15:149. Abstract.

131. Falkson G, Holcroft C, Gelman RS, et al. Ten-year follow-up study of premenopausal women with metastatic breast cancer: an Eastern Coop-

erative Oncology Group study. *J Clin Oncol* 1995;13:1453–1458.

132. Diamandidou E, Buzdar AU, Smith T, et al. Treatment-related leukemia in breast cancer patients treated with 5-fluorouracil, doxorubicin, cyclophosphamide (FAC) combination adjuvant chemotherapy. *J Clin Oncol* 1996;14:2722–2730.

133. Carter C, Allen C, Henson D. Relation of tumor size, lymph node status, and survival in 24, 740 breast cancer cases. *Cancer* 1989;56:181–187.

134. Sedlacek SM, Horowitz KB. The role of progestins and progesterone receptors in the treatment of breast cancer. *Steroids* 1984;44:467–484.

135. Buchanan RB, Blamey RW, Durrant KR, et al. A randomized comparison of tamoxifen with surgical oophorectomy in premenopausal patients with advanced breast cancer. *J Clin Oncol* 1986;4:1326–1330.

136. Ingle JN, Krook JE, Green SJ, et al. Randomized trial of bilateral oophorectomy versus tamoxifen in premenopausal women with metastatic breast cancer. *J Clin Oncol* 1986;4:178–185.

137. Escher GC, Heber JM, Woodard HQ, et al. Newer steroids in the treatment of advanced mammary carcinoma. In: White A, ed. *Symposium on steroids in experimental and clinical practice*. Philadelphia: P Blakiston, 1951:375–378.

138. Nathanson IT, Engel LL, Kennedy BJ, et al. Screening of steroids and allied compounds in neoplastic disease. In: White A, ed. *Symposium on steroids in experimental and clinical practice*. Philadelphia: P Blakiston, 1951:379–405.

139. Lundgren S. Progestins in breast cancer treatment. A review. *Acta Oncol* 1992;31:709–722.

140. Kaufmann M, Jonat W, Kleeberg U, et al. Goserelin, a depot gonadotropin-releasing hormone agonist in the treatment of premenopausal patients with metastatic breast cancer. German Zoladex Trial group. *J Clin Oncol* 1989;7:1113–1119.

141. Kaufmann M, Jonat W, Schachner-Wunschmann E, et al. The depot GnRH analogue goserelin in the treatment of premenopausal patients with metastatic breast cancer—a 5-year experience and further endocrine therapies. Cooperative German Zoladex Study group. *Onkologie* 1991;14:22–24.

142. Jonat W, Howell A, Blomqvist C, et al. A randomized trial comparing two doses of the new selective aromatase inhibitor anastrozole (Arimidex) with megestrol acetate in postmenopausal patients with advanced breast cancer. *Eur J Cancer* 1996;32A:404–412.

143. Buzdar AU, Jonat A, Howell A, et al. Anastrozole, a potent and selective aromatase inhibitor, versus megestrol acetate in postmenopausal women with advanced breast cancer: results of an overview analysis of two phase III trials. *J Clin Oncol* 1996;14:2000–2011.

Inflammatory Breast Cancer

S. EVA SINGLETARY
AMAN U. BUZDAR

*I*nflammatory breast cancer (IBC) is a highly malignant form of breast cancer. As early as 1814, Sir Charles Bell (1) said that "When a purple color is on the skin over the tumor it is a very unpropitious beginning." The term *inflammatory breast cancer* was initially used in 1924 by Lee and Tannenbaum (2), who likened the appearance of the inflamed areas to erysipelas. Others have since confirmed the unique, rapidly fatal nature of IBC (3–7). Today, with prompt diagnosis and multimodality therapy, the outlook for patients with IBC has improved and 30% to 48% remain free of disease for more than 10 years (8).

Epidemiology

IBC represents 1% to 6% of all cases of breast cancer in the United States (3,4,9). Studies showed that the median age of women with this disease is 52 years, which is similar to the average age for women with invasive ductal breast cancer in general (2–4,6,10,11). Rarely, IBC is found in men. Treves (12) reported that 3 (2%) of 131 men with breast cancer had features consistent with IBC.

Pregnancy and lactation were thought to be associated with IBC in some early studies (13–15). However, Taylor and Meltzer (3) found that only 1 of 38 patients with IBC developed the disease during pregnancy, and Haagensen (4) reported that only 4 of 89 patients with IBC were pregnant or lactating.

Staging System

The most widely used cancer staging system is the tumor-node-metastasis (TNM) system of the American Joint Committee on Cancer (16) and the International Union Against Cancer (17), which designates IBC as a T4 (stage IIIB) breast carcinoma. In the Columbia Clinical Classification System (4), stage C disease is defined by edema of less than one third of the breast skin, skin ulceration, chest wall fixation, axillary node fixation, or axillary nodes larger than 2.5 cm in diameter; and stage D disease is characterized by two or more of these "grave signs." The Institut Gustave-Roussy has used its own system (18), Poysee Evolutive (PEV), which differs from the TNM staging system by including tumor growth characteristics and signs of inflammation. The PEV categories are described as follows: PEV 0, a tumor without recent increase in volume and without inflammatory signs; PEV 1, a tumor showing marked increase in volume for a period of 2 months but without inflammatory signs; PEV 2, a tumor in which the overlying breast tissue, particularly the skin, is affected by subacute inflammation and edema involving less than half of the breast surface; and PEV 3, a tumor with acute or subacute inflammation and edema involving more than half of the breast surface.

Diagnosis

The diagnosis of IBC continues to be based on three clinical findings: 1) erythema (associated with increased heat), 2) skin edema or peau d'orange (exaggerated hair follicle pits secondary to tumor blockage of the lymphatics), and 3) wheals or ridging of the skin (indicating that the lymphatics have filled with tumor cells) (Fig. 9-1). A history of rapid onset (within 3 months) is often used to distinguish IBC from locally advanced breast carcinoma with secondary clinical lymphatic invasion.

The description of primary IBC versus secondary IBC is controversial. Taylor and Meltzer (3) defined primary IBC as the simultaneous development of inflammatory skin changes and carcinoma in a previously normal breast, whereas secondary IBC was referred to as the development of inflammatory changes in a breast that already contained cancer. Haagensen (4) and Sherry et al (10) urged colleagues to discontinue using the term *secondary IBC* because neglected locally advanced breast carcinoma may have a better clinical course than true IBC. However, the results of retrospective studies by Piera et al (19) and others (20,21) suggest that primary and secondary IBC patients may have similar outcomes when treated with the same modalities.

Another controversy concerns whether histologic evidence of dermal lymphatic involvement is necessary for the diagnosis of IBC. Anecdotal reports (22,23) indicate that patients with documented histologic dermal lymphatic invasion have a worse prognosis than do those

FIGURE **9-1**

Clinical signs of inflammatory carcinoma in situ of the breast include rapid onset of (*A*) subtle erythema or (*B*) violaceous erythema, (*C*) skin ridging, and (*D*) peau d'orange secondary to dermal lymphatic tumor involvement.

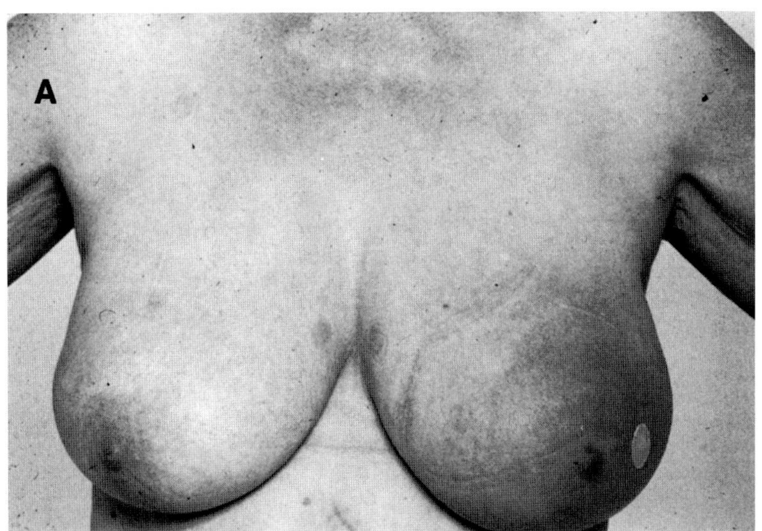

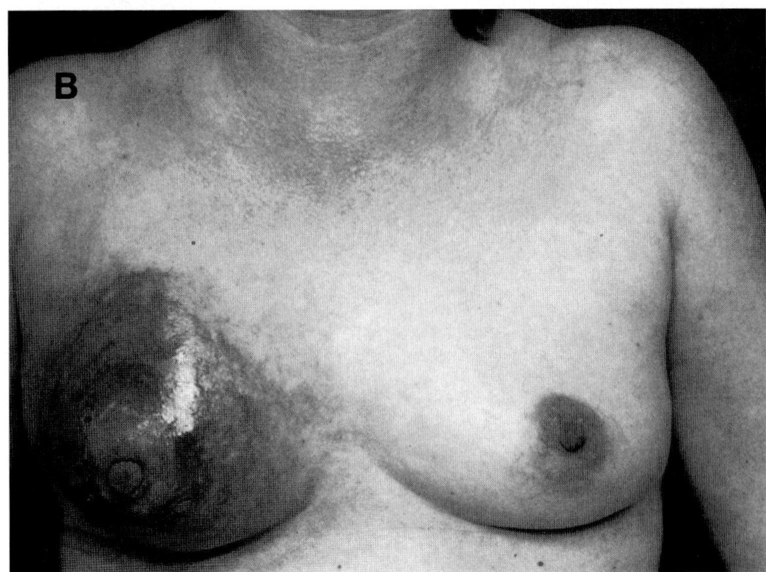

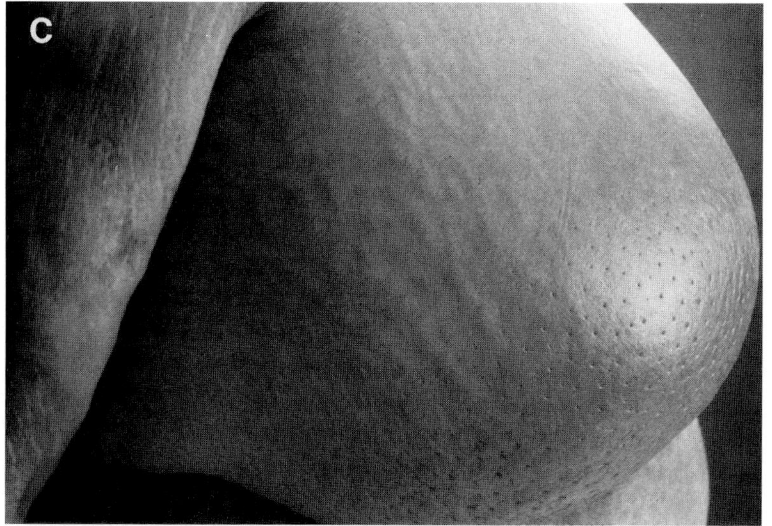

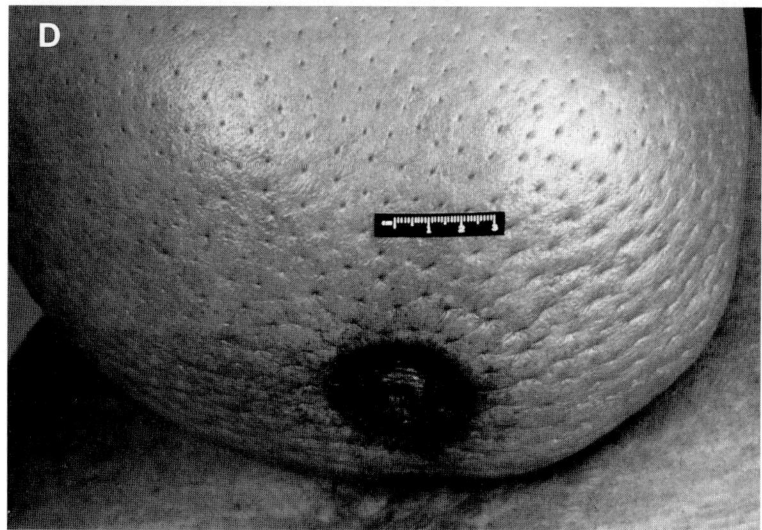

FIGURE **9-1**

Continued

without such histologic findings. In contrast, Lucas and Mesa-Perez (24) found that patients with clinical signs of IBC had a median survival time of 14 months regardless of histologic skin involvement. In that study, a subset of patients with occult IBC (histologic evidence of dermal lymphatic disease without clinical signs) had the best median survival time (40 months). Unfortunately, this study also included locally advanced breast carcinomas, and patients were treated with a variety of modalities. Analysis of Surveillance, Epidemiology, and End Results (SEER) program data for patients who received chemotherapy plus surgery and radiation therapy revealed that those who had both clinical and pathologic diagnoses of IBC had a 3-year survival rate of 34%, compared with a 60% rate for patients with only clinical features of IBC

and 52% for those with only a histologic diagnosis (9). To resolve this issue, future studies should include a skin biopsy before therapy to assess whether dermal lymphatic invasion has occurred. In addition, even though IBC is more likely than other types of breast cancer to test negative for estrogen and progesterone receptors (25–28), receptor status should also be assessed to identify patients who may benefit from hormonal therapy.

Treatment

The dismal results of surgical treatment alone for IBC (Table 9-1) (2–4,29–33) led to the philosophy that surgery was contraindicated for this disease. Thus, the policy on treatment of

T A B L E   **9-1**

Five-Year Survival Rate and Median Duration of Survival for Patients with Inflammatory Breast Cancer Treated by Radical or Simple Mastectomy Alone

Authors	Total No. of Patients	5-Year Survival Rate (%)	Median Survival Duration (mo)
Lee and Tannenbaum (2)	4	0	15
Taylor and Meltzer (3)	6	0	21
Treves (29)	114	3.5	NA
Byrd and Stevenson (30)	12	0	16
Donegan (31)	12	0	18.5
Haagensen (4)	30	3	19
Robbins et al (32)	4	0	12
Bozzetti et al (33)	8	0	12

NA = not available.

T A B L E   **9-2**

Five-Year Survival Rate and Median Duration of Survival for Patients with Inflammatory Breast Cancer Treated by Combined Radiation Therapy and Surgery

Authors	Total No. of Patients	5-Year Survival Rate (%)	Median Survival Duration (mo)
Lee and Tannenbaum (2)	4	0	24
Meyer et al (36)	47	2	28
Chris (37)	7	0	13
Rogers and Fitts (38)	20	5	21
Dao and McCarthy (39)	6	0	13
Richards and Lewison (40)	11	0	14
Barber et al (41)	50	10	25
Donegan (31)	9	0	16
Droulias et al (7)	5	20	29

IBC has evolved to radical irradiation alone. From 1948 to 1972 at The University of Texas M. D. Anderson Cancer Center, a protracted irradiation technique, first with orthovoltage and subsequently with cobalt-60 irradiation, was used to deliver doses up to 100 Gy over 10 to 14 weeks. This experience was first reported in 1965 (34). In 47 treated patients, a locoregional recurrence rate of 40.5% and a 5-year survival rate of 12% were observed (34). An updated report in 1976 (35) showed only 7 (10%) of 69 patients were alive at 5 years. In 1972, an accelerated fractionation technique was introduced; it delivered 74 Gy to the breast over 5.5 weeks in twice-daily treatments. Of 11 patients treated with irradiation alone, the locoregional failure rate was 27%, and the disease-free survival rate at 24 months was 27%.

The disappointing survival results associated with irradiation alone or irradiation combined with surgery (Table 9-2) (4,7,31,36–41) provided the rationale for using systemic chemotherapy as the first-line approach in IBC patients as soon as active drugs became available. The regimen used at M. D. Anderson Cancer Center from 1973 to 1981 was a combination of 5-fluorouracil, doxorubicin, and cyclophosphamide (FAC). After a median of three courses of chemotherapy, a mastectomy or definitive irradiation (twice-daily fractionation) was performed; maintenance chemotherapy continued for 2 years. In 63 patients with a recorded response, induction chemotherapy resulted in a complete response in 13%, a partial response in 57%, and a minor response in 23%. The 5-year disease-free survival rate was 25%, and the overall survival rate was 33% (8).

Because of a locoregional relapse in 25% of these patients and an interruption of systemic therapy for 9 to 10 weeks in patients treated with irradiation only, a standard mastectomy was included beginning in 1982 for all patients with operable disease. Vincristine and prednisone (VP) were added to the FAC combination chemotherapy (FACVP). After three cycles of FACVP, patients underwent mastectomy, which was followed by eight cycles of FACVP and then irradiation. In 1987 at M. D. Anderson, we began using an alternative chemotherapy regimen of methotrexate and vinblastine (MV) before surgery if the patient's disease did not respond to three cycles of FACVP (42). If the tumor still had not responded after two cycles of MV, irradiation was performed followed by mastectomy. If the tumor responded to MV, the patient underwent a mastectomy followed by four more cycles of MV chemotherapy.

A recent analysis of the combined experience (1973–1993) of 172 consecutive patients at M. D. Anderson who received induction chemotherapy for IBC demonstrated that the clinical response to chemotherapy is significantly related to disease-free and overall survival rates (43). The 5-year disease-free and overall survival rates were 63% and 70%, respectively, for the 21 patients who had a complete response, and 37% and 44% for the 106 patients with a partial response, and only 7% and 12% for the 45 patients with a nonsignificant response. The amount of residual tumor found on histologic examination of the mastectomy specimen was also highly predictive of overall and disease-free survival. For the 38 patients with less than $1\,cm^3$ of residual tumor in the mastectomy specimen after induction chemotherapy, the 5-year disease-free and overall survival rates were 59% and 71%, respectively, as compared to 27% and 31% in 87 patients with more than $1\,cm^3$ of remaining tumor. Factors that did not affect survival were age (≤50 years versus >50), estrogen receptor status, initial nodal stage, biopsy-proved dermal lymphatic invasion, and specific chemotherapy protocol.

The effect of the addition of mastectomy to chemotherapy plus radiation therapy on overall and disease-free survival depended on the patient's response to induction chemotherapy. Patients who had a clinical complete response or partial response to induction chemotherapy and were treated with mastectomy in addition to chemotherapy and irradiation had improved overall and disease-free survival rates compared with those patients with a complete or partial response who underwent only chemotherapy plus irradiation. Five-year overall and disease-free survival rates were 60% and 53%, respectively, for patients treated with mastectomy compared to 34% and 31% for patients who were treated with only chemotherapy and irradiation. Patients who had no significant response to induction chemotherapy demonstrated no improvement in overall or disease-free survival rates when mastectomy was added to chemotherapy plus irradiation (43).

Fields et al (44) also reported an improvement in relapse-free survival rates in 53 patients undergoing mastectomy as part of their treatment compared with 52 patients having no surgery. Locoregional recurrences occurred in 45% overall (19% of patients treated with mastectomy versus 70% of patients without surgery), with 90% of these relapses occurring within 2 years of treatment. Similarly, the results of the study by Brun et al (45) of attempts to conserve the breast by substituting interstitial irradiation for mastectomy in patients who experienced substantial tumor reduction with chemotherapy showed that local recurrence occurred in 7 of 13 patients treated conservatively, as compared with only two local relapses in 10 patients who had a mastectomy. Other advantages of including mastectomy as part of the combined-modality therapy are the abilities to obtain important information on histologic response to induction chemotherapy and to allow the use of a lower dose of radiation afterward (46–49). In patients who have a good tumor response to chemotherapy and who may attain long-term survival, avoiding late complications from high-dose radiation is of substantial benefit. For patients who fail to respond to chemotherapy, mastectomy serves only as a palliative tumor-debulking measure.

The major obstacle in improvement of survival has been the large percentage of patients who have a poor response to chemotherapy (25% of 172 patients in the M. D. Anderson series [43]). An analysis of 45 patients with IBC from a National Cancer Institute study indicated that a higher number of chemotherapy cycles combined with hormonal synchronization until maximal clinical response was achieved resulted in a 98% response rate and that 55% of patients had a clinically complete response (50). Thus far, relapses have occurred in 21 patients (47%), with a median time to progression of 23 months and a median survival duration of 36 months. This survival duration is similar to that observed in other studies that used chemotherapy before local therapy (Table 9-3) (1,28,45,51–58).

Our current protocol is to evaluate whether paclitaxel (Taxol), which has demonstrated activity against metastatic breast disease despite a history of prior anthracycline chemotherapy exposure, can provide a better crossover tumor response (Fig. 9-2).

Another strategy in the treatment of IBC explores the use of high-dose chemotherapy

T A B L E **9-3**

Five-Year Survival Rate and Median Duration of Survival for Patients with Inflammatory Breast Cancer Treated by Initial Chemotherapy and Local Modalities

Authors	Treatment	Total No. of Patients	5-Year Survival Rate (%)	Median Survival Duration (mo)
DeLena et al (50)	CT + RT ± CT	36	NA	25
Krutchik et al (51)	CT + RT + CT	32	NA	24
Pouillart et al (52)	CT + RT + CT	77	NA	34
Zylberberg et al (53)	CT + S + CT ± RT	15	70	>56
Keiling et al (54)	CT + S + CT	41	63	NA
Israel et al (55)	CT + S + CT	25	62	NA
Brun et al (44)	CT + RT + S + CT	26	NA	31
Thoms et al (11)	CT + S + CT + RT	61	35	NA
Fields et al (56)	CT + S + RT + CT	37	44	49
Rouesse et al (57)	CT + RT + CT + H	91	40	36
	CT + RT + CT + H	97	55	NA
Maloisel et al (28)	CT + S + CT + RT + H	43	75	46

CT = chemotherapy; RT = radiation therapy; S = surgery; H = hormonal therapy; NA = not available.

INFLAMMATORY CARCINOMA OF BREAST

F I G U R E **9-2**

M. D. Anderson Cancer Center's current strategy for the treatment of patients with inflammatory carcinoma of the breast. CR = complete response; PR = partial response; <PR = less than partial response; FAC = 5-fluorouracil, doxorubicin, and cyclophosphamide; XRT = radiation therapy.

and autologous stem cell support. In a review of five trials (a total of 56 women) of either single- or multiple-drug chemotherapy followed by autologous bone marrow transplantation (ABMT) for IBC and other stage III breast cancers, Antman et al (59) reported that 79% (44/56) of the patients had achieved a complete response after induction chemotherapy but before ABMT and that 89% were in complete remission after ABMT. Complete remission was maintained in 54% (30/56 patients); follow-up duration was 1 to 37 months. The mortality rate associated with the treatment was 4%. In a review of four studies of combination chemotherapy plus ABMT in 53 previously untreated IBC and metastatic breast cancer patients (some of whom had adjuvant therapy), 47% (25/53) of the patients achieved a complete response either before or after ABMT, and the overall response rate was 75%. The complete remission rate was maintained in 17% (9/53 patients) for 4 to 86 months following ABMT.

The mortality rate associated with the treatment was 9%.

The ABMT approach is still investigational, but these limited data indicate that it warrants further evaluation. A randomized study is under way at M. D. Anderson for IBC patients who have four or more positive axillary lymph nodes after preoperative chemotherapy but are rendered disease free by surgery. The trial involves the use of standard FAC or FAC followed by two cycles of high-dose chemotherapy (cyclophosphamide, etoposide, and cisplatin) and either ABMT or peripheral stem cell support.

The need to develop more effective treatment strategies for patients with IBC is clear. Because there is urgent need to further improve therapy for IBC, patients should be treated as part of clinical studies whenever feasible.

The current recommendation for patients not treated in research studies includes preoperative FAC for three cycles followed by mastectomy in patients with tumor downstaging, then postoperative FAC for six cycles, followed by radiation therapy (60).

REFERENCES

1. Bell C. *A system of operative surgery*, vol. 2. Hartford, CT: Hale & Hosmer, 1814:136.

2. Lee B, Tannenbaum N. Inflammatory carcinoma of the breast: a report of twenty-eight (28) cases from the breast clinic of Memorial Hospital. *Surg Gyncol Obstet* 1924;39:580–595.

3. Taylor G, Meltzer A. Inflammatory carcinoma of the breast. *Am J Cancer* 1938;33:33–49.

4. Haagensen C. Inflammatory carcinoma. In: Haagensen C, ed. *Diseases of the breast.* 2nd ed. Philadelphia: WB Saunders, 1971:576–584.

5. Lucas F, Perez-Mesa C. Inflammatory carcinoma of the breast. *Cancer* 1978;41:1595–1605.

6. Stocks L, Patterson FMS. Inflammatory carcinoma of the breast. *Surg Gynecol Obstet* 1976; 143:885–889.

7. Droulias S, Sewell C, McSweeney M, Powell RW. Inflammatory carcinoma of the breast: a correlation of clinical, radiologic, and pathologic findings. *Ann Surg* 1976;184:217–222.

8. Singletary SE, Ames FC, Buzdar AU. Management of inflammatory breast cancer. *World J Surg* 1994;18:87–92.

9. Levine PH, Steinhorn SC, Ries LG, Aron JL. Inflammatory breast cancer: the experience of the Surveillance, Epidemiology, and End Results (SEER) program. *J Natl Cancer Inst* 1985; 74:291–297.

10. Sherry M, Johnson D, Page DI, et al. Inflammatory carcinoma of the breast: clinical review and summary of the Vanderbilt experience with multimodality therapy. *Am J Med* 1985;79: 355–364.

11. Thoms WN, McNeese MD, Fletcher GH, et al. Multimodal treatment for inflammatory breast cancer. *Int J Radiat Oncol Biol Phys* 1989;17: 739–745.

12. Treves N. Inflammatory carcinoma of the breast in the male patient. *Surgery* 1953;34:810–820.

13. Klotz ID. *Uber mastitis carcinomatosa gravidarum et lactantium.* Halle, Germany: Lyske, 1869:30.

14. Von Volkmann R. *Brust Krebse. Beitrage Zur Chirugie.* Leipzig, Germany: Breitkopf & Hartel, 1875:319 334.

15. Schumann EA. A study of carcinoma mastitoides. *Ann Surg* 1911;54:69–77.

16. Beahrs O, Henson D, Hatter R, eds. *Manual for staging of cancer.* 3rd ed. Philadelphia: JB Lippincott, 1988:145–150.

17. Hermanek P, Sobin LH, eds. *TNM classification of malignant tumors: UICC international union against cancer.* 4th ed. Berlin: Springer, 1987: 93–99.

18. Denoix P. The Institut's contribution to the definition of factors guiding the choice of treatment and phase I development. *Recent Results Cancer Res* 1970;32:3–11.

19. Piera J, Alonso M, Ojeda M. Locally advanced breast cancer with inflammatory component: a clinical entity with poor prognosis. *Radiat Oncol* 1986;7:199–204.

20. McBride C, Hortobagyi G. Primary inflammatory carcinoma of the female breast: staging and treatment possibilities. *Surgery* 1985;98:792–797.

21. Henderson M, McBride C. Secondary inflammatory breast cancer: treatment options. *South Med J* 1988;81:1512–1516.

22. Ellis DL, Teitelbaum SL. Inflammatory carcinoma of the breast: a pathologic definition. *Cancer* 1974;33:1045–1047.

23. Saltzstein SL. Clinically occult inflammatory carcinoma of the breast. *Cancer* 1974;34:382–388.

24. Lucas FV, Mesa-Perez C. Inflammatory carcinoma of the breast. *Cancer* 1978;41:1595–1605.

25. DeLarue JC, May-Levin F, Mouriesse H, et al. Oestrogen and progesterone cytosolic receptors in clinically inflammatory tumors of the human breast. *Br J Cancer* 1981;44:911–916.

26. Harvey H, Lipton A, Lawrence BV, et al. Estrogen receptors in inflammatory breast carcinoma. *J Surg Oncol* 1982;21:42–44.

27. Paradiso A, Tommasi S, Brandi M, et al. Cell kinetics and hormonal receptor status in inflammatory breast carcinoma: comparison with locally advanced disease. *Cancer* 1989;64:1922–1927.

28. Maloisel F, Dufour P, Bergerat JP, et al. Results of initial doxorubicin, 5-fluorouracil, and cyclophosphamide combination chemotherapy for inflammatory carcinoma of the breast. *Cancer* 1990;65:851–855.

29. Treves N. The inoperability of inflammatory carcinoma of the breast. *Surg Gynecol Obstet* 1959;109:240–242.

30. Byrd B Jr, Stevenson S Jr. Management of inflammatory breast cancer. *South Med J* 1960;53:945–948.

31. Donegan W. Staging and end results. In: JS Spratt, WL Donegan, eds. *Cancer of the breast.* Philadelphia: WB Saunders, 1967:117–161.

32. Robbins GF, Shah J, Rosen P, et al. Inflammatory carcinoma of the breast. *Surg Clin North Am* 1974;54:801–810.

33. Bozzetti F, Saccozzi R, DeLena M, Salvadori B. Inflammatory cancer of the breast: analysis of 114 cases. *J Surg Oncol* 1981;18:355–361.

34. Fletcher GH, Montague ED. Radical irradiation of advanced breast cancer. *J Roentgenol* 1965;93:573–584.

35. Barker JL, Nelson JA, Montague ED. Inflammatory carcinoma of the breast. *Radiology* 1976;121:173–176.

36. Meyer AC, Dockerty MB, Harrington SW. Inflammatory carcinoma of the breast. *Surg Gynecol Obstet* 1948;87:417–424.

37. Chris SM. Inflammatory carcinoma of the breast: a result of 20 cases and a review of the literature. *Br J Surg* 1950;38:163–174.

38. Rogers CS, Fitts WT. Inflammatory carcinoma of the breast: a critique of therapy. *Surgery* 1956;39:367–370.

39. Dao TL, McCarthy JD. Treatment of inflammatory carcinoma of the breast. *Surg Gynecol Obstet* 1957;105:289–294.

40. Richards G, Lewison E. Inflammatory carcinoma of the breast. *Surg Gynecol Obstet* 1961;113:729–732.

41. Barber KW, Dockerty MB, Clagett OT. Inflammatory carcinoma of the breast. *Surg Gynecol Obstet* 1961;112:406–410.

42. Koh EH, Buzdar AU, Ames FC, et al. Inflammatory carcinoma of the breast: result of a combined-modality approach—M. D. Anderson Cancer Center experience. *Cancer Chemother Pharmacol* 1990;27:94–100.

43. Fleming RYD, Asmar L, Buzdar AU, et al. Effectiveness of mastectomy by response to induction chemotherapy for control in inflammatory breast cancer. *Ann Surg Oncol* 1997;4:452–461.

44. Fields JN, Kuske RR, Perez CA, et al. Prognostic factors in inflammatory breast cancer, univariate and multivariate analyses. *Cancer* 1989;63:1225–1232.

45. Brun B, Otmezguine Y, Feuilhade F, et al. Treatment of inflammatory breast cancer with combination chemotherapy and mastectomy versus breast conservation. *Cancer* 1988;161:1096–1103.

46. Hagelberg RS, Jolly PC, Anderson RP. Role of surgery in the treatment of inflammatory breast carcinoma. *Am J Surg* 1984;148:125–131.

47. Moore MP, Ihde JK, Crowe JP, et al. Inflammatory breast cancer. *Arch Surg* 1991;126:304–306.

48. Schafer P, Alberto P, Forni M, et al. Surgery as part of a combined modality approach for inflammatory breast carcinoma. *Cancer* 1987;59:1063–1067.

49. Knight CD, Martin JK, Welch JS, et al. Surgical considerations after chemotherapy and radiation therapy for inflammatory breast cancer. *Surgery* 1986;99:385–391.

50. Swain SM, Lippman ME. Treatment of patients with inflammatory breast cancer. In: DeVita V Jr, Hellman S, Rosenberg S, eds. *Cancer: principles and practice of oncology.* Philadelphia: JB Lippincott, 1989:129–150.

51. DeLena M, Zucali R, Viganotti G, et al. Combined chemotherapy-radiotherapy approach in a locally advanced (T3-T4) breast cancer. *Cancer Chemother Pharmacol* 1978;1:53–59.

52. Krutchik AN, Buzdar AU, Blumenschein GR, et al. Combined chemoimmunotherapy and radiation therapy of inflammatory breast cancer. *J Surg Oncol* 1979;11:325–332.

53. Pouillart P, Palangie T, Joure M. Cancer inflammatoire du sein traite par une association de chimotherapie et d'irradiation. *Bull Cancer (Paris)* 1981;68:171–196.

54. Zylberberg B, Salat-Baroux J, Ravina JH, et al. Initial chemoimmunotherapy in inflammatory carcinoma of the breast. *Cancer* 1982;49: 1537–1543.

55. Keiling R, Guiochot N, Calderoli H, et al. Preoperative chemotherapy in the treatment of inflammatory breast cancer. In: Wagener DJT, Blijham GH, Smeets JBE, Wils JA, eds. *Primary chemotherapy in cancer medicine.* New York: Alan R. Liss, 1985:95–104.

56. Israel L, Breau JL, Morere J-F. Two years of high dose cyclophosphamide and 5-fluorouracil followed by surgery after three months for acute inflammatory breast carcinomas: a phase II study of 25 cases with a median follow-up of 35 months. *Cancer* 1986;57:24–28.

57. Fields JN, Perez C, Kuske R, et al. Inflammatory carcinoma of the breast: treatment results in 107 patients. *Int J Radiat Oncol Biol Phys* 1989; 17:249–255.

58. Rouesse J, Sarrazin D, Spielman M, et al. Treatment of inflammatory cancer of the breast: combined chemotherapy and radiotherapy—a study of 270 women treated at the Institut Gustave-Roussy. *Bull Cancer (Paris)* 1989;76:87–92.

59. Antman K, Bearman SI, Davidson N, et al. Dose intensive therapy in breast cancer: current status. In: Gale RP, Champlin RE, eds. *New strategies in bone marrow transplantation.* New York: Alan R. Liss, 1990:423–426.

60. Singletary SE. Inflammatory breast cancer. In: Cameron JL, ed. *Current surgical therapy.* St Louis: Mosby Year Book, 1992:608–611.

CHAPTER 10

Lobular Carcinoma In Situ

S. EVA SINGLETARY

escribed histologically in 1941 by Foote and Stewart (1), lobular carcinoma in situ (LCIS) develops from the inner cuboidal cell layer of the terminal duct–lobular acini (2,3). Microscopically, LCIS is defined by the disorderly proliferation of epithelial cells to the extent that more than 50% of the acini are filled and distended (4,5). Although the proliferating cells are usually enlarged and have loss of cohesion, these cells have a bland, homogeneous appearance with rarely any mitosis or necrosis. When these changes are less developed with no more than 50% of the acini involved or incompletely filled, the term *atypical lobular hyperplasia* should be used (5). LCIS is usually associated with diploid DNA morphology (6), low proliferative rates (7), and the lack of amplification or overexpression of c-*erb* B-2 (8,9). Because of its low-grade nature and anticipated favorable clinical outcome, the term *lobular neoplasia* has been advocated. However, this term is imprecise and unclear in meaning, so today use of the original terminology of LCIS is preferred (10).

The diagnosis of LCIS is usually made incidentally from a biopsy specimen obtained from a patient with a palpable mass or a mammographic abnormality. When discovered within biopsy specimens of tissue containing microcalcifications, LCIS is often adjacent to, but not necessarily contained within, the area of calcifications (11–13). Because routine screening mammography has become more accepted as a standard of care, the number of diagnostic biopsies has also increased, leading to a slight increase in the incidence of LCIS (14). LCIS has been detected in approximately 2.5% of all breast biopsy specimens (14–16).

At the time of diagnosis, most patients with LCIS are premenopausal and in their late 40s (17–22). This finding suggests the hypothesis that LCIS is estrogen dependent and may regress after menopause. Although LCIS may be more likely to be estrogen receptor positive (23,24), approximately one fourth to one third of cases are found in postmenopausal women, including those not on estrogen replacement therapy (25,26).

LCIS occurs 12 times more frequently in white women than in black women, whereas Japanese women have a much lower incidence (21,27,28). Similar to invasive breast carcinoma, a family history of breast cancer is found in 15% to 20% of women with LCIS (17,22,27–29). No relationship to a history of abortion and LCIS has been confirmed (30).

In the past, treatment of the ipsilateral breast in patients with LCIS alone has varied from biopsy only to total mastectomy, sometimes including axillary node dissection (22). Today, LCIS is considered to be a marker of increased risk for the development of breast cancer rather than necessarily as a site of origin for cancer. This philosophy is based on the following observations: 1) The lifetime risk of subsequent development of an invasive breast carcinoma following a biopsy revealing LCIS is as high as 20% to 30% overall; 2) this risk is equally divided between the two breasts (10%–15% risk per breast, or approximately 0.5%–1.0% per year from the time of the initial diagnosis of LCIS) (Table 10-1) (5,10,20,22,30–35); and 3) 50% to 65% of invasive carcinomas subsequent to a diagnosis of LCIS are ductal rather than lobular in histology (30). Further evidence that LCIS itself is not always a precursor to an invasive process is that

T A B L E   **10-1**

Risk and Mortality of Subsequent Invasive Breast Carcinoma Following Diagnosis of Lobular Carcinoma In Situ

Series	No. of Evaluable Patients	Mean Follow-up (yr)	Ipsilateral Carcinoma Intact Breast	Contralateral Carcinoma Intact Breast	No. of Deaths
Page et al (5)	39	18	6/39 (15%)	4/39 (10%)	3
Haagensen et al (10)	295	16.3	33/281 (12%)	27/276 (10%)	11
McDivitt et al (20)	48	—	9/40 (23%)	4/47 (9%)	2
Singletary (22)	45	10	2/13 (15%)	1/27 (4%)	2
Rosen et al (30)	84	24	19/83 (23%)	19/83 (23%)	16
Wheeler et al (31)	35	15.7	1/25 (4%)	3/32 (9%)	2
Andersen (32)	52	15	9/46 (20%)	4/47 (9%)	6
Carson et al (33)	65	6.9	3/51 (6%)	0/60 (0%)	0
Hutter and Foote (34)	49	—	10/40 (25%)	4/46 (9%)	2
Salvadori et al (35)	99	4.8	5/78 (6%)	0/99 (0%)	0
Total	811	13.8	97/696 (14%)	66/756 (9%)	44 (5%)

most subsequent carcinomas occur 10 to 15 years after the initial diagnosis, with 40% detected more than 20 years later (30). The extent of LCIS within the biopsy specimen (17,30) or a personal or family history of breast carcinoma (5,30) has not been conclusively shown to add further to this risk. In contrast, a family history of breast cancer doubles the risk of breast cancer following a biopsy revealing atypical lobular hyperplasia (eight times the risk of the general population), approaching the risk of LCIS alone (5).

LCIS represents a bilateral diffuse process, with multicentricity noted in more than 60% of mastectomy specimens (18,36–38) and bilaterality in 18% to 69% (21,27,36–41). LCIS treatment options include lifelong observation of both breasts with mammography and physical examination, bilateral total mastectomies with consideration of breast reconstruction (Fig. 10-1), or participation in clinical prevention trials such as hormone/growth factor regulation with tamoxifen or retinoid analogues (22,42). Ipsilateral total mastectomy, radiation therapy, and re-excision of the original biopsy site to obtain clear margins are not indicated because all genetically identical breast tissue (i.e., both breasts) is at increased risk for breast carcinoma. Routine contralateral biopsy in the absence of standard indications, such as an abnormal finding on physical examination or by mammography, is not justified because the likelihood of finding a lesion requiring treatment (invasive carcinoma or ductal carcinoma in situ)

is small (<5%). The clinical significance of contralateral LCIS may be negligible, and negative biopsy results have never been clearly shown to be associated with reduced risk (43–45). As with excisional biopsy, subcutaneous mastectomy that leaves significant residual breast tissue may not reduce the risk substantially and may, in fact, give a false sense of security to the patient and physician (46). Thus, if surgery is elected for LCIS alone, the preferred choice is bilateral total mastectomy (22,39,47–49). Because the incidence of axillary nodal metastases associated with LCIS alone is less than 1%, an axillary node dissection offers no benefit (22,36,50). With major advances in breast reconstruction, particularly the use of autogenous flaps, reconstructive surgery at the time of mastectomy should be considered for most patients, unless the additional procedure increases the operative risk or the patient has already indicated that the procedure is unnecessary for her quality of life (51).

With the option of nonoperative observation, it is imperative that both the patient and the physician fully understand the lifelong commitment to careful surveillance of the breasts with physical examinations and yearly mammography (17,22,33,52). The combined data from 811 patients with LCIS in 10 follow-up series showed a 5% mortality rate from breast cancer with mean time intervals from the diagnosis of LCIS of 5 to 24 years (see Table 10-1). Thus, the purpose of observation is to detect a subsequent breast carcinoma at an early stage

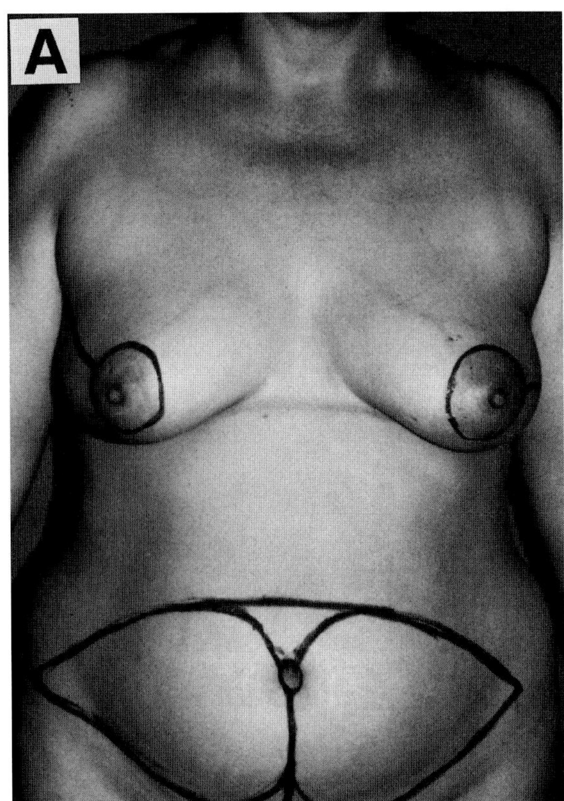
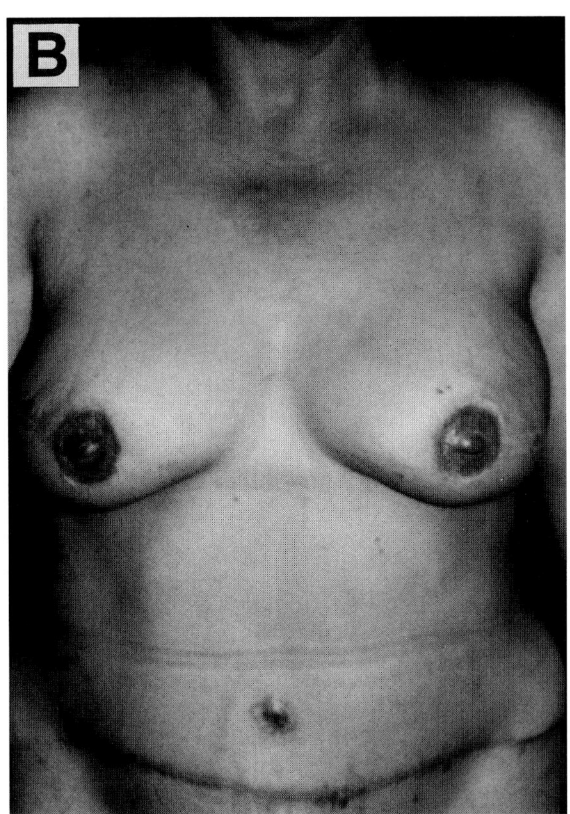

FIGURE 10-1

A. A 50-year-old woman with lobular carcinoma in situ of the right breast chose to have bilateral prophylactic total mastectomies with immediate reconstruction. *B.* The breast mounds were created with autogenous tissue using the transverse rectus abdominis myocutaneous flap (TRAM), the so-called "tummy tuck" method. With this technique, a large area of the abdominal skin and fat is outlined and raised with a portion of the rectus muscle and its blood supply. The flap can then be tunneled under the skin or directly transferred by a free microvascular anastomosis of the inferior epigastric to the axillary thoracodorsal vessels. Nipple reconstruction was performed 3 months later using double-opposing tab flaps from nearby skin of the breast mound. The areola was created by tattooing.

so that the diagnosis will not significantly have an adverse affect on the patient's chances of survival. The decreased breast cancer mortality observed in mammographic screening trials supports this approach (53–55).

For patients in whom LCIS is associated with another primary ipsilateral breast carcinoma, treatment is based on the stage and histology of the non-LCIS breast carcinoma (22). Local recurrence rates after breast preservation surgery and irradiation reveal no significant difference by histology of the primary tumor and may instead be related to whether histologically clear margins of the non-LCIS lesion were

actually achieved (56–58). Prophylactic mastectomy of the contralateral breast may be appropriate in a very select group of patients, such as those who need or elect to have an ipsilateral mastectomy and desire to remove the other breast for their perceived emotional well-being (22,59).

REFERENCES

1. Foote FW, Stewart FW. Lobular carcinoma in situ: a rare form of mammary carcinoma. *Am J Pathol* 1941;17:491–495.

2. Tobon H, Price HM. Lobular carcinoma in situ: some ultrastructural observations. *Cancer* 1972; 30:1082–1091.

3. Gad A, Azzopardi JG. Lobular carcinoma of the breast: a special variant of mucin-secreting carcinoma. *J Clin Pathol* 1975;28:711–716.

4. Rosen PP. Lobular carcinoma in situ and intraductal carcinoma of the breast. *Monogr Pathol* 1984;25:59–105.

5. Page DL, Kidd TE, Dupont WD, et al. Lobular neoplasia of the breast: higher risk for subsequent invasive cancer predicted by more extensive disease. *Hum Pathol* 1991;22:1232–1239.

6. Ludwig AS, Okagaki T, Richart RM, Lattes R. Nuclear DNA content of lobular carcinoma in situ of the breast. *Cancer* 1973;31:1553–1560.

7. Meyer JS. Cell kinetics of histologic variants of in situ breast carcinoma. *Breast Cancer Res Treat* 1986;7:171–180.

8. Porter PL, Garcia R, Moe R, et al. c-*erb* B-2 oncogene protein in situ and invasive lobular breast neoplasia. *Cancer* 1991;68:331–334.

9. Schimmelpenning H, Eriksson ET, Pallis L, et al. Immunohistochemical c-*erb* B-2 proto-oncogene expression and nuclear DNA content in human mammary carcinoma in situ. *Am J Clin Pathol* 1992;97(suppl 1):S48–S52.

10. Haagensen CD, Lane N, Lattes R, Bodian C. Lobular neoplasia (so-called lobular carcinoma in situ) of the breast. *Cancer* 1978;42:737–769.

11. Hutter RVP, Snyder RE, Lucas JC, et al. Clinical and pathologic correlation with mammographic findings in lobular in situ. *Cancer* 1969; 23:826–839.

12. Pope TL, Fechner RE, Wilhelm MC, et al. Lobular carcinoma in situ of the breast: mammographic features. *Radiology* 1988;168:63–66.

13. Beute BJ, Kalisher L, Hutter RVP. Lobular carcinoma in situ of the breast: clinical, pathologic, and mammographic features. *AJR* 1991;157: 257–265.

14. Mackarem G, Yacoub LK, Lee AKC, et al. Effects of screening on detection of lobular carcinoma in situ of the breast: nonspecificity of mammography and physical examination. *Breast Dis* 1994;7:339–345.

15. Schwartz GF, Feig SA, Rosenberg AL, et al. Staging and treatment of clinically occult breast cancer. *Cancer* 1984;53:1379–1384.

16. Giordano JM, Klopp CT. Lobular carcinoma in situ: incidence and treatment. *Cancer* 1973;31: 105–109.

17. Haagensen CD. Lobular neoplasia (lobular carcinoma in situ). In: Haagensen CD, ed. *Diseases of the breast.* 3rd ed. Philadelphia: WB Saunders, 1986:192–241.

18. Benfield JR, Jacobson M, Warner NE. In situ lobular carcinoma of the breast. *Arch Surg* 1965;91:130–135.

19. Farrow JH. Clinical considerations and treatment of in situ lobular breast cancer. *AJR Am J Roentgenol* 1968;102:652–656.

20. McDivitt RW, Hutter RVP, Foote FW Jr, Stewart FW. In situ lobular carcinoma. *JAMA* 1967; 201:96–100.

21. Newman W. In situ lobular carcinoma of the breast. *Ann Surg* 1963;157:591–599.

22. Singletary SE. Lobular carcinoma in situ of the breast: a 31-year experience at The University of Texas M. D. Anderson Cancer Center. *Breast Dis* 1994;7:157–163.

23. Giri DD, Dundas SAC, Nottingham JF, Underwood JCE. Oestrogen receptors in benign epithelial lesions and intraductal carcinomas of the breast. *Histopathology* 1989;15:575–584.

24. Bur ME, Zimarowski MJ, Schnitt SJ, et al. Estrogen receptor immunohistochemistry in CIS of the breast. *Cancer* 1992;69:1174–1181.

25. Hutter RVP. The management of patients with lobular carcinoma in situ of the breast. *Cancer* 1984;53:798–802.

26. Rosen PP, Senie RT, Farr GH, et al. Epidemiology of breast carcinoma: age, menstrual status, and exogenous hormone usage in patients with lobular carcinoma in situ. *Surgery* 1979;85: 219–224.

27. Farrow JH. Current concepts in the detection and treatment of the earliest of early breast cancers. *Cancer* 1970;25:468–477.

28. Rosner D, Bedwani RN, Vana J, et al. Noninvasive breast carcinoma: results of a national survey by the American College of Surgeons. *Ann Surg* 1980;192:139–147.

29. Davis N, Baird RM. Breast cancer in association with lobular carcinoma in situ: clinicopathologic review and treatment recommendation. *Am J Surg* 1984;147:641–645.

30. Rosen PP, Lieberman PH, Braun DW, et al. Lobular carcinoma in situ of the breast: detailed analysis of 99 patients with average follow-up of 24 years. *Am J Surg Pathol* 1978;3:225–251.

31. Wheeler JE, Enterline HT, Roseman JM, et al. Lobular carcinoma in situ of the breast: long-term follow-up. *Cancer* 1974;34:554–563.

32. Andersen JA. Lobular carcinoma in situ of the breast: an approach to rational treatment. *Cancer* 1977;39:2597–2602.

33. Carson W, Sanchez-Forgach E, Stomper P, et al. Lobular carcinoma in situ: observation without surgery as an appropriate therapy. *Ann Surg Oncol* 1994;1:141–146.

34. Hutter RVP, Foote FW. Lobular carcinoma in situ. *Cancer* 1969;24:1081–1085.

35. Salvadori B, Bartoli C, Zurrida S, et al. Risk of invasive cancer in women with lobular carcinoma in situ of the breast. *Eur J Cancer* 1991;27:35–37.

36. Carter D, Smith RRL. Carcinoma in situ of the breast. *Cancer* 1977;40:1189–1193.

37. Dall'Olmo CA, Ponka JL, Horn RC, Rui R. Lobular carcinoma of the breast in situ: are we too radical in its treatment? *Arch Surg* 1975;110:537–542.

38. Ringberg A, Palmer B, Linell F. The contralateral breast at reconstructive surgery after breast cancer operation: a histopathological study. *Breast Cancer Res Treat* 1982;2:151–161.

39. Urban JA. Biopsy of the "normal" breast in treating breast cancer. *Surg Clin North Am* 1969;49:291–301.

40. Rosen PP, Braun DW, Lyngholm B, et al. Lobular carcinoma in situ of the breast: preliminary results of treatment by ipsilateral mastectomy and contralateral breast biopsy. *Cancer* 1981;47:813–819.

41. Sunshine JA, Moseley HS, Fletcher WS, Krippaehne WW. Breast carcinoma in situ: a retrospective review of 112 cases with a minimum of 10 year follow-up. *Am J Surg* 1985;150:44–51.

42. Nayfield SG, Karp LG, Dorr FA, Kramer BS. Potential role of tamoxifen prevention of breast cancer. *J Natl Cancer Inst* 1991;83:1450–1459.

43. Balch CM, Singletary SE, Bland KI. Clinical decision-making in early breast cancer. *Ann Surg* 1993;217:207–225.

44. Baker RR, Kuhajda FP. The clinical management of a normal contralateral breast in patients with lobular breast cancer. *Ann Surg* 1989;210:444–448.

45. Walt AJ, Simm M, Swanson GM. The continuing dilemma of lobular carcinoma in situ. *Arch Surg* 1992;127:904–916.

46. Goodnight JE, Quagliana JM, Morton DL. Failure of subcutaneous mastectomy to prevent the development of breast cancer. *J Surg Oncol* 1984;26:198–201.

47. Osborne MP, Hoda SA. Current management of lobular carcinoma in situ of the breast. *Oncology* 1994;8:45–54.

48. Frykberg ER, Santiago F, Betsill WL, O'Brien PH. Lobular carcinoma in situ of the breast. *Surg Gynecol Obstet* 1987;164:285–301.

49. Swain SM. Lobular carcinoma in situ: incidence, presentation, guidelines to treatment. *Oncology* 1989;3:35–51.

50. Rosen PP. Axillary lymph node metastases in patients with occult noninvasive breast carcinoma. *Cancer* 1980;46:1298–1306.

51. Singletary SE. Surgical concepts in lobular carcinoma in situ. *Breast Surg Index Rev* 1993;1:1, 19.

52. Frykberg ER, Bland KI. Management of in situ and minimally invasive breast carcinoma. *World J Surg* 1994;18:45–57.

53. Shapiro S, Venet W, Strax P, et al. Ten-to-fourteen year effect of screening on breast cancer mortality. *J Natl Cancer Inst* 1982;46:1298–1303.

54. Tabar L, Fagerberg CJG, Gad A, et al. Reduction in mortality from breast cancer after mass screening with mammography. *Lancet* 1985;1:829–832.

55. Seidman H, Gelb SK, Silverberg E, et al. Survival experience in the Breast Cancer Detection Demonstration Project. *CA Cancer J Clin* 1987;37:258–290.

56. Kurts JM, Jacquamier J, Torhorst J, et al. Conservation therapy for breast cancers other than infiltrating ductal carcinoma. *Cancer* 1989;63:1630–1635.

57. Schnitt SJ, Connolly JL, Recht A, et al. Influence of infiltrating lobular histology on local tumor control in breast cancer patients treated with conservative surgery and radiotherapy. *Cancer* 1989;64:448–454.

58. Schnitt SJ, Abner A, Gelman R, et al. The relationship between microscopic margins of resection and the risk of local recurrence in patients with breast cancer treated with breast conserving surgery and radiation therapy. *Cancer* 1994;74:1746–1751.

59. Singletary SE, Taylor SH, Guinee VF. Occurrence and prognosis of contralateral carcinoma of the breast. *J Am Coll Surg* 1994;178:390–396.

CHAPTER 11

Breast Cancer in the Elderly

S. EVA SINGLETARY

$\mathscr{T}$he probability of breast cancer developing is highest in older women. Data from the Surveillance, Epidemiology, and End Results study (1) reveal that for women 80 to 84 years old, the breast cancer incidence is as high as 435 per 100,000; in contrast, the incidence is 212 per 100,000 in women 50 to 54 years old. Whether a woman survives breast cancer depends on the biology of the tumor, the immune defenses of the patient, and the appropriateness of the intervention by the physician. Controversy over the management of breast cancer in the elderly has been generated by the following ingrained beliefs:

1. Elderly patients more often have locally advanced disease at the time of initial presentation.
2. Elderly patients have more indolent disease.
3. Elderly patients have a limited life expectancy from comorbid conditions other than breast cancer.
4. Elderly patients cannot tolerate standard treatment.

However, in a review of 184 women older than 69 years who received treatment for locoregional breast cancer between 1976 and 1985 at The University of Texas M. D. Anderson Cancer Center, the majority of elderly women whose breast cancer had been treated appropriately remained free of disease and maintained a good quality of life (2). Therefore, the myths surrounding the treatment of the elderly need to be examined.

Myth 1. Elderly Patients More Often Have Locally Advanced Disease at the Time of Initial Presentation

Mueller et al (3), in a review of 3558 breast cancer patients, reported that stage I disease was equally common in all age groups. The limitation of the study was that 25% of the elderly patients did not undergo staging at the time of diagnosis. Other investigators noted a higher proportion of locally advanced tumors among elderly patients (4–6). Most patients in these series were classified as having stage III disease because of the large size of the primary tumor rather than the presence of regional (matted axillary nodes) or positive supraclavicular nodes. In the M. D. Anderson Cancer Center series (2), on clinical examination, 66 (36%) of the elderly patients had primary tumors 2 cm or smaller (T1), 81 (44%) had tumors larger than 2 cm but no larger than 5 cm (T2), and 15 (8%) had tumors larger than 5 cm (T3). Only 22 (12%) had skin ulceration or dermal lymphatic involvement (peau d'orange) of the breast (T4). The axilla was described as clinically negative (N0) in 131 (71%), contained palpable, movable lymph nodes (N1) in 35 (19%), and contained fixed or matted lymph nodes (N2) in only 18 (10%). Based on the current American Joint Committee on Cancer staging system (7), 61 (33%) of patients had stage I disease (T1, N0), 85 (46%) had stage II (T1, N1; T2, N0-1; T3, N0-1), and 38 (21%) had stage III (T3, N2; T4, N0-2).

Presentation with a locally advanced tumor is often attributed to a delay in seeking treatment by an individual. However, recent studies indicated that the medical profession also may substantially contribute to this delay. In a review of 1680 women with breast cancer treated in 17 community hospitals, Chu et al (8) found that elderly patients with breast lumps were less likely to undergo mammography or biopsy or to be referred for consultation. Makuc et al (9) found that older women were also less likely than younger women to have had a recent clinical examination of their breasts by their physician or to have been instructed in breast self-examination. In the M. D. Anderson Cancer Center series (2), 157 (85%) of the women detected their breast cancer by self-examination; only 22 (12%) of tumors were discovered by a physician. Only 5 (3%) of the women had a screening mammogram with a positive result. Although elderly women are often accused of delaying seeking a diagnosis, 78% sought medical attention within 2 months of the onset of symptoms.

Myth 2. Elderly Patients Have More Indolent Disease

The presumption that elderly patients have less aggressive biologic forms of breast cancer has been based on reports of a higher frequency of low-grade tumors (10,11); of more indolent histologic subtypes such as medullary, colloid, and tubular carcinomas (12); and of estrogen receptor–positive lesions in elderly patients (13). It has also been postulated that the gradual involution of immunity that occurs with aging may offer an immunologic advantage in reducing the likelihood of immunofacilitating mechanisms of tumor enhancement (suppressor T cells) (14).

Other studies challenged this concept of indolent disease in the elderly (3,15). Although 80% of breast cancers in women over age 75 have been reported to be estrogen receptor positive (13), the prognostic significance of this is uncertain. In patients with axillary nodal metastases or locally advanced disease, estrogen receptor status has been observed to have no prognostic significance (15,16). Furthermore, data suggest that estrogen receptor positivity in node-negative breast cancer may reflect growth rate rather than metastatic potential, and therefore serves as a predictor only of the pattern of

recurrence (predominantly bone) and a longer disease-free interval (15,16). In addition, the growth rate of a breast cancer (tumor doubling time) may not remain constant over time.

In the M. D. Anderson Cancer Center series (2), of 104 women with known estrogen receptor status, 82 (79%) were estrogen receptor positive (≥10 fmol). Invasive ductal carcinoma was the predominant histologic type (84%). Pure noninvasive disease was detected in 5 patients and other histologic types in 24 (colloid or mucinous, 13; invasive lobular, 5; Paget's disease, 3; papillary, 2; and tubular, 1). Recurrent breast cancer occurred in 47 patients (26%); 10 experienced locoregional relapse (on the chest wall or within the intact breast) only, 24 had distant metastases only, and 13 had both. The median interval between diagnosis and distant relapse was 33 months. The most common presentations or sites of distant metastases were simultaneous multiple sites in 40%, bone in 27%, and visceral organs in 24%. After distant recurrence, the median survival time was 11 months.

Stoll (17) defined "shower of metastases" as the involvement in rapid succession of at least two or three major sites of recurrence or metastasis (local, osseous, or visceral), followed by death within 18 months of the appearance of the first metastasis. In his series of 1141 breast cancer patients, recurrence developed in 755 patients. A "shower of metastases" occurred in 55% (50/91) of all women with recurrences before the age of 40 but in only 26% (23/90) of women older than 70. However, the proportion of patients whose first recurrence occurred at least 3 years after treatment was similar in all age groups.

Myth 3. Elderly Patients Have a Limited Life Expectancy from Comorbid Conditions Other Than Breast Cancer

Satariano et al (18) reported that the comorbid conditions present in elderly women with breast cancer are similar to those found in women in the general population. Arthritis, cardiovascular disease, and hypertension were the predominant health problems for women with or without breast cancer in their study. Similarly, Koch et al (19) found the likelihood of patients with breast cancer dying of other causes similar to that of the sex-matched and age-matched population.

The assumption that elderly patients have concurrent health problems that override the life-threatening risks from breast cancer has frequently resulted in less aggressive treatment of breast cancer. Greenfield et al (20) discovered that only 58.9% of women over age 50 with moderate to severe comorbid conditions received appropriate therapy for breast cancers, whereas 81.3% of women with no or only minor comorbidity received appropriate therapy. After adjustment for stage of disease and comorbidity, age remained a significant predictor of treatment. Only 83% of patients aged 70 or older with stage I or II disease and minimal comorbidity were treated appropriately, whereas 95.6% of similar patients aged 50 to 69 received appropriate treatment (20).

At the time of breast cancer diagnosis in the M. D. Anderson Cancer Center series (2), the most frequent comorbid conditions under active treatment were hypertension (48%), cardiovascular disease (23%), and arthritis (26%). Although 27% of elderly patients had no other major health problems requiring treatment and 91% were totally mobile, two or more comorbid conditions were present in 29%. Over a 16-year follow-up period (median, 106 months for living patients), there were 101 deaths. Forty percent of these deaths were from breast cancer and 60% from other causes (Fig. 11-1). The breast cancer–specific survival rate was 79% at 7 years. The most common known cause of non-cancer-related death was cardiovascular disease.

As life expectancy increases in the elderly population, physicians must recognize that physiologic and chronologic age often do not coincide. Treatment should be guided by an acceptable benefit-risk ratio that allows for quality and quantity of life.

Myth 4. Elderly Patients Cannot Tolerate Standard Treatment

Based on the assumption that older individuals cannot tolerate surgery, surgeons may be reluctant to perform standard surgical procedures on the elderly. In a study of 4050 operations, Turnbull et al (21) found the operative mortality rate in patients over age 70 (4.8%) to be similar to that in patients of all ages (3.4%). For breast cancer surgery in elderly patients, most series reported an operative mortality rate of 1% or less, and the primary morbidity appears to be related to short-term wound complications that respond to conservative management (6,22–24). In the M. D. Anderson Cancer Center series (2), total mastectomy with axillary node dissection (including three radical mastectomies) was performed in 82% of elderly patients. Only 18 patients had breast preservation surgery. Seven patients had total mastectomy without node dissection for debulking, and nine patients received no surgical intervention because of advanced disease and poor performance status. Only three postoperative deaths occurred (at 5 days, 7 days, and 23 days). Each of these deaths was related to myocardial infarction. Only 24% of the remaining patients who had surgery

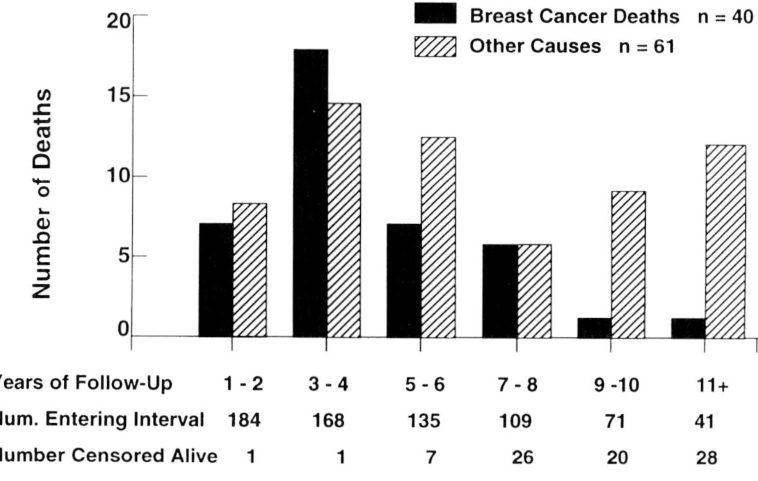

FIGURE 11-1

Cause of 101 deaths by years of follow-up in 184 women age 70 years or older with locoregional breast cancer.

experienced complications. The most common postsurgical problems were related to the wound: infection in 14 patients, hematoma in 5, and minor flap necrosis in 8.

As randomized clinical trials have not shown a survival difference between standard mastectomy and breast preservation surgery plus radiotherapy, the option to preserve the breast should also be discussed with the elderly patient (25,26). Radiation can decrease the likelihood of local recurrence following breast preservation and is well tolerated by the elderly (27). In the M. D. Anderson Cancer Center study, radiation therapy was given to 30% of patients: 10 preoperatively and 44 postoperatively. Complications from the radiation were recorded in fewer than 5%.

As indicated, elderly patients with breast cancer treated by standard therapy can attain a survival rate equal to that of younger patients with breast cancer. The physician must remember, however, to treat the patient and not just the disease. In elderly patients with significant comorbid conditions and limited life expectancy, the magnitude of the surgical procedure must be adjusted. The randomized National Surgical Adjuvant Breast and Bowel Project trial B-04 showed that axillary node dissection in patients with clinically negative axillae does not affect survival (28). Only 20% of patients in the non-axillary-dissection group required a subsequent therapeutic node dissection for clinical evidence of axillary disease. Thus, in elderly patients with operable tumors who are at high risk for complications of general anesthesia, a partial or total mastectomy under local anesthesia without axillary dissection is appropriate.

Recently, the antiestrogen tamoxifen was proposed as an alternative to surgery. Overall response rates to tamoxifen have ranged from 49% to 68%; complete responses were noted in 27% to 40% of patients (29–31). Clinical trials that compared tamoxifen to surgery did not show a survival difference (32–34). However, the median follow-up time for these studies was short (≤3 years). Horobin et al (31) demonstrated that at a minimum follow-up time of 5 years, 70 (62%) of 113 patients aged 70 or older with locoregional breast cancer did not achieve disease control with tamoxifen alone. The incidence of local relapses continued to increase over time; thus, caution is necessary when using tamoxifen as the sole primary treatment. In patients able to undergo standard surgery with acceptable risks, tamoxifen may be more appropriate in the adjuvant setting (35) or as a preoperative induction therapy for those with locally advanced disease.

The role of chemotherapy in elderly breast cancer patients has yet to be fully explored. Most chemotherapy protocols have had age limits of 65 or 70 years, the requirement of normal renal function, or an arbitrary dose reduction in patients older than 60 (36,37). Nineteen studies conducted by the Eastern Cooperative Oncology Group (ECOG) of cancer chemotherapy for eight tumor types (breast cancer excluded) demonstrated that toxicity and response rates were identical in younger patients and in those 70 years or older (38). A subsequent ECOG study of 92 patients aged 65 to 90 who had advanced breast carcinoma and were treated with combination cyclophosphamide, methotrexate, and 5-fluorouracil with dose adjustments based on creatinine clearance revealed no significant age trends in toxicity, response, or cycle-by-cycle reduction of chemotherapy dose (39). In the M. D. Anderson Cancer Center series of elderly patients (2), combination chemotherapy was used as an adjuvant in only eight patients (4%). Eleven additional patients (6%) received preoperative chemotherapy for initially unresectable disease. Seven of the 11 patients were disease free at the time of writing. No major toxicities from the chemotherapy occurred in any of the 19 patients. Thus, for elderly patients with estrogen receptor–negative or hormone-resistant breast carcinomas, the use of chemotherapy should be based on physiologic parameters (renal, liver, and marrow function) and performance status rather than on chronologic age (40–42).

Conclusions

Elderly women have the same right as their younger counterparts to take part in decisions about their health care. Women with breast cancer, regardless of age, should be informed of treatment options and the advantages and disadvantages of each choice as it applies to their individual circumstance. In patients with poor performance status and known limited life expectancy, clinical judgment should be used as to the approach that will provide the best quality of life for the maximum duration with acceptable risks.

REFERENCES

1. Ries LAB, Hankey BF, Edwards BK, eds. *Cancer statistics review, 1973-1987.* NIH publication no. 90-2789. Washington, DC: National Cancer Institute, 1990.

2. Singletary SE, Shallenberger R, Guinee VF. Breast cancer in the elderly. *Ann Surg* 1993; 218:667–671.

3. Mueller CB, Ames F, Anderson GD. Breast cancer in 3558 women: age as significant determinant in the rate of dying and causes of death. *Surgery* 1978;83:123–131.

4. Davis SJ, Karrer FW, Moor BJ, et al. Characteristics of breast cancer in women over 80 years of age. *Am J Surg* 1985;150:655–658.

5. Herbsman H, Feldman J, Seldera J, et al. Survival following breast cancer surgery in the elderly. *Cancer* 1981;47:2358–2363.

6. Hunt KE, Fry DE, Bland KI. Breast carcinoma in the elderly patient. *Am J Surg* 1980;140: 339–342.

7. Chu J, Diehr P, Feigl P, et al. The effect of age on the care of women with breast cancer in community hospitals. *J Gerontol* 1987;42:185–190.

8. Makuc DM, Fried VM, Kleinman JC. National trends in the use of preventive health care by women. *Am J Public Health* 1989;79:21–26.

9. American Joint Committee on Cancer. *Manual for staging of cancer.* 3rd ed. Philadelphia: JB Lippincott, 1988:145–150.

10. Berg JW, Robbins GF. Modified mastectomy for older poor risk patients. *Surg Gynecol Obstet* 1961;11:631–634.

11. Taylor SG, Gelman RS, Falkson G, Cummings FJ. Combination chemotherapy compared to tamoxifen as initial therapy for stage IV breast cancer in elderly women. *Ann Intern Med* 1986; 104:455–461.

12. Rosen PP, Lesser ML, Kinne DW. Breast carcinoma at the extremes of age: a comparison of patients younger than 35 years and older than 75 years. *J Surg Oncol* 1985;28:90–96.

13. Von Rosen A, Gardelin A, Auer G. Assessment of malignancy potential in mammary carcinomas in elderly patients. *Am J Clin Oncol* 1987; 10:61–64.

14. Ershler WB. Why tumors grow more slowly in old people. *J Natl Cancer Inst* 1986;77:837–839.

15. Adami H-O, Graffman S, Lindgren A, Sallstrom J. Prognostic implications of estrogen receptor content in breast cancer. *Breast Cancer Res Treat* 1985;5:293–300.

16. Qazi R, Chuang J-LC, Drobyski W. Estrogen receptors and the pattern of relapse in breast cancer. *Arch Intern Med* 1984;144:2365–2367.

17. Stoll BA. Does the malignancy of breast cancer vary with age? *Clin Oncol* 1976;2:73–80.

18. Satariano WA, Ragheb NE, Dupuis MH. Comorbidity in older women with breast cancer: an epidemiologic approach. In: Yancik R, Yates JW, eds. *Cancer in the elderly: approaches to early detection and treatment.* New York: Springer, 1989:71–103.

19. Koch M, Hanson J, Gaedke H, Wilson D. Competing causes of death in breast cancer patients. In: Paterson AHG, Lees AW, eds. *Proceedings of the second international symposium on fundamental problems in breast cancer.* Alberta, Canada: 1986:265–272. Norwell, MA: Kluwer, 1986.

20. Greenfield S, Blanco DM, Elashoff RM, Ganz PA. Patterns of care related to age of breast cancer patients. *JAMA* 1987;20:2766–2770.

21. Turnbull AD, Gundy E, Howland WS, Beattie EJ Jr. Surgical mortality among the elderly. An analysis of 4050 operations (1970–1974). *Clin Bull* 1978;8:139–142.

22. Amsterdam E, Birkenfeld S, Gilad A, Krispin M. Surgery for carcinomas of the breast in women over 70 years of age. *J Surg Oncol* 1987;35: 180–183.

23. Kesseler HJ, Seton JZ. The treatment of operable breast cancer in the elderly female. *Am J Surg* 1978;135:664–666.

24. Svastics E, Sulyok Z, Besnyak I. Treatment of breast cancer in women older than 70 years. *J Surg Oncol* 1989;41:19–21.

25. Fisher B, Redmond C, Poisson R, et al. Eight-year results of a randomized clinical trial comparing total mastectomy and lumpectomy with or without irradiation in the treatment of breast cancer. *N Engl J Med* 1989;320:822–828.

26. Veronesi U, Salvadore B, Luini A, et al. Conservative treatment of early breast cancer. Long-term results of 1232 cases treated with quadrantectomy, axillary dissection and radiotherapy. *Ann Surg* 1990;211:250–259.

27. Kantorowitz DA, Poulter CA, Sischy B. Conservative surgery and radiotherapy in elderly women. *Int J Radiat Oncol Biol Phys* 1988;15: 263–270.

28. Fisher B, Redmond C, Fisher ER, et al. Ten-year results of a randomized clinical trial comparing radical mastectomy and total mastectomy with or without radiation in the treatment of breast cancer. *N Engl J Med* 1985;312:665–673.

29. Akhtar SS, Allan SG, Rodger A, et al. A 10-year experience of tamoxifen as primary treatment of breast cancer in 100 elderly and frail patients. *Eur J Surg Oncol* 1991;17:30–35.

30. Bradbeer JW, Kyngdon J. Primary treatment of breast cancer in elderly women with tamoxifen. *Clin Oncol* 1983;9:31–34.

31. Horobin JM, Preece PE, Dewar JA, et al. Long-term follow-up of elderly patients with locoregional breast cancer treated with tamoxifen only. *Br J Surg* 1991;78:213–217.

32. Bates T, Riley DL, Houghton J, et al. Breast cancer in elderly women: a Cancer Research Campaign trial comparing treatment with tamoxifen and optimal surgery with tamoxifen alone. *Br J Surg* 1991;78:591–594.

33. Gazet J-C, Ford HT, Coombes RC, et al. Prospective randomized trial of tamoxifen versus surgery in elderly patients with breast cancer. *Eur J Surg Oncol* 1994;20:207–214.

34. Robertson JFR, Todd JH, Ellis IO, et al. Comparison of mastectomy with tamoxifen for treating elderly patients with operable breast cancer. *BMJ* 1988;297:511–514.

35. Castiglione M, Gelber RD, Goldhirsch A (International Breast Cancer Study Group). Adjuvant systemic therapy for breast cancer in the elderly: competing causes of mortality. *J Clin Oncol* 1990;8:519–526.

36. Bonadonna G, Valagussa P. Dose response effect of adjuvant chemotherapy in breast cancer. *N Engl J Med* 1981;304:10–15.

37. *Compilation of experimental cancer therapy protocol summaries.* NIH publication no. 81-1116. Washington, DC: National Cancer Institute, 1981:1–51.

38. Begg CB, Carbone PP. Clinical trials and drug toxicity in the elderly. *Cancer* 1983;2:1986–1992.

39. Gelman RS, Taylor SG IV. Cyclophosphamide, methotrexate, and 5-fluorouracil chemotherapy in women more than 65 years old with advanced breast cancer. The elimination of age trends in toxicity by using doses based on creatinine clearance. *J Clin Oncol* 1984;2:1404–1413.

40. Christman K, Muss HB, Case DL, Stanley V. Chemotherapy of metastatic breast cancer in the elderly. The Piedmont Oncology Association experience. *JAMA* 1992;268:57–62.

41. Martin LM, Le Pechoux C, Calitchi E, et al. Management of breast cancer in the elderly. *Eur J Cancer* 1994;30A:590–596.

42. Muss HB. The role of chemotherapy and adjuvant therapy in the management of breast cancer in older women. *Cancer* 1994;74:2165–2171.

Pregnancy, Hormone Replacement Therapy, and Reproductive Factors

FRANKIE ANN HOLMES

The pregnant patient newly diagnosed with breast cancer never fails to emotionally affect even the most seasoned oncologist. Although pregnant breast cancer patients require highly specialized, integrated multidisciplinary care, all physicians—generalists as well as specialists—should be aware of the current options for therapy. It is the generalist physicians to whom these women first turn, and the generalists often influence which subspecialists the women see.

Incidence of Breast Cancer During Pregnancy: Good News and Bad News

The good news is that breast cancer during pregnancy is rare. Table 12-1 shows results from some of the reported series in which incidence figures were calculated (1–15). The most widely quoted series is White's review of the world literature (4), showing an incidence of 2.8% of all breast cancers and about 1 of every 3333 deliveries. Others looked at the incidence of breast cancer during pregnancy by focusing on only fertile patients younger than 40 years who are at risk for both pregnancy and breast cancer. In that subset, the incidence of breast cancer

during pregnancy or lactation is higher, ranging from 1.5% to 26% (5,8–12). This wide range is the result of differences in the cutoff age chosen by various authors. In these historical series, the younger the cutoff age, the more likely a woman with breast cancer was to be pregnant. If breast cancer occurred at a young age, the likelihood of a concurrent pregnancy was high. *Lactation* is defined as the period from delivery to 6 to 12 months after delivery regardless of whether the patient actually breast-feeds. As Donegan (16) observed, in view of the known long natural history of breast cancer, 1 year to several years for a tumor to reach 1 cm in diameter, the distinction between breast cancers diagnosed during pregnancy and those diagnosed during lactation is somewhat arbitrary. One can assume that in all lactating women in these series, the tumor was present during pregnancy.

The bad news is that breast cancer during pregnancy is certain to become more common. The incidence of breast cancer increased 32% from 1980 to 1987. Recently, this trend has stabilized or even reversed (17). In 1994 there were approximately 182,000 new cases of breast cancer and 46,000 deaths from breast cancer, the same as in 1993 (18). However, increasing numbers of women defer or delay childbearing (19). Both of these reproductive behaviors increase the risk of breast cancer (20,21). In addition, the incidence of breast cancer increases with age. While breast cancer is distinctly uncommon in women in their 20s

Portions of this chapter are reprinted from Holmes FA. Breast cancer during pregnancy. *Cancer Bull* 1994;46: 400-411. Copyright 1994, The University of Texas M. D. Anderson Cancer Center, Houston, Texas. Used with permission.

and 30s, a substantial majority of patients are affected in their 40s (22,23). Many career women will be in their 40s during their first pregnancy. Cognizant of these data, even perinatal nursing journals are addressing the issue of breast cancer during pregnancy (24).

Diagnosis and Staging

Two cardinal rules must be followed in the evaluation of a breast problem in a pregnant patient: First, ignore the pregnancy and evaluate the problem; second, keep the fetus out of the evaluations. During pregnancy, the physiologic changes in the breast are almost as striking as those in the uterus. The nipple enlarges, and the glandular tissue of the breast increases and begins to differentiate. The breast feels engorged and is tender on pal-

pation. Against this background, examination of the breast is difficult. However, the most common presentation of breast cancer during pregnancy is a painless lump discovered by the patient.

Differential Diagnosis

The differential diagnosis of a breast mass in a pregnant woman is similar to that in a non-pregnant patient. In one illuminating series, Byrd et al (6) reviewed 134 pregnant or lactating women who had undergone surgery for a mass in the breast. Pregnant women accounted for 86 patients (64%) in the series. Of the 134 tumors, 105 (78%) were benign. Of the benign tumors, 37% were nonmalignant neoplasms, such as adenofibroma, lipoma, papilloma, or cystosarcoma phyllodes; 34% were cystic disease; 22% were other breast

T A B L E **12-1**

Incidence of Breast Cancer During Pregnancy and Lactation from Selected Series

Study[a]	Years Accrued	No. of Patients	Average Age, Yr (Range)[b]	Percentage of All Breast Cancers	Percentage of All Breast Cancers Occurring During Pregnancy or Lactation in Potentially Fertile Women	Incidence per Number of Deliveries
Harrington (1937)	1910–33	92	37	2.0	NA	NA
Lewison (1954)	1932–51	46	NA	NA	NA	1/1360
White (1955)[a]	1850–1953	1413	38[c]	2.8	NA	1/3333
Treves (1958)[a]	1937–49	108	≤35	NA	19.6	NA
Byrd (1962)	1925–60	29	34	2.5	NA	NA
Rissanen (1968)[a]	1940–61	33	34.6 (25–42)	0.9	NA	NA
Crosby (1971)[a]	1932–65	29 135 <35 yr	38 (26–54)	1.1	NA 1.5	NA NA
Applewhite (1973)[a]	1948–67	2689 (655 <45 yr)	34	2.0	8.3 (in women ≤45 yr)	NA
Riberio (1977)	1941–69	88	? (21–47)	0.3	2.8 (in women ≤45 yr)	NA
Noyes (1982)[a]	1945–77	32	≤30	0.9	26 (in women ≤30 yr)	NA
Nugent (1985)	1970–80	19	32 (26–37)	1.4	11 (in women <40 yr)	NA
King (1985)	1950–80	60	35 (22–44)	NA	NA	NA

Modified from Wallach et al (14) and van der Vange et al (15).

NA = not available.

[a] Denotes that both pregnant and lactating patients were included.

[b] Age range not available for all series.

[c] Age known in 55% of series of 1375 patients [White 1955 (4)].

changes of pregnancy, such as lobular hyperplasia or galactocele; and 7% were inflammation or abscess. Not noted in Byrd's series, but reported by others, is the phenomenon of infarction of a fibroadenoma or hyperplastic breast tissue stimulated to grow rapidly during pregnancy (25). Only 22% of the tumors in Byrd et al's series were malignant. This percentage was identical to the percentage of malignant tumors among all the breast masses removed during the 5-year period preceding publication of Byrd et al's results (1956–1961). Thus, a breast lump in a pregnant woman is not more likely to be malignant than is a breast lump in a nonpregnant woman.

Complete Physical Examination and Biopsy

Standard evaluation of a breast mass in a pregnant woman begins with a complete examination of the breast and the lymph node basins of the breast. Complete breast examination is a standard part of all gynecologic and obstetric evaluations. If a painless mass alone is discovered, it should be evaluated by fine-needle aspiration or ultrasonography to determine whether it is cystic or solid (26,27). If the mass is cystic, it should be aspirated and the aspirate should be sent for cytologic evaluation. While the occurrence of intracystic carcinomas (28) is infrequent, so is breast cancer during pregnancy. If no fluid is obtained or a mass persists after aspiration, an incisional or excisional biopsy should be performed, and the tissue should be sent for histopathologic evaluation and estrogen (ER) and progesterone receptor (PR) assays. Biopsy is necessary because although fine-needle aspiration is a reliable method of diagnosing malignancy, it cannot differentiate invasive from noninvasive masses (29).

Hormone Receptor Determination

Only limited studies of hormone receptor data are available in the literature (11,27,30–32). The majority of young patients have hormone receptor–negative tumors (33). When determination of ER status is performed by the ligand-binding method, there is a concern that false-negative results may occur in premenopausal women because of competitive inhibition by the high circulating levels of endogenous estrogens (34). However, determination of ER by

enzyme immunoassay (EIA) (35) or immunocytochemical assay (ICA) (36) avoids this problem by using a monoclonal antibody that recognizes both the occupied and the unoccupied form of the receptor. A second theoretical concern is that the high levels of circulating estrogens will downregulate ERs and PRs. Other evaluations for research purposes include flow cytometry with determination of DNA index and S-phase fraction and evaluation for HER-2/*neu* oncogene (37). However, these latter data do not contribute information necessary for decisions about treatment.

Diagnostic Imaging and Laboratory Studies

The use of mammography for evaluation of breast masses in pregnant women is somewhat controversial. Liberman et al (38) noted that the exposure to the human embryo from a standard bilateral mammography study with craniocaudal and mediolateral oblique views of both breasts using low-dose screen-film technique and shielding of the pelvis is less than 50 mrad (500 μGy). In contrast the dose estimated to cause intrauterine death in preimplantation mouse embryos is 10 rad (100 mGy) or higher, that is, 200-fold higher. Thus, the radiation risk to the fetus is minimal (39). However, the increased density of the breast makes accurate interpretation difficult (40). Even when the mammogram shows no signs of cancer, the physician should obtain an accurate histopathologic diagnosis. Thus, obtaining a mammogram may only delay appropriate management. Mammography, may, however, be useful to document occult disease in the contralateral breast.

Metastatic Workup

If invasive malignancy is confirmed, the patient needs evaluation for systemic disease as a prelude to initiation of local therapy. Evaluation for systemic disease includes a thorough physical examination with attention to the contralateral breast and all draining nodal basins. Standard laboratory evaluations include a hemogram, liver function studies, and cancer markers such as carcinoembryonic antigen (CEA) and CA 15-3. Radiographic and scintigraphic imaging should be done only if justified by clinical and laboratory findings. A chest radiograph may be safely performed, since the maximum dose to the uterus will be less than

50 mrad (reported doses range from 0.2–43.0 mrad) (39). If blood test results are abnormal, an ultrasound of the liver or radiographs of specific symptomatic bones may be obtained. Radiographs of the lumbosacral spine will expose the uterus to 51 to 126 mrad (41). Although a bone scan may be performed in a pregnant patient by using special precautions such as hydration and insertion of a Foley catheter (42), bone scans rarely provide evidence of metastases in an asymptomatic patient with normal laboratory findings.

Dental Evaluation

The patient's dentition should always be evaluated. Pregnancy causes hypertrophy of the gums, and the ensuing periodontal disease that occurs in some patients—not the loss of calcium—is the basis for the "old wives' tale" about loss of one tooth for each live birth. In a patient who may need chemotherapy, good dental health is important to prevent oral complications of chemotherapy.

Effect of Concomitant Pregnancy and Breast Cancer on Outcome—The Basis for Selection of Therapy

Effect on the Patient

In 1880, Samuel Gross's vivid description of breast cancer during pregnancy entrenched the notion that pregnancy has a negative effect on the course of breast cancer (43): "When, however, carcinoma appears during pregnancy or during lactation, its growth is wonderfully rapid and its course is excessively malignant. . . ." Beatson's treatise on castration as an effective therapy undoubtedly galvanized this notion (44). However, critical review of the available data in the literature does not support the concept of a uniformly dismal outcome.

Tables 12-2 and 12-3 show the 5- and 10-year survival rates from reported series by nodal status (Table 12-2) and stage (Table 12-3) (1,3,6–10,12,13,45–50). Note that most series include both pregnant and lactating patients. Only total survival, not disease-free survival, rates are reported. Three conclusions are obvious from Table 12-2. First, patients with nodal involvement had dismal outcomes. Second, for patients without nodal involvement,

5- and 10-year survival rates were reasonable in most series. Third, the majority of patients in most series, 60% to 85%, had nodal involvement. A number of authors commented on the unusually high percentage of pregnant patients with involved lymph nodes compared to their nonpregnant patients. Delay in diagnosis may explain this.

Delay in Diagnosis

Table 12-4 (6,8,10,15,51) shows results from selected series in which the timeliness of diagnosis and treatment of patients with breast cancer was reviewed. Delays of 6 months to 1 year were common and were the result of both patient and physician judgments. Zemlickis et al (52), in a 1992 case-control study from the Princess Margaret Hospital in Canada, compared the stage at presentation of breast cancers in a group of 118 pregnant patients to a control group of 3949 women younger than 48 years diagnosed during the same time period. The pregnant patients were less likely to have stage I or II disease and more likely to have stage IV disease (52). In Canada, unlike the United States, access to medical care is universal, so delays were probably not due to problems accessing medical care. The authors concluded that pregnant patients are at a higher risk of presenting with advanced disease because pregnancy impedes early detection.

Overall Outcome Is Similar

Peters (51), Nugent and O'Connell (12), Petrek (49), and Zemlickis et al (52) compared outcomes in pregnant patients with those in control patients matched by age and stage and found no differences. Nugent and O'Connell (12) and others (8,11,23,51) suggested that the worse outcome of pregnant patients is related to the young age of the patients and not to pregnancy. Earlier series unfairly compared young pregnant women with series that included predominantly postmenopausal women, the majority of whom have more indolent disease.

Three series found worse outcomes for pregnant patients than for nonpregnant patients even when patients were matched by age and stage (15,50,53). Guinee et al (50) reviewed records of 407 patients who were 20 to 29 years old at the time of diagnosis of breast cancer and who were treated at one of nine cancer centers in the United States or Europe collaborating in

T A B L E   12-2

Five and 10-Year Survival Rates for Pregnant or Lactating[a] Breast Cancer Patients in Selected Series by Nodal Status

Study	Years Accrued	No. of Patients	Survival Rate			Comments
			Overall	Node Neg	Node Pos	
Harrington (1937)	1910–33	92 P + L	5 yr: NA 10 yr: NA	62% 40%	6% 3%	N0 = 14 (15%) N+ = 78 (85%)
Haagensen (1967)	1915–50	48 P + L	5 yr: 31% 10 yr: 0%	83% NA	NA NA	N0 = 6: 31 patients had radical mastectomy
White (1955)	≤1948	27 P + L	5 yr: NA 10 yr: NA	73% 26%	6% 0%	N0 = 11 (41%); N+ = 16 (59%); personal series
Byrd (1962)	1925–60	24 P + 5 L	5 yr: 55% 10 yr: NA	100% 80%	28% 6%	N0 = 11 (38%) N+ = 18 (62%); 3 had metastases
Holleb and Farrow (1962)	1920–53	45 P 72 L	5 yr: NA 5 yr: NA	58% 68%	21% 13%	N0: P = 26%, L = 28% vs 54% N0 in subsequent pregnancy
Miller (1962)	1921–55	45	5 yr: NA 10 yr: NA	47% 20%	16% 3%	N0 = 15 (33%) N+ = 30 (67%)
Crosby (1971)	1932–65	29 P + L	5 yr: 46% 10 yr: 36%	NA NA	NA NA	5-yr survival: P = 33%, L = 50%; 5 patients (17%) had metastases; 0 aborted
Applewhite (1973)	1948–67	48 P + L	5 yr: 25% 10 yr: 15%	56% 22%	18% 13%	N0 = 9 (19%) N+ = 39 (81%)
Clark (1978)	1931–75	121 P 80 L	10 yr: 22% 10 yr: 32%	35% 69%	22% 18%	Total series: N0 = 25%, N+ = 39%, N? = 36%
Nugent (1985)	1970–80	19 P	5 yr —	100%	50%	N0 = 4 (21%); N+ = 14 (74%); stage IV = 1 (5%) w/ 0% 5 yr S
King (1985)	1950–80	63 P	5 yr: 53% 10 yr: 49%	82% 71%	33% 33%	N0 = 24 (38%); N+ = 39 (62%); includes stage IV
Petrek (1991)	1960–80	12 P + 44 L	5 yr: 61% 10 yr: 45%	82% 77%	47% 25%	N0 = 22 (39%); N+ = 34 (61%); 30% had adj chemo
Guinee (1994)	1978–88	26 P	5 yr: 40%	NA	NA	N0 = 9 (35%); N = 11 (42%); N? = 6 (23%) 50% had adj chemo; 11 had abortions

P = pregnant; L = lactating; NA = not available; N0 = node negative; N+ = node positive; N? = unknown nodal status; adj chemo = adjuvant chemotherapy; S = survival.

[a]Lactation refers to the period from delivery until 6–12 months after delivery regardless of whether the patient actually breast-fed.

the International Cancer Patient Data Exchange Systems between January 1, 1978, and December 31, 1988 (Table 12-5) (50). Only 26 patients were pregnant at the time of diagnosis. Complete data were available for only 291 patients, 20 of whom were pregnant at the time of diagnosis of breast cancer. These data show that the risk of dying from breast cancer was inversely related to the length of time between diagnosis of breast cancer and date of the most recent previous pregnancy, with the highest risk in patients who were pregnant at diagnosis. For each additional year up to 4 years between the most recent previous pregnancy and the diagnosis of breast cancer, the risk of dying of breast cancer decreased by 15%. Patients diagnosed with breast cancer 4 or more years after the most recent pregnancy had a risk of dying of breast cancer not statistically different from that for patients who had never been pregnant. While the authors did not speculate on possible causes for these findings, subsequent letters (54,55) and a report (56) suggested that some aspect of the immunosuppressive effects of pregnancy may be contributory.

On balance, most of the available data support the conclusion that, when matched by age and stage with nonpregnant breast cancer patients, pregnant patients with breast cancer do not have worse outcomes.

TABLE 12-3

Five and 10-year Survival Rates for Pregnant or Lactating[a] Breast Cancer Patients in Selected Series by TNM Staging[b]

Study	Years Accrued	No. of Patients	Survival Rate				Comments
			Stage I	Stage II	Stage III	Stage IV	
Rissanen (1968)	1940–61	33	5 yr: 80%	8/10[c]	2/13[c]	0%	Only 2 patients were lactating
			10 yr: 80%	7/9[c]	2/9[c]	0%	
Riberio (1977)	1941–69	88	5 yr: 90%	37%	15%	0%	% Survival matched by age and stage *Pregnant* v *Not* 5 yr: 38 45 10 yr: 24 29
			10 yr: 90%	21%	10%	0%	

[a] Lactation refers to the period from delivery until 6–12 months after delivery regardless of whether or not the patient actually breast-fed.

[b] In this staging system, stage I means tumor confined to breast; II, breast and lymph nodes; III, any T4 regardless of nodes; IV, distant metastases.

[c] Data presented as number of living patients at specified time interval versus those at risk.

TABLE 12-4

Delays in Diagnosis of Breast Cancer in Selected Series

Study	Delays in Pregnant Patients (Months)			Delays in Nonpregnant Patients			Difference in Total Delay Between Pregnant and Nonpregnant Patients
	Total	Patient	Doctor	Total	Patient	Doctor	
Westberg (1946)	9	6	3	6	4	2	3
Applewhite (1973)	11	>6 (in 36%)	2.2	4	18% > 6	0.6 m	7 range: 2 days to 24 months
Byrd (1962)	6 (average)						
Bunker, Peters (1962)[a]	>6 (in 50%)						
Peters (1968)	15 (stage IV)			9 (stage IV)			
Riberio (1977)	10						

[a] Data from van der Vange and van Donegan.

Other Myths About Pregnancy and Breast Cancer

Some authors suggested an increased incidence of inflammatory cancer in pregnancy. However, a review of available data by Zinns (57) and other more recent reports (27,31) showed no differences in reported histologic types between pregnant and nonpregnant patients. Peters (51) initiated the concept of worse prognosis in the second trimester of pregnancy. No other studies, however, replicated this finding (52).

Effect on the Fetus

Metastases to the placenta or fetus are uncommon. A 1989 review found only 45 documented cases of placental metastases and 7 cases of fetal metastases. None of these seven were in patients with breast cancer (58). In 1994, Salamon et al (59) described microscopic metastases to the placenta that were not detectable on gross examination, in a patient with brain and liver metastases from an invasive ductal carcinoma diagnosed approximately 12.5 months earlier. This pattern of normal findings on gross

T A B L E **12-5**

Tumor Size, Nodal Status, Chemotherapy, 5-Year Overall Survival, and Risk of Breast Cancer in 291 Patients by Time from Most Recent Pregnancy to Diagnosis of Breast Cancer[a]

| | Time from Most Recent Pregnancy to Diagnosis of Breast Cancer | | | | |
Risk factor	Never Pregnant (n = 139)	Pregnant at Diagnosis (n = 26)	0–12 Months (n = 40)	13–48 Months (n = 51)	≥49 Months (n = 35)
Tumor size, cm					
≤2	36%	8%	17%	34%	37%
>2–5	27%	35%	35%	29%	31%
>5	7%	19%	10%	8%	3%
Unknown	30%	38%	38%	29%	29%
No. of Positive Lymph Nodes					
0	47%	35%	28%	35%	37%
1–3	26%	19%	22%	26%	29%
≥4	20%	23%	35%	27%	17%
Unknown	7%	23%	15%	12%	17%
Received Chemotherapy, %	50%	50%	65%	53%	49%
5-yr Overall Survival	74%	40%	n	65%	n
RR of Breast Cancer Death (95% CI)					
Unadjusted	1.0	3.26 (1.81–5.87)	1.89 (1.09–3.29)	1.59 (0.96–2.63)	0.66 (0.31–1.39)
Adjusted[b]	1.0	2.83 (1.24–6.45)	1.88 (0.88–3.98)	1.09 (0.54–2.19)	0.54 (0.19–1.54)

RR = relative risk; CI = confidence interval.

[a] Modified from Guinee et al.[50] (50)

[b] Adjusted for tumor size and number of involved axillary lymph nodes.

examination but extensive microscopic disease is reminiscent of the behavior of the lobular subtype of carcinoma in the breast, although this patient apparently did not have this subtype. Detailed sectioning revealed that adenocarcinoma was present only within the intervillous (maternal) space, not in the chorionic villi (fetal space). Salamon et al (59) recommended careful evaluation of the placenta for evidence of invasion of the chorionic villi. They postulated a higher risk of neonatal metastatic disease if invasion of the chorionic villi is observed.

Zemlickis et al (52) at the Princess Margaret Hospital assessed fetal outcomes by evaluation of detailed delivery records available for 62 of 85 deliveries (83 live births, 2 stillbirths) from patients diagnosed with breast cancer between 1958 and 1987 (out of a total of 118 pregnant patients with breast cancer). Sixty of the 62 deliveries were live births. Of these 60, there was a statistically lower mean birth weight compared to matched control birth weights. The mean gestational age was also lower

because of preterm deliveries (22 cesarean sections, 18 of which were to expedite cancer treatment), compared to matched control ages. The ratio of stillbirths to live births (2/85, 2.4%) was numerically greater than the general figure in Ontario (11.1 stillbirths/1000 total births, 1.1%). However, the small sample size precludes any meaningful conclusions. Earlier, Clark and Reid (48) observed a higher incidence of spontaneous abortions in patients with breast cancer diagnosed during pregnancy than in patients with breast cancer diagnosed during lactation or later (14% versus 1% and 7%, respectively).

Therapy Decisions

Local Therapy

In 1943, when Haagensen and Stout developed their criteria for operability of breast cancer, they noted that none of the 20 patients who developed breast cancer during pregnancy or lactation were cured and declared this subset of patients categorically inoperable (45). However, after several subsequent pregnant or lactating patients who had mastectomy performed by Haagensen and Stout's colleagues during pregnancy or lactation were observed to have longer survival times, Haagensen reversed his decision (45).

For pregnant patients with localized breast cancer (stages I–III) the usual criteria for conservative therapy versus modified radical mastectomy pertain (60). Both standard modified radical mastectomy and lumpectomy with axillary dissection are acceptable methods of local control. However, if the patient chooses lumpectomy, definitive local irradiation should be deferred until after delivery. The doses of internally scattered radiation have been calculated in experimental situations (15). Throughout the initial 12 weeks of pregnancy, when the fetus is still within the true pelvis, a tumor dose of 5000 cGy will expose the fetus to 10 to 15 cGy. Later in gestation, when the fetus is high in the abdomen, some fetal areas may receive as much as 200 cGy. Although some authors question whether there is any safe dose of radiation to the fetus, Brent (61) extensively reviewed this area and defined 5 cGy as a relatively safe upper limit of fetal exposure. There is no reason to risk exposure to the embryo or fetus in a non-life-threatening situation.

Anesthetic Considerations

In experienced hands, general anesthesia can be safely administered to the pregnant patient (62–64). When surgery is performed in the second and third trimesters, careful attention must be paid to proper positioning of the patient so as to avoid uterine compression of the vena cava. Other effects of pregnancy include increased blood volume and coagulability, decreased lung capacity, and slow gastric emptying (64). In Byrd et al's classic surgical series (6) of 86 pregnant patients, all patients had general anesthesia for breast biopsy, and a radical mastectomy was performed if the diagnosis was carcinoma. There were no maternal deaths, and only one fetal death occurred. They reported this as a 0.75% mortality. (However, in the denominator they erroneously included 48 women who were lactating. The actual rate should have been reported as 1.2% or 1 of 86 pregnant women, which is not

significantly different.) Even that one death, however, seems somewhat peripherally related to the procedure since it occurred 3 weeks after the biopsy when the patient, who was peri-menopausal and who had a negative pregnancy test twice before excision of a cystic lesion, had a spontaneous abortion.

"Therapeutic" Abortion?

As noted earlier, Gross's (43) description of breast cancer during pregnancy led to a general principle that the hormonal changes of pregnancy must contribute to the cancer's rapid growth. The apparently worse outcome of this subset of patients with breast cancer supported a consensus for therapeutic abortion. However, although controlled clinical trials are not possible in this situation, most published series did not consistently show improved survival rates for patients who had spontaneous or therapeutic abortion (see Addendum) (7,13,46,48,65). Adair's study (65), which showed an apparent benefit for therapeutic abortion, considered both patients who were pregnant at the time of diagnosis and patients who subsequently became pregnant after treatment of breast cancer. These are entirely different patient groups, as discussed later. In some series, patients who continued the pregnancy fared better than did those who terminated the pregnancy. Although Clark and Reid (48) and King et al (13) specifically stated that selection of abortion was not biased for patients with more advanced disease, this bias is a valid concern in the interpretation of retrospective study results. However, two other issues are relevant to the question of therapeutic abortion: the age of the patient, discussed already, and the hormone receptor status of the tumor.

Hormone Receptor Determination

Since the late 1970s tumors have been analyzed for hormone receptors as a guide to prognosis and therapy. As noted earlier, women younger than 50 years tend to have hormone receptor–negative tumors (33). Initially this finding was thought to reflect limitations of the ligand-binding technique in which endogenous estrogen blocked the ability of the radiolabeled ligand to bind to and "detect" the receptor. However, as discussed previously, the more modern EIAs and ICAs use monoclonal antibodies that detect the receptor whether or not it is bound by endogenous estrogen. Earlier studies by the ligand-binding technique (12), as well as more recent studies using the ICA (30), confirmed the excess of estrogen receptor–negative tumors in women younger than 50 years. Thus, there is no justification for termination of pregnancy or castration as an adjunct to therapy.

When Is Abortion Indicated?

Abortion may be indicated in patients with rapidly progressive disease, such as inflammatory breast cancer or metastatic breast cancer. In the case of inflammatory cancer, the chance for long-term survival depends on immediate initiation of combination chemotherapy. As discussed later, the use of combination chemotherapy in the second and third trimesters is associated with a low to absent probability of fetal malformations or death (66,67). In the first trimester, however, the risks are higher. In the case of metastatic disease, the goal of therapy is effective palliation. While 3% to 5% of patients with metastatic disease continue unmaintained remissions for 10 or more years, the median survival time in large series is 2 to 3 years (68). The patient and the child's father must consider the probability that the mother will not live to parent her child.

In summary, except in unique circumstances, Byrd et al's advice (6) continues to be timely: "better terminate the disease than terminate the pregnancy."

Chemotherapy

In an era when health professionals advise most pregnant patients to limit caffeine consumption and abstain from alcohol and nicotine, it is paradoxical for other health professionals to talk about the use of antineoplastic agents during pregnancy. In the early years of our chemotherapy program for pregnant patients with breast cancer, some nurses refused to administer antineoplastic agents to pregnant patients. However, despite solid theoretical reasons for avoiding these agents during pregnancy, the incidence of serious complications from administration of chemotherapy during pregnancy is quite low.

Effects of Chemotherapy on the Fetus

Doll et al (66) extensively reviewed the literature of fetal injury related to intrauterine expo-

sure and found that, except for aminopterin, the use of chemotherapy agents was not associated with the frequency of adverse outcomes that would be predicted. One special problem with aminopterin and other analogues of methotrexate is sequestration in third spaces such as ascites, pleural effusions, and amniotic fluid. However, there are only limited data about the extent to which chemotherapy drugs cross the placenta and enter the fetal circulation (69,70). It is known, however, that the expression of P-glycoproteins is high in uterine and placental tissue. These proteins function as drug efflux pumps for xenobiotic substances and may exclude many drugs from the fetus (71,72). The experience at M. D. Anderson Cancer Center with administration of chemotherapy to pregnant patients shows that fetal hair growth is normal even though the mother has alopecia (73). The risk of major teratogenesis is highest during the first trimester, when organogenesis occurs. The most critical portion of this trimester, when the embryo is exquisitely sensitive to multiple system malformation, is from the week 2 to week 4 (days 14–28) from conception, only 5% of the total duration of pregnancy (61). Major malformations in this period are often spontaneously aborted, as noted by Doll et al (66), because of the narrow range between lethal fetal toxicity and no discernible effect. In the second and third trimesters, there is little risk of serious teratogenicity; however, there is a risk of impaired fetal growth and functional development, spontaneous abortion, premature labor, and major organ toxicity. Note that in the normal population of pregnant patients without cancer, the background incidence of spontaneous abortion is 30% to 50%, and the incidence of major and minor congenital malformations is 3% and 9%, respectively (61).

Clinical Studies

For the adjuvant or palliative treatment of patients with breast cancer, the Breast Medical Oncology Department of The University of Texas M. D. Anderson Cancer Center uses the standard combination of fluorouracil, doxorubicin, and cyclophosphamide (FAC) (67). Although antimetabolites such as fluorouracil are generally believed to be associated with a higher risk for fetal complications than are alkylators, we have not observed complications. We never administer methotrexate to pregnant patients. Other centers also utilize doxorubicin-based combinations (74,75). Preliminary results of our small series have been presented in abstract form (67). From 1989 to 1992, we treated 11 patients who had concomitant breast cancer and pregnancy. The median age was 34 years (range, 24–37). The distribution of patients by stage was as follows: stage II, 4 patients; stage III, 5; and stage IV, 2. Three patients had preoperative chemotherapy followed by mastectomy; six patients had postmastectomy chemotherapy. The remaining two patients had metastatic disease at the time of presentation so mastectomy was not indicated. The maximum number of chemotherapy courses given was 7; the median was 4 (range, 1–7). Ten normal infants were delivered. The eleventh infant was spontaneously delivered during a period of maternal neutropenia and fever and experienced respiratory distress. However, his peripheral blood counts were normal (i.e., appropriately elevated), and he recovered uneventfully. At the time of this writing two children were older than 4 years; all children had reached normal developmental milestones.

Aviles et al (76) at the University of Mexico evaluated long-term outcomes of 43 children of mothers with hematologic malignancies who were treated with chemotherapy during pregnancy. At the time of the report, the median age of the children was 9 years (range, 3–19). Nineteen mothers (44%) received chemotherapy during the first trimester, and most received antimetabolites and alkylators. Comprehensive evaluations of the children included physical examination, hemogram, cytogenetic studies, bone marrow aspiration and biopsy, determination of immunoglobulin levels and stimulated lymphocyte responses to various mitogens, Wechsler intelligence testing, and the Bender-Gestalt test. There were no instances of physical or intellectual dysfunction or cytogenetic abnormalities.

In 1985, Mulvihill at the University of Pittsburgh Genetics Institute established a national registry for patients exposed to chemotherapy in utero (77). The database also includes a summary of all cases published in all languages since 1950. Although data on the initial patients are scanty, more complete data have been obtained on recent patients. These data show that many pregnant women exposed to chemotherapy, particularly if within the second

and third trimesters, generally had normal children. This registry provides an important opportunity to document outcomes in these patients. I strongly recommend that all physicians who administer chemotherapy to pregnant patients register their patients.

Management of Chemotherapy Complications in the Pregnant Patient

The usual acute and subacute complications of chemotherapy include nausea, vomiting, stomatitis, neutropenia with fever, and alopecia.

Emesis can be effectively prevented by a number of agents. We used diphenhydramine, promethazine (Phenergan), and lorazepam in our series. However, ondansetron (Zofran) was used to control hyperemesis gravidarum without adverse consequences in two patients in weeks 11 and 30 to 33 of pregnancy (78,79). Ondansetron is classified as pregnancy category B, which means that no teratogenicity has been seen in animal studies and isolated human cases but that controlled studies in humans have not been done. Prevention of nausea and vomiting is important because dehydration, especially in the last trimester, is permissive for preterm labor.

Accurate dosing of the patient becomes difficult as the patient's body weight increases during pregnancy. We generally use body weight at the time of diagnosis to calculate the initial chemotherapy dose and adjust dose on the basis of nadir granulocyte counts on day 14. We aim for a nadir granulocyte count between 500 and 1000 cells/μL and the absence of fever, infection, serious stomatitis, or other gastrointestinal symptoms such as diarrhea or abdominal cramping. Unless patients have metastatic disease with involvement of the bone marrow, thrombocytopenia is not a serious concern. Anemia may be important if the patient had anemia before pregnancy. However, a physiologic anemia occurs during the first trimester as a result of the increased plasma volume and should not alarm the oncologist.

In all patients, prompt management of fever during neutropenia is important. For pregnant patients whose chemotherapy will continue after delivery, the timing of the last cycle before delivery is important. We generally administer the last chemotherapy treatment before delivery, no later than 6 weeks before the estimated due date (at 32–33 weeks). In the one patient in our series who was neutropenic, the neonate experienced respiratory distress that resolved completely; his white blood cell count was appropriately elevated (67).

For patients whose chemotherapy continues postpartum, special arrangements are needed to help the patient deal with the newborn's around-the-clock needs. Although many patients tolerate chemotherapy quite well, some patients receiving chemotherapy experience chronic fatigue, which will be exacerbated in the pregnant patient if sleep is limited and irregular.

Lactation

If chemotherapy is initiated in the second trimester, patients are not usually able to breast-feed. For patients who must continue to receive chemotherapy after delivery, lactation is contraindicated. Antineoplastic agents are excreted in the milk. There is one case report of cytopenia in a breast-fed neonate whose mother was receiving cyclophosphamide (80,81).

Fertility

The ovary appears to be more resistant to chemotherapy than the testes do (82,83). However, in both sexes, the incidence of chemotherapy-induced sterility increases with age and cumulative dose of alkylating agents (83,84). Shalet (85) observed the following correlation between the age of the patient and the total dose of cyclophosphamide received before the onset of amenorrhea: older than 40 years, 5.2 g; 30 to 39 years, 9.3 g; and 20 to 29 years, 20.4 g. Doxorubicin probably contributes to the risk of infertility, but the antimetabolite fluorouracil does not. Richards et al (86) reported that 37% and 97%, respectively, of patients

younger than and older than 40 years became amenorrheic after adjuvant cyclophosphamide, methotrexate, and fluorouracil. Hortobagyi et al (87) reported the age-related incidence of amenorrhea during chemotherapy as well as the probability of resumption of menses after completion of chemotherapy in a subset of premenopausal patients treated with adjuvant FAC at M. D. Anderson Cancer Center (Table 12-6). Over half of all patients younger than 40 who became amenorrheic resumed menses after completion of chemotherapy. In a 1990 review of 227 consecutive patients who were 35 years or younger and were treated with the same doxorubicin-based combination for a median of 12 months, the status of menstrual function was known in 56%. Of these, 59% had no amenorrhea, 32% had temporary amenorrhea, and 11% had permanent amenorrhea (31). In pregnant patients with breast cancer, in whom the median age is approximately 32 to 34 years, a majority of patients will retain fertility after chemotherapy treatment with standard doses of FAC. However, all patients must be cautioned about the possibility of permanent amenorrhea and premature menopause.

Two pharmacologic strategies to prevent chemotherapy-induced sterility have been evaluated: oral contraceptives and the gonadotropin agonists. The working hypothesis was that the ovary would be suppressed in a manner similar to suppression of the adrenal gland during administration of exogenous corticosteroids. Neither of these approaches was completely protective (88).

The science of infertility medicine has advanced considerably, and a number of options may be available in the future for the patient who becomes infertile because of

TABLE **12-6**

Incidence of Amenorrhea by Age in Patients Treated with FAC Adjuvant Chemotherapy at M. D. Anderson Cancer Center

Age, Years	Percentage Patients Who Became Amenorrheic During Chemotherapy	Percentage of Patients Who Resumed Menses After Chemotherapy
<30	0	—
30–39	33	50
40–49	96	"few"
≥50	100	

Data from Hortobagyi GN, Buzdar AU, Marcus CE, et al. Immediate and long-term toxicity of adjuvant chemotherapy regimens containing doxorubicin in trials at M. D. Anderson Hospital and Tumor Institute. *Monogr Natl Cancer Inst* 1986;1:105–109.

F = fluorouracil; A = doxorubicin; C = cyclophosphamide.

chemotherapy but who wants to become pregnant. First, efforts are ongoing to develop techniques to harvest and cryopreserve the patient's own oocytes, analogous to sperm banking (88). Second, if the patient's own ova are no longer available, ova may be donated by family or others. The patient is given hormonal stimulation to prepare the uterus, and the donor ova are fertilized in vitro with the husband's (or other donor) sperm. The viable 8- to 12-cell pre-embryos are transferred to the patient's uterus. Successful pregnancy with this technique was achieved in a patient rendered menopausal from her adjuvant chemotherapy (89). In 1994, investigators in London discussed the use of fetal ova as a donor source (90).

Pregnancy After Breast Cancer

Effect of Pregnancy on Risk of Recurrence

The recommendations about pregnancy after breast cancer emanate from the same "forces of intuitive conviction" (91) who advocate therapeutic abortion as an adjuvant to treatment of breast cancer. The obvious concern is that the significant rise in sex hormones, particularly estrogen, during pregnancy will stimulate recurrent cancer.

Most of the historical series of patients with breast cancer antedate the use of cytotoxic chemotherapy, and most institutes do not routinely employ castration as a therapeutic maneuver. Thus, there is substantial information on the outcome of patients who become pregnant after a diagnosis of breast cancer. Danforth (92) reviewed this issue in detail in 1991, with critical commentary by Epstein and Henderson (91) and Wood (93). Approximately 25% of women who develop breast cancer are of reproductive age. Nearly one third (7% of all women who develop breast cancer) of these women of reproductive age will have one or more pregnancies subsequently, and 70% of these pregnancies will occur within 5 years of treatment. The available data do not show that subsequent pregnancy hastens or induces recurrence. Epstein and Henderson (91) noted that the numbers of patients are too small to rule out an effect, but the studies do suggest that if there is any effect, it is very small. In two series, patients who had subsequent pregnancies had higher survival rates than those who did not. The most important prognostic factors were the nodal status and the stage.

How Reliable Are Available Data?

Conversely, Petrek (94) argued that the available data are based on only a small subset of patients who become pregnant after a diagnosis of breast cancer. First, she noted that as pregnancy is not a disease, it is not coded in hospital or tumor registries. Patients may not always report a subsequent pregnancy to the physician who treated the breast cancer. Thus, it may be difficult to determine the total number of patients at risk. Second, Petrek reviewed the data from her own institution, Memorial Sloan-Kettering Cancer Center, over a 30-year period. She found only 41 patients with stage I and II cancer who became pregnant after a diagnosis of breast cancer. Assuming the above estimate of a 7% pregnancy rate for women younger than 40 years, and accounting for the age distribution of patients seen during that era, Petrek estimated that at least 450 women would have had a subsequent pregnancy. She concluded that while existing data do not suggest that subsequent pregnancy increases the risk of recurrence, these data are based on a nonrandom, and perhaps positively biased sampling of 10% or fewer of the total patients at risk who did have a good outcome.

The Finnish Studies: Population Registry Data—Complete, Accurate

However, subsequent to these two reviews, Sankila et al (95) from Finland reported the results of a population-based matched survival study designed to assess the risk of death from breast cancer in breast cancer patients relative to whether they did or did not have a subsequent pregnancy producing a live birth. Because medicine is socialized, reports of all diagnoses of cancer and all death certificates in which cancer is mentioned are required to be sent to the centralized Finnish Cancer Registry. Additionally, since 1967, all citizens have been given a unique personal identification number. This study used the Finnish Cancer Registry to identify 2536 women who were diagnosed with breast cancer between 1967 and 1990 and were younger than 40 years at the time of diagnosis. Linking the patients' unique personal identification numbers to the Central Population Register, Sankila et al determined the dates of births of the patients' biologic children. Information on abortions and stillbirths was not available. Of these 2536 women, 95 (3.7%) had a child before the end of

1990. These 95 patients were matched for stage, age, and year of diagnosis with one to six control subjects chosen from the remaining patients. Appropriate control subjects could not be found for four patients. The results showed that control patients had a 4.8-fold higher risk of death compared with patients who had a subsequent pregnancy. The authors acknowledged one possible confounding issue. Patients were matched with data from the time of diagnosis. However, to assess the actual effect of the pregnancy on survival, it would have been more accurate to match patients at the time of delivery, which ranged from 10 to 154 months after diagnosis. This was not possible with their database. The authors hypothesized that patients who felt and did well had children, whereas those who were affected by recurrence did not. They termed this the "healthy mother effect." Note that the rate of pregnancy in this group of women was accurately determined and was approximately 4%. There are at least two possible explanations for this relatively low rate. Patients with breast cancer may not decide to have children at the same rate as those who have not had breast cancer. In addition, in earlier eras physicians usually cautioned against subsequent pregnancy.

M. D. Anderson Cancer Center's Experience

Sutton et al (31) reviewed the M. D. Anderson experience with patients who were 35 or younger at the time of diagnosis and became pregnant after adjuvant chemotherapy with FAC. Of 227 consecutive breast cancer patients, 25 patients had 33 pregnancies. The median interval between the completion of chemotherapy and pregnancy was 12 months (range, 0–87). Ten pregnancies were terminated, 2 spontaneously aborted, and 19 resulted in normal, full-term infants; 2 patients were still pregnant at the time of the report. The incidence of recurrence was 46% and 28%, respectively, in patients who did not become pregnant and those who had subsequent pregnancies. Similarly, 38% of patients without subsequent pregnancies, but only 12% of subsequently pregnant patients had died at the time of publication.

Conclusion: Should I? When?

The two questions all patients ask are "Should I become pregnant?" and "When?" (92). Given the lack of any demonstrable effect of pregnancy on the risk of recurrence, the "Should I?" question compels the patient and physician to address openly the probability of recurrence and to consider how recurrence would affect any future children. Patients with a low risk of recurrence (those with stage I or II disease with fewer than three involved axillary lymph nodes) can be advised that because of their favorable prognosis, it is probable that if they do conceive, they will live to mother their children. Patients with high-risk breast cancer (stage II with four or more involved axillary lymph nodes, stage III, and stage IV) have a less favorable prognosis and should be advised that the probability of living to parent their children is low.

As regards "When?," Danforth endorsed the standard 2- to 3-year waiting period after diagnosis before conceiving. Epstein and Henderson (91) disagreed and suggested that for patients with low-risk breast cancers, waiting only wastes time. In the current therapeutic era, many patients receive adjuvant chemotherapy for early-stage breast cancer. Certainly this will impose a minimum 6-month interval between the end of treatment and conception.

Lactation After Previous Breast Surgery and Irradiation

Harris's group (96) noted that the usual administered radiation dose of 4600 cGy injures the glandular and ductal tissue, causing atrophy of the lobules and perilobar and periductal fibrosis which inhibit the normal physiology of lactation. They noted reports of successful lactation in 24% of a sample of 52 patients who became pregnant after conservative surgery and breast irradiation. However, in their own experience at the Joint Center for Radiation Therapy in 23 patients with 30 live births after surgery and irradiation for breast cancer, few women reported being able to lactate. Dow et al (96) advised patients not to attempt breastfeeding because they fear that the disruptions of the ductal system will cause mastitis.

Two other investigators, however, observed lactation in a few patients who had lumpectomy and irradiation (97,98). Location of the incision was important. Not surprisingly, circumareolar incisions are associated with absence of lactation, because they interrupt multiple ducts. Radial incisions may disrupt fewer ducts but may be cosmetically inferior.

Pregnancy After Transverse Rectus Abdominis Myocutaneous Flap Breast Reconstruction

Many women opt for breast reconstruction after mastectomy. The use of autogenous tissue for reconstruction has become a particularly attractive alternative because of recent reports of adverse consequences of silicone-filled breast implants. The transverse rectus abdominis myocutaneous (TRAM) flap, which uses skin and muscle from the abdominal area to reconstruct a breast, is one approach to breast reconstruction. Since patients who undergo a TRAM flap reconstruction lose an important component of abdominal support, concerns are raised when these patients become pregnant. In 1993, surgeons at M. D. Anderson reported a pregnancy that occurred after TRAM flap reconstruction, and reviewed the literature about this situation (99). Nine cases of pregnancy after TRAM flap breast reconstruction have been reported since the technique was first described in 1981. None of the patients had problems with abdominal wall integrity during pregnancy, and all but one patient had full-term spontaneous vaginal deliveries. One patient had a spontaneous abortion at 6 weeks' gestation unrelated to the abdominal-wall integrity. Two patients, including the patient in the case report, had postpartum abdominal bulges that did not require repair. These limited data indicate that normal pregnancy and delivery are possible after TRAM flap breast reconstruction.

Hormone Replacement Therapy

Hormone Replacement Therapy After Breast Cancer

An even more difficult question than pregnancy after breast cancer in this era is the question of hormone replacement therapy after menopause, whether natural or chemotherapy induced, for patients with a history of breast cancer. Hormone replacement therapy should address the four major areas affected by estrogen deficiency: vasomotor and neurocognitive/neuropsychiatric function, genitourinary tract (dyspareunia and frequent urinary tract infections), bones, and the cardiovascular system (100). A full review of this topic is beyond the scope of this chapter. A comprehensive review

by a proponent of hormone replacement therapy was published in 1993 (101). Since then, a handful of papers have addressed this issue. Eden et al (102) performed a case-control study of combined estrogen-progestin replacement therapy in 90 women who had been treated for breast cancer, most of whom had node-negative disease. The median time from diagnosis to initiation of estrogens was 5 years (range, 0–25 years). The ER status of the primary tumor was known in only 22 patients (24%); 12 tumors were ER positive and 10 were ER negative. In this select group, only 6 patients had a recurrence (7%) compared to 30 (17%) of 180 control subjects who did not use estrogens. The ER status of the primary was known in only 2 of the 6 patients whose disease recurred. One tumor was ER negative; one was ER positive. The median duration of estrogen use was only 1.5 years (range, 0.3–12.0). Despite the small numbers of patients and the limited follow-up time, the authors concluded that short-term use of estrogens posed little risk of breast cancer recurrence.

Is Previous Hormone Replacement Therapy a Risk Factor for Development of Breast Cancer?

Two trials comparing the use of hormone replacement therapy in women with and without breast cancer were published in 1995. The trials reached opposite conclusions.

Population Case-Control Study: No

Stanford et al (103) performed a population-based case-control study comparing 537 patients with breast cancer diagnosed between January 1 and June 30, 1988, with a random control group of 492 women without a history of breast cancer. These authors found no association between breast cancer risk and the use of either estrogen alone or estrogen with progestin. In addition, long-term use from 8 to 20 years was not associated with an increased risk of breast cancer. In an accompanying editorial, Adami and Persson (104) noted two limitations of this study. First, patients with in situ carcinoma were included. In situ disease was not used as an end point in most other studies because it does not inevitably progress to invasive disease. Second, the power of the study was only sufficient to reveal a substantially increased risk of 2.5-fold or higher after long-term therapy, so although there was certainly no major excess risk, a small but biologically illuminating and clinically important excess risk could not be ruled out. Adami and Persson noted that a Swedish study, to be completed by 1996, of over 3000 women who were given combined estrogen and progestin replacement therapy should provide additional information. These authors also referenced a report suggesting that breast cancer occurring in patients receiving estrogen replacement therapy has a more favorable prognosis than do tumors that arise in the absence of hormone replacement therapy. The reader is cautioned that this concept that tumors arising during hormone replacement therapy are less aggressive was also erroneously believed to be true of the initial endometrial cancers induced by tamoxifen.

Cohort Study: Yes, Increased Risk

In contrast to the findings of Stanford et al (103), Colditz et al (105) reported a 30% to 46% increase in the risk of breast cancer in women receiving hormone replacement therapy in a cohort of nurses registered in the Nurses' Health Study followed from 1976 through 1992. The report was based on 725,550 person-years of follow-up of menopausal women. Risk increased by age and number of years of hormone use after 5 years of use. Moreover, this study excluded cancer in situ, and as noted in the accompanying editorial by Davidson (106), the death rate from breast cancer paralleled the incidence of it. This suggested that these cancers were clinically important, that is, not less aggressive. Little increase in risk was noted for women of any age who used estrogen or estrogen and progestin for less than 5 years. Both the Stanford and the Colditz studies observed that the addition of progestin did not neutralize the increased risk of breast cancer. Colditz et al (105) noted that the lack of an increased risk of breast cancer in younger women might relate only to the short time since menopause and the correspondingly shorter periods of use.

Breast Cancer During Estrogen Replacement Therapy: Therapeutic Withdrawal

For patients diagnosed with stage I, II, or III breast cancer who decide to use hormone replacement therapy and subsequently develop metastatic disease, estrogen withdrawal may provide clinically meaningful palliation. Dhodapkar et al (107) evaluated and Pritchard and Sawaka (108) reviewed the use of withdrawal as a therapeutic manipulation in three patients with a history of primary breast cancer who developed metastatic disease while using estrogens and a fourth patient who was using estrogens who presented with diffuse bone metastases and a breast mass. Withdrawal of estrogens caused disease regression lasting 2 to 3 years in all four patients.

Use of Megestrol Acetate for Tamoxifen-Induced Hot Flashes

Loprinzi et al (109) evaluated the use of a 6-week course of megestrol acetate to ameliorate climacteric symptoms in a double-blind, randomized, placebo-controlled study of 97 women with a history of breast cancer who had "bothersome" hot flashes. Eighty-one percent of the patients were receiving tamoxifen. They found an 83% reduction in hot flash scores with megestrol acetate compared with a 27% reduction with placebo. However, this study was not designed to look at long-term consequences such as disease recurrence and effect on lipid profile. Progestins can "blunt, block, or even overwhelm estrogenic effects, particularly on lipoproteins" (110). Conversely, Powles et al (111) gave conjugated estrogens (Premarin, 0.625 mg daily) to 35 women experiencing menopausal symptoms caused by adjuvant tamoxifen for stage I, II, or III primary breast cancer. In five women, the dose needed to control hot flashes was 1.25 mg daily. Nearly 70% (24/35) of the women had total or partial relief of symptoms. At a mean follow-up time of 43 months, one patient each had a relapse with local and distant metastases at 68 and 27 months, respectively. Powles et al (111) concluded that concomitant use of tamoxifen and estrogens did not compromise the effectiveness of either treatment.

Need for Further Data

All of the previously mentioned investigators and many practicing oncologists echo Epstein and Henderson's thoughts that "the jury is not in" (91) on the relationship between hormone replacement therapy and breast cancer risk. A large-scale randomized (inter)national trial should be designed to answer this question. At the National Cancer Institute of the United States, an open meeting was held in November 1993 to address this issue. In a succinct review of this meeting, Cobleigh et al (112) made a clarion call for a national trial. As of late 1995, no national protocol has emerged. Since 1993, investigators at the M. D. Anderson Cancer Center have been conducting a randomized, placebo-controlled trial using conjugated estrogens (Premarin) 0.625 mg daily for 5 years with escalation of the dose to 1.25 mg daily based on serum follicle-stimulating hormone (FSH) levels. Patients must be confirmed to be post-menopausal by serum FSH levels and must have had either stage I or II breast cancer. Patients for whom the hormonal status of the original tumor was ER negative or unknown are eligible at 2 and 10 years after diagnosis, respectively. Unfortunately, patients whose original tumor was ER positive are not eligible. This study has two objectives: first, to evaluate the effect of estrogen replacement therapy on maintenance of bone mineral density, and second, to evaluate the effect of estrogen replacement therapy on recurrence rates. Lipid profiles and fibrinogen levels will also be followed serially. Because this issue is emotionally charged for both physicians and patients, accrual has been very slow. The issue of hormone replacement therapy after breast cancer challenges the international oncology community to address the other side of the coin, the consequences of adjuvant therapies in women whose lives have been spared or prolonged.

Reproductive Factors and the Risk of Breast Cancer

Pregnancy Before Age 30

The landmark study of the International Union Against Cancer (UICC) in 1962 (113) showed an increased incidence of breast cancer in nulliparous patients and in patients who became pregnant after age 30. Layde et al (20) confirmed the importance of age at first full-term pregnancy but showed that the increased risk of breast cancer was confined only to pre-menopausal breast cancer. After age 50, women who had had a full-term pregnancy at any age had a lower risk of breast cancer than nulliparous women had. Vatten and Kvinnsland (114) showed that parity of four or more pro-

vided a lifelong protective effect against breast cancer [relative risk (RR) adjusted for age and age at first birth, 0.73; 95% confidence interval (CI), 0.54–0.98] independent of the protection afforded by early first term birth. However, they showed that the effects of parity varied by age. Nulliparous women had a lower risk (RR, 1.65; 95% CI, 1.18–2.31) of breast cancer than did women whose first pregnancy occurred after age 34 (RR, 1.77; 95% CI, 1.04–3.00) even after adjustment for parity. Nulliparous women also had a lower risk of breast cancer than did women of low parity (one to three births) before age 45. However, sometime between ages 45 and 49, these risks reversed, and women of any parity had a lower risk of breast cancer than did nulliparous women, an occurrence Vatten and Kvinnsland (114) termed a "crossover effect." Kalache et al (115) suggested that the age of the most recent pregnancy is more important than the age at the first pregnancy. However, Vatten and Kvinnsland's data (114) did not support this. While reproductive decisions will not be made on the basis of these data, health-care providers should be aware of this information in light of recent trends in breast cancer incidence and age at the time of first pregnancy.

Does Pregnancy Cause a Transient Increase in the Risk of Developing Breast Cancer?

Guinee et al's study discussed earlier (50) suggested that recent pregnancy adversely affects the survival of women diagnosed with breast cancer. Bruzzi et al (116) and Williams et al (117) observed that a full-term pregnancy causes a short-term increase in the risk of developing breast cancer. However, Williams et al (117) acknowledged that both their and Bruzzi's results could have been influenced by selection bias in the control groups. Vatten and Kvinnsland (114), in a prospective cohort study of 29,981 Norwegian women, found no evidence of a transient increase in the risk of developing breast cancer subsequent to pregnancy.

Proposed Protective Alternative to Early Pregnancy

Based on data showing that combination oral contraceptives have reduced the risk of endometrial and ovarian cancer, Pike's group (118) developed a contraceptive program to reduce breast cell proliferation, and thus limit the opportunities for the occurrence and accumulation of potentially neoplastic genetic damage, by reducing the sex steroid levels that stimulate breast cell proliferation. The gonadotropin-releasing hormone agonist leuprolide acetate in depot form is given monthly to suppress ovarian hormone production. To prevent menopausal symptoms, a low dose of conjugated estrogens (Premarin, 0.625 mg) is used orally for 6 of every 7 days. Every fourth 28-day cycle, medroxyprogesterone acetate, 10 mg, is given orally for 13 days to protect the uterus from the potentially neoplastic effects of unopposed estrogen. The estimated benefit from 10 years of this is a greater than 50% reduction in the lifetime risk of breast cancer.

In a pilot study to test the tolerability and other metabolic effects of this regimen, 21 patients with a fivefold or greater risk of breast cancer were randomized to either the control arm, 7 patients, or the treatment arm, 14 patients (118). Only two side effects required medication changes: Vaginal dryness was relieved by increasing the conjugated estrogen dose to 0.9 mg, and loss of bone mineral density was stopped by addition of low doses of androgen. Although the study is too small and premature, a marked reduction in mammographic parenchymal density was observed after 12 months in the patients in the treatment arm. This was interpreted as an intermediate end point, that is, obvious evidence of reduced breast cell proliferation. From the clinician's perspective, this decrease in mammographic parenchymal density would also translate into more effective detection of any new mass by physical and radiographic examination of the breast.

Lactation

Early study findings suggested that lactation is protective against breast cancer (119). However, later studies showed that it is the pregnancy, not the lactation, that had the protective effect. A 1994 analysis (120) showed that lactation provides a small measure of protection against breast cancer. The benefits of breast-feeding to the newborn and mother are well described. This is one more reason to recommend it.

Oral Contraceptive Use

A related issue is whether oral contraceptive use is a risk factor for subsequent breast cancer. In a review of 44 epidemiologic studies conducted from 1974 through 1991, La Vecchia (121) showed there was no consistent association for "ever use" of oral contraceptives and breast cancer risk. However, in 19 of the 20 trials that focused on long-term use in "young" (defined heterogeneously as 20–34 years, 30–44 years, "premenopause," or younger than 35, 40, or 45 years) women, he noted an increased relative risk of breast cancer. Two meta-analyses evaluating duration-related effects of oral contraceptive use before first full-term pregnancy reached the same conclusions (122,123). However, in their compendious analysis, Prentice and Thomas (122) reviewed all aspects of collateral effects of oral contraceptives in nine trials addressing oral contraceptive use before first full-term pregnancy and found inconsistent results precluding any definitive conclusions in this area. The most dramatic and well-characterized studies are from Sweden, where Olsson et al (124,125) found a significant relationship between early use of oral contraceptives and increased risk of breast cancer in women aged 30 to 40 years. These women tended to have larger tumors with more frequent lymph node involvement and higher indices of cell proliferation (124). Of interest, in women who had used oral contraceptives at an early age who had a history of breast cancer in first-degree relatives, indices of cell proliferation (S-phase fraction and ploidy) were not higher than those in similar women without a family history. Olsson et al (125) independently showed that HER-2/*neu* oncogene is amplified more frequently in women who used oral contraceptives at an early age.

However, there are a number of confounding factors. The most obvious is that early use of oral contraceptives delays the age of first childbirth and decreases parity, two known risk factors for breast cancer (126). Herbst and Berek (126) further showed that in women aged 20 to 44 years, the apparent increase in risk of breast cancer with extended use of oral contraceptives before the first pregnancy is directly related to parity. Only the nulliparous women have an increased relative risk of breast cancer. Second, the formulations of the agents used before 1980 contained higher doses of steroid hormones than do preparations currently used. Thus, results from an earlier era may not be applicable. This is an area that merits continued evaluation.

Abortions: No Convincing Data

In 1981, Pike et al (127) reported that women younger than 33 years who had a first-trimester abortion before the first full-term pregnancy had a 2.4-fold greater risk of breast cancer compared with women who had not had spontaneous or induced abortions. Since that time, a number of studies supporting and refuting Pike et al's finding have appeared (124,128–132). These studies also addressed other aspects of this issue such as spontaneous versus induced abortions and abortions in women with a family history of breast cancer. The case-control study from Rosenberg et al (132) at Boston University compared 3200 women with breast cancer with 4844 control subjects and found that the risk of breast cancer was not related to the number of spontaneous or induced abortions. In 1993, Louise Brinton (128) at the National Cancer Institute's Division of Cancer Etiology concluded that the available data on the relationship between abortion and breast cancer were not convincing. Her own study of breast cancer risk factors including abortion was nearing completion in 1993 but no results have been published as of December 1995.

Lehrer et al (133) noted an interesting twist to this issue, however. They identified a polymorphism in the ER gene that, in association with a history of spontaneous abortion, is correlated with an increased incidence of ER-positive breast cancer in middle-aged and older women. The incidence of ER-negative breast cancers is not affected. The single point mutation in the B allele of the ER gene does not result in an amino acid change in the ER protein, so the investigators interpreted this to mean that another mutation that segregates with the mutated allele is responsible for the spontaneous abortions in these patients.

Conclusions

Review of the available data suggests that the outcome of breast cancer occurring during pregnancy is not worse than the outcome in the nonpregnant patient. The options for treatment of breast cancer during pregnancy are somewhat limited. Radiotherapy should not be given during pregnancy; however, chemotherapy may be administered after the first trimester with reasonable safety to mother and fetus. Surgery may be performed safely at any time. All therapies require close coordination of care between the medical oncologist, surgeon, and maternal-fetal specialist. Abortion has not been shown to improve outcomes. The relationship of previous and subsequent reproductive events and hormonal therapies to outcomes was reviewed. Pregnancy after the diagnosis of breast cancer does not worsen survival. Conflicting data exist regarding the influence of hormone replacement therapy after breast cancer on the risk of recurrence. A national or international trial is sorely needed to address this issue.

Acknowledgments

The author appreciates the secretarial assistance of Judy Dillon and editorial assistance of Stephanie Deming.

REFERENCES

1. Harrington SW. Carcinoma of the breast: results of surgical treatment when the carcinoma occurred in the course of pregnancy or lactation and when pregnancy occurred subsequent to operation (1910–1933). *Ann Surg* 1937;106:690–700.

2. Lewison EF. Breast cancer and pregnancy or lactation. *Surg Gynecol Obstet* 1954;99:417–424.

3. White TT. Prognosis of breast cancer for pregnant and nursing women. Analysis of 1,413 cases. *Surg Gynecol Obstet* 1955;100:661–666.

4. Treves N, Holleb AI. A report of 549 cases of breast cancer in women 35 years of age or younger. *Surg Gynecol Obstet* 1958;107:271–283.

5. White TT. Carcinoma of the breast in the pregnant and the nursing patient. Review of 1375 cases. *Am J Obstet Gynecol* 1955;69:1277–1286.

6. Byrd BF, Bayer DS, Robertson JC, Stephenson SE. Treatment of breast tumors associated with pregnancy and lactation. *Ann Surg* 1962;155:940–947.

7. Rissanen PN. Carcinoma of the breast during pregnancy and lactation. *Br J Cancer* 1968;22:663–668.

8. Crosby CH, Barclay THC. Carcinoma of the breast: surgical management of patients with special conditions. *Cancer* 1971;28:1628–1636.

9. Applewhite RR, Smith LR, DiVincenti F. Carcinoma of the breast associated with pregnancy and lactation. *Ann Surg* 1973;39:101–104.

10. Riberio GG, Palmer MK. Breast carcinoma associated with pregnancy: a clinician's dilemma. *BMJ* 1977;2:1524.

11. Noyes RD, Spanos WJ, Montague ED. Breast cancer in women aged 30 and under. *Cancer* 1982;49:1302–1307.

12. Nugent P, O'Connell TX. Breast cancer and pregnancy. *Arch Surg* 1985;120:1221–1224.

13. King RM, Welch JH, Martin JK Jr, Coulam CB. Carcinoma of the breast associated with pregnancy. *Surg Gynecol Obstet* 1985;160:228–232.

14. Wallach MK, Wolf JA Jr, Bedwinek J, et al. Gestational carcinoma of the female breast. *Curr Probl Cancer* 1983;7:1–58.

15. van der Vange N, van Donegan JA. Breast cancer and pregnancy. *Eur J Surg Oncol* 1991;17:1–8.

16. Donegan WL. Breast cancer and pregnancy. *Obstet Gynecol* 1977;50:244–252.

17. Garfinkel L. Evaluating cancer statistics. *CA Cancer J Clin* 1994;44:5–6.

18. Boring CC, Squires TS, Tong T, Montgomery S. Cancer statistics 1994. *CA Cancer J Clin* 1994;44:7–27.

19. National Center for Health Statistics. *Advance report of final natality statistics, 1989. Monthly vital statistics report*, vol. 50 (suppl). Publication no. (PHS) 92-1120. Washington, DC: Government Printing Office, 1991:1.

20. Layde PM, Webster LA, Baughman AL, et al. The independent associations of parity, age at first full term pregnancy, and duration of breast-feeding with the risk of breast cancer. Cancer and Steroid Hormone Study Group. *J Clin Epidemiol* 1989;42:963–973.

21. White E. Projected changes in breast cancer incidence due to the trend toward delayed childbearing. *Am J Public Health* 1987;77:495–497.

22. Mueller CB, Ames F, Anderson GD. Breast cancer in 3558 women: age as a significant determinant in the rate of dying and causes of death. *Surgery* 1978;83:123–132.

23. Adami H-O, Malker B, Holmberg L, et al. The relation between survival and age at diagnosis in breast cancer. *N Engl J Med* 1986;315:559–563.

24. Preftakes DK. Breast cancer and pregnancy: implications for perinatal care and fetal outcomes. *J Perinat Neonat Nurs* 1994;7:31–41.

25. Jimenez JF, Ryals RO, Cohen C. Spontaneous breast infarction associated with pregnancy presenting as a palpable mass. *J Surg Oncol* 1986;32:174–178.

26. Bottles K, Taylor RN. Diagnosis of breast masses in pregnant and lactating women by aspiration cytology. *Obstet Gynecol* 1985;66(3 suppl):76S–78S.

27. Tobon H, Horowitz LF. Breast cancer during pregnancy. *Breast Dis* 1993;6:127–134.

28. Roth JA, Feinberg M, McAvoy JM. Carcinoma arising in the wall of a breast cyst during pregnancy. *Ann Surg* 1977;185:247–250.

29. Bibbo M, Underhill S. Cytology of fine needle aspiration. In: Harris JR, Hellman S, Henderson IC, Kinne DW, eds. *Breast diseases.* 2nd ed. Philadelphia: JB Lippincott, 1991:297–300.

30. Elledge RM, Ciocca DR, Langone G, McGuire WL. Estrogen receptor, progesterone receptor, and HER-2/neu protein in breast cancers from pregnant patients. *Cancer* 1993;71:2499–2506.

31. Sutton R, Buzdar AU, Hortobagyi GN. Pregnancy and offspring after adjuvant chemotherapy in breast cancer patients. *Cancer* 1990;65:847–850.

32. Wolin M, Giuliano A, Glaspy J. Breast cancer in pregnancy: the UCLA experience. *Proc Am Soc Clin Oncol* 1990;9:45. Abstract 171.

33. Clark GM, Osborne CK, McGuire WL. Correlations between estrogen receptor, progesterone receptor, and patient characteristics in human breast cancer. *J Clin Oncol* 1984;2:1102–1109.

34. Sarrif AM, Durant JR. Evidence that estrogen-receptor-negative, progesterone-receptor-negative breast and ovarian carcinoma contain estrogen receptor. *Cancer* 1981;48:1215–1220.

35. Holmes FA, Fritsche HA, Loewy JW, et al. Measurement of estrogen and progesterone receptors in human breast tumors: enzyme immunoassay versus binding assay. *J Clin Oncol* 1990;8:1025–1035.

36. McClelland RA, Berger U, Millar LS, et al. Immunocytochemical assay for estrogen receptor in patients with breast cancer: relationship to a biochemical assay and to outcome of therapy. *J Clin Oncol* 1986;4:1171–1176.

37. McGuire WL, Tandon AK, Allred DC, et al. How to use prognostic factors in axillary node-negative breast cancer patients. *J Natl Cancer Inst* 1990;82:1006–1015.

38. Liberman L, Giess CS, Dershaw DD, et al. Imaging of pregnancy-associated breast cancer. *Radiology* 1994;191:245–248.

39. Wagner LK, Lester RG, Saldana LR. The amount of radiation absorbed by the conceptus. In: *Exposure of the pregnant patient to diagnostic*

radiations. A guide to medical management. Philadelphia: JB Lippincott, 1985:52.

40. Max MH, Lamer TW. Breast cancer in 120 women under 35 years old. *Am Surg* 1984;50: 23–25.

41. Imaging modalities during pregnancy. In: Cunningham FG, MacDonald PC, Leveno KJ, et al, eds. *Williams obstetrics.* 19th ed. Norwalk, CT: Appleton & Lange, 1993:981–989.

42. Baker J, Ali A, Groch MW, et al. Bone scanning in pregnant patients with breast carcinoma. *Clin Nucl Med* 1987;12:519–524.

43. Gross SW. *A practical treatise on tumors of the mammary gland: embracing their histology, pathology, diagnosis, and treatment.* New York: D Appleton, 1880:146.

44. Beatson GT. On the treatment of inoperable cases of carcinoma of the mamma: suggestions for a new method of treatment with illustrative cases. *Lancet* 1886;2:104–107.

45. Haagensen CD. Cancer of the breast in pregnancy and during lactation. *Am J Obstet Gynecol* 1967;98:141–149.

46. Holleb AI, Farrow JH. The relation of carcinoma of the breast and pregnancy in 283 patients. *Surg Gynecol Obstet* 1962;115:65–71.

47. Miller HK. Cancer of the breast during pregnancy and lactation. *Am J Obstet Gynecol* 1962; 83:602–611.

48. Clark RM, Reid J. Carcinoma of the breast in pregnancy and lactation. *Int J Radiat Oncol Biol Phys* 1978;4:693–698.

49. Petrek JA, Dukoff R, Rogatko A. Prognosis of pregnancy-associated breast cancer. *Cancer* 1991;67:869–872.

50. Guinee VF, Olsson H, Möller T, et al. Effect of pregnancy on prognosis for young women with breast cancer. *Lancet* 1994;343:1587–1589.

51. Peters MV. The effect of pregnancy in breast cancer. In: Forrest APM, Kunkler PB, eds. *Prognostic factors in breast cancer.* Edinburgh: E & S Livingstone, 1968:65–81.

52. Zemlickis D, Lishner M, Degendorger P, et al. Maternal and fetal outcome after breast cancer in pregnancy. *Am J Obstet Gynecol* 1992;166: 781–787.

53. Tretli S, Kvalheim G, Thoresen S, Host H. Survival of breast cancer patients diagnosed during pregnancy or lactation. *Br J Cancer* 1988;58: 382–384.

54. Oliver RTD. Pregnancy and breast cancer. *Lancet* 1994;344:471–472. Letter.

55. Stewart THM. Pregnancy and breast cancer. *Lancet* 1994;344:1235–1236. Letter.

56. Tafuri A, Alterink J, Moller P, et al. T cell awareness of paternal alloantigens during pregnancy. *Science* 1995;270:630–633.

57. Zinns JS. The association of pregnancy and breast cancer. *J Reprod Med* 1979;22:297–301.

58. Dildy G, Moise K, Carpenter R, et al. Maternal malignancy metastatic to the products of conception: a review. *Obstet Gynecol Surv* 1989;44: 535–540.

59. Salamon MA, Sherer DM, Devereux N, et al. Placental metastases in a patient with recurrent breast carcinoma. *Am J Obstet Gynecol* 1994;171: 573–574.

60. Kinne DW. Primary treatment of breast cancer. In: Harris JR, Hellman S, Henderson IC, Kinne DW, eds. *Breast diseases.* 2nd ed. Philadelphia: JB Lippincott, 1991:356–359.

61. Brent RL. The effect of embryonic and fetal exposure to x-ray, microwaves, and ultrasound: counseling the pregnant and nonpregnant patient about these risks. *Semin Oncol* 1989;16: 347–368.

62. Kim Y, Pomper J, Goldberg ME. Anesthetic management of the pregnant patient with carcinoma of the breast. *J Clin Anesth* 1993;5:76–78.

63. Diaz JH. Perioperative management of the pregnant patient undergoing nonobstetric surgery. Part I. Indications for surgery and direct and indirect effects of anesthetics on fetal well-being. *Anesth Rev* 1991;18:21–22.

64. Saunders CM, Baum M. Breast cancer and pregnancy: a review. *J R Soc Med* 1993;86:162–165.

65. Adair EA. Cancer of the breast. *Surg Clin North Am* 1953;33:313–327.

66. Doll DC, Ringenberg S, Yarbro JW. Antineoplastic agents and pregnancy. *Semin Oncol* 1989; 16:337–346.

67. Theriault R, Walters R, Holmes F, et al. Management of breast cancer (BC) during pregnancy. *Proc Am Soc Clin Oncol* 1992;11:86. Abstract 171.

68. Hortobagyi GN, Frye D, Buzdar AU, et al. Complete remissions in metastatic breast cancer: a thirteen year follow-up report. *Proc Am Soc Clin Oncol* 1988;7:37. Abstract 143.

69. Roboz J, Gleicher N, Wu K, et al. Does doxorubicin cross the placenta? *Lancet* 1979;2: 1382–1383. Letter.

70. Karp GI, von Oeyen P, Valone F, et al. Doxorubicin in pregnancy: possible transplacental passage. *Cancer Treat Rep* 1983;67:773–777.

71. Arceci RJ, Croop JM, Horwitz SB, Housman D. The gene encoding multidrug resistance is induced and expressed at high levels during pregnancy in the secretory epithelium of the uterus. *Proc Natl Acad Sci USA* 1988;85:4350–4354.

72. Weinstein RS, Kuszak JR, Kluskens LF, Coon JS. P-glycoproteins in pathology: the multidrug resistance gene family in humans. *Hum Pathol* 1990;21:34–48.

73. Theriault RL, Stallings CB, Buzdar AU. Pregnancy and breast cancer: clinical and legal issues. Clinical case reports from MD Anderson Cancer Center. *Am J Clin Oncol* 1992;15:535–539.

74. Willemse PHB, van der Sijde R, Sleijfer DTh. Combination chemotherapy and radiation for stage IV breast cancer during pregnancy. *Gynecol Oncol* 1990;36:281–284.

75. Barni S, Ardizzola A, Zanetta G, et al. Weekly doxorubicin chemotherapy for breast cancer in pregnancy. A case report. *Tumori* 1992;78:349–350.

76. Aviles A, Diaz Maqueo JC, Talavera A. Growth and development of children of mothers treated with chemotherapy during pregnancy: current status of 43 children. *Am J Hematol* 1991;36:243–248.

77. Randall T. National registry seeks scarce data on pregnancy outcomes during chemotherapy (News). *JAMA* 1993;269:323.

78. Guikontes E, Spantideas A, Diakakis J. Ondansetron and hyperemesis gravidarum. *Lancet* 1992;340:1223. Letter.

79. World MJ. Ondansetron and hyperemesis gravidarum. *Lancet* 1993;341:185. Letter.

80. Beely L. Drugs and breast feeding. *Clin Obstet Gynecol* 1981;8:291–295.

81. Sutcliffe SB. Treatment of neoplastic disease during pregnancy: maternal and fetal effects. *Clin Invest Med* 1985;8:333–338.

82. Klein CE, Glode M. Options for preserving fertility in the chemotherapy patient. *Contemp Oncol* 1993;48–56.

83. Gradishar WJ, Schilsky RL. Ovarian function following radiation and chemotherapy for cancer. *Semin Oncol* 1989;16:425–436.

84. Damewood MD, Grochow LB. Prospects for fertility after chemotherapy or radiation for neoplastic disease. *Fertil Steril* 1986;45:443–459.

85. Shalet SM. Effects of cancer chemotherapy on gonadal function of patients. *Cancer Treat Rev* 1980;7:1419–1520.

86. Richards MA, O'Reilly SM, Howell A, et al. Adjuvant cyclophosphamide, methotrexate, and fluorouracil in patients with axillary node-positive breast cancer: an update of the Guy's/Manchester trial. *J Clin Oncol* 1990;8:2032–2039.

87. Hortobagyi GN, Buzdar AU, Marcus CE, Smith TE. Immediate and long-term toxicity of adjuvant chemotherapy regimens containing doxorubicin in trials at M. D. Anderson Hospital and Tumor Institute. *Monogr Natl Cancer Inst* 1986;1:105–109.

88. Jones SE, Stringer CA, Dorr RT, Senzer NN. Cancer and pregnancy. In: *American Society of Clinical Oncology (ASCO) educational book.* Chicago: ASCO and Bostrom Corp, 1991:228–236.

89. Sauer MV, Paulson RJ, Lobo RA. Successful pre-embryo donation in ovarian failure after treatment for breast carcinoma. *Lancet* 1990;335:723. Letter.

90. Farley JC, Gregory SS, Quinn M, et al. Harvesting fetal ovaries. *Time* 1994;143:19.

91. Epstein RJ, Henderson IC. The Danforth article reviewed: the jury is in. *Oncology* 1991;5:30–31.

92. Danforth DN Jr. How subsequent pregnancy affects outcome in women with a prior breast cancer. *Oncology* 1991;11:21–30.

93. Wood WC. The Danforth article reviewed. *Oncology* 1991;5:35.

94. Petrek JA. Pregnancy safety after breast cancer. *Cancer* 1994;74:528–531.

95. Sankila R, Heinävaara S, Hakulinen T. Survival of breast cancer patients after subsequent term pregnancy: "healthy mother effect." *Am J Obstet Gynecol* 1994;170:818–823.

96. Dow KH, Harris JR, Roy C. Pregnancy after breast-conserving surgery and radiation therapy for breast cancer. *Monogr Natl Cancer Inst* 1994;16:131–137.

97. Higgins S, Haffty B. Pregnancy and lactation after breast-conserving therapy for early stage breast cancer. *Cancer* 1994;73:2175–2180.

98. Tralins A. Is lactation possible after breast irradiation? *Proc Am Soc Clin Oncol* 1993;12:77. Abstract 109.

99. Miller MJ, Ross ME. Pregnancy following breast reconstruction with autogenous tissue (case report). *Cancer Bull* 1993;45:546–548.

100. Theriault RL, Sellin RV. Estrogen-replacement therapy in younger women with breast cancer. *Monogr Natl Cancer Inst* 1994;16:149–152.

101. DiSaia PJ. Hormone-replacement therapy in patients with breast cancer. A reappraisal. *Cancer* 1993;71(4 suppl):1490–1500.

102. Eden JA, Bush T, Nand S, et al. A case-control study of combined continuous estrogen-progestin replacement therapy among women with a personal history of breast cancer. *Menopause* 1995;2:67–72.

103. Stanford JL, Weiss NS, Voigt LF, et al. Combined estrogen and progestin hormone replacement therapy in relation to risk of breast cancer in middle-aged women. *JAMA* 1995;274:137–142.

104. Adami HO, Persson I. Hormone replacement and breast cancer. A remaining controversy? *JAMA* 1995;274:178–179. Editorial.

105. Colditz GA, Hankison SE, Hunter DJ, et al. The use of estrogens and progestins and the risk of breast cancer in postmenopausal women. *N Engl J Med* 1995;332:1589–1593.

106. Davidson NE. Hormone-replacement therapy—breast versus heart versus bone. *N Engl J Med* 1995;332:1638–1639. Editorial.

107. Dhodapkar MV, Ingle JN, Ahmann DL. Estrogen replacement therapy withdrawal and regression of metastatic breast cancer. *Cancer* 1995; 75:43–46.

108. Pritchard KI, Sawaka CA. Menopausal estrogen replacement therapy in women with breast cancer. *Cancer* 1995;75:1–3.

109. Loprinzi CL, Michalak JC, Quella SK, et al. Megestrol acetate for the prevention of hot flashes. *N Engl J Med* 1994;331:347–352.

110. Effects of estrogen or estrogen/progestin regimens on heart disease risk factors in postmenopausal women. The Postmenopausal Estrogen/Progestin Interventions (PEPI) Trial. The Writing Group for the PEPI Trial. *JAMA* 1995;273:199–208.

111. Powles TJ, Hickish T, Casey S, et al. Hormone replacement after breast cancer. *Lancet* 1993; 342:60–61. Letter.

112. Cobleigh MA, Berris RF, Bush T, et al. Estrogen replacement therapy in breast cancer survivors. A time for change. *JAMA* 1994;272:540–545.

113. MacMahon B, Cole P, Lin TM, et al. Age at first birth and breast cancer risk. *Bull World Health Organ* 1970;43:209–221.

114. Vatten LJ, Kvinnsland S. Pregnancy-related factors and risk of breast cancer in a prospective study of 29,981 Norwegian women. *Eur J Cancer* 1992;28A:1148–1153.

115. Kalache A, Maguire A, Thompson SG. Age at last full-term pregnancy and risk of breast cancer. *Lancet* 1993;341:33–36.

116. Bruzzi P, Negri E, La Vecchia C, et al. Short term increase in risk of breast cancer after full term pregnancy. *BMJ* 1988;297:1096–1097.

117. Williams EMI, Jones L, Vessey MP, McPherson K. Short term increase in risk of breast cancer associated with full term pregnancy. *BMJ* 1990; 300:578–579.

118. Spicer DV, Krecker EA, Pike MC. The endocrine prevention of breast cancer. *Cancer Invest* 1995; 3:495–504.

119. MacMahon B, Lin TM, Lowe CR, et al. Lactation and cancer of the breast. A summary of an international study. *Bull World Health Organ* 1970; 42:185–194.

120. Newcomb PA, Storer BE, Longnecker MP, et al. Lactation and a reduced risk of premenopausal breast cancer. *N Engl J Med* 1994;330:81–87.

121. La Vecchia C. Oral contraceptives and breast cancer. Review article. *Breast* 1992;2:76–81.

122. Prentice RL, Thomas DB. On the epidemiology of oral contraceptives and disease. *Adv Cancer Res* 1987;49:285–401.

123. Romieu I, Berlin JA, Colditz G. Oral contraceptives and breast cancer. *Cancer* 1990;66: 2253–2263.

124. Olsson H, Ranstam J, Baldetorp B, et al. Proliferation and DNA ploidy in malignant breast tumors in relation to early oral contraceptive use and early abortions. *Cancer* 1991;67:1285–1290.

125. Olsson H, Borg A, Fernö M, et al. Her-2/neu and INT2 proto-oncogene amplification in malignant breast tumors in relation to reproductive factors and exposure to exogenous hormones. *J Natl Cancer Inst* 1991;83:1483–1487.

126. Herbst AL, Berek JS. Contraceptive choices for women with medical problems. Impact of contraception on gynecologic cancers. *Am J Obstet Gynecol* 1993;168:1980–1985.

127. Pike MC, Henderson BE, Casagrande JT, et al. Oral contraceptive use and early abortion as risk factors for breast cancer in young women. *Br J Cancer* 1981;43:72–76.

128. Parkins T. Does abortion increase breast cancer risk? (News). *J Natl Cancer Inst* 1993;35:1987–1988.

129. Andrieu N, Clavel F, Gairard B, et al. Familial risk of breast cancer and abortion. *Cancer Detect Prev* 1994;18:51–55.

130. Parazzini F, La Vecchia C, Negri E. Spontaneous and induced abortions and risk of breast cancer. *Int J Cancer* 1991;48:816–820.

131. Parazzini F, La Vecchia C, Negri E, et al. Menstrual and reproductive factors and breast cancer in women with family history of the disease. *Int J Cancer* 1992;51:677–681.

132. Rosenberg L, Palmer JR, Kaufman DW, et al. Breast cancer in relation to the occurrence and time of induced and spontaneous abortion. *Am J Epidemiol* 1988;127:981–989.

133. Lehrer S, Schmutzler RK, Rabin JM, et al. An estrogen receptor genetic polymorphism and a history of spontaneous abortions—correlation with estrogen receptor positive breast cancer but not in women with estrogen receptor negative breast cancer or women without cancer. *Breast Cancer Res Treat* 1993;26:175–180.

Addendum: Effect of Interruption of Pregnancy on Outcome of Breast Cancer

Study	Years Accrued	No. of Patients	Normal Delivery			Therapeutic Abortion			Comments
			No. of Patients	% Survival 5 Yr	10 Yr	No. of Patients	% Survival 5 Yr	10 Yr	
Adair (1953)	NA	59	36	44	NA	23	70	NA	25 pregnant at diagnosis, 34 pregnant after treatment for cancer. Only node-positive patients benefited from abortion
Holleb (1962)	1962	24	12	33	NA	12	17	NA	Patients operated on during first trimester
Rissanen (1968)	1940–61	31	20*	50	NA	7*	43	NA	*4 other patients (totalling 31) were stage IV (1 aborted, 3 delivered); all were dead at 5 yr
Clark (1978)	1931–75	121	93	29	23	13	15	8	12% spontaneously aborted; 1 infant was stillborn. Abortion was not biased for more advanced disease
King (1985)	1950–80	63	35*	67	NA	18*	53	NA	*10 other patients (4 normal delivery, 6 aborted) were stage IV; only 1 alive at 5 yr. For stage I patients: 5-yr survival rate = 88% for normal delivery (n = 18) and 33% for abortion (n = 4)

NA = not available.

Index